Electronystagmography/ Videonystagmography (ENG/VNG)

Second Edition

Electronystagmography/ Videonystagmography (ENG/VNG)

Second Edition

Devin L. McCaslin, PhD

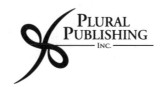

PLURAL
PUBLISHING
INC.

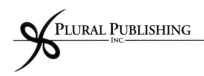

5521 Ruffin Road
San Diego, CA 92123

e-mail: information@pluralpublishing.com
Website: https://www.pluralpublishing.com

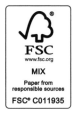

Copyright ©2020 by Plural Publishing, Inc.

Typeset in 11/13 Palatino by Flanagan's Publishing Services, Inc.
Printed in the United States of America by McNaughton & Gunn, Inc.

Library of Congress Cataloging-in-Publication Data:

Names: McCaslin, Devin L. (Devin Lochlan), author.
Title: Electronystagmography/videonystagmography (ENG/VNG) / Devin L. McCaslin.
Other titles: ENG/VNG | Electronystagmography and videonystagmography | Core clinical concepts in audiology.
Description: Second edition. | San Diego, CA : Plural Publishing, Inc., [2020] | Series: Core clinical concepts in audiology | Preceded by ENG/VNG / Devin L. McCaslin. c2013. | Includes bibliographical references and index.
Identifiers: LCCN 2019032347 | ISBN 9781635500813 (paperback) | ISBN 1635500818 (paperback)
Subjects: MESH: Electronystagmography | Oculomotor Muscles--physiology | Eye Movements--physiology | Vestibule, Labyrinth--physiopathology | Vestibular Diseases--diagnosis | Ocular Motility Disorders--pathology
Classification: LCC RE748 | NLM WW 410 | DDC 617.7/62--dc23
LC record available at https://lccn.loc.gov/2019032347

Contents

Foreword

I had been doing ENG at Ohio State for a couple of years when my department chairman said to me, "Charlie (he always called me 'Charlie'), why don't you write a book about this?"

I said, "But . . . but . . . Doctor Saunders (I always called him 'Doctor Saunders'), I've only been doing ENG for a couple of years."

He said, "Very good, Charlie. I'll put you in touch with my publisher."

His publisher did agree to publish the book, but first I had to get a physician to be co-author. My first choice was Hugh Barber of Sunnybrook Hospital in Toronto. He conducted the most elegant dizziness clinic I've ever attended. Patients came to him from all over Canada and many were desperate. He entered the exam room trailing a retinue of fellows and residents and other hangers-on like me and spent considerable time with each patient—probing, inquiring, listening, reassuring—and many of them were in tears when we left. Once outside, he went over his findings, diagnosis, and treatment plan with us, and his clinical acumen often blew us away.

So I called him up and said, "Doctor Barber (I always called him 'Doctor Barber'), would you perhaps agree to be co-author with me on a book about ENG?"

To my great surprise, he said, "Sure, Charlie (he always called me 'Charlie'), let's give it a go." So began a collaboration that lasted for three decades.

Our book, *Manual of Electronystagmography*, was published in 1976, reissued as a second edition in 1980, and dropped by the publisher in 1983. Thereafter it seemed to have a life of its own. Del Bloem of ICS Medical published a paperback edition for many years, and I've heard there were bootleg versions as well. In those days, I conducted ENG courses and attendees would sometimes ask me to autograph their copies of the book, often tattered and held together with rubber bands. By then, *Manual of Electronystagmography* had gotten seriously out of date. Eye movements were recorded on strip charts and nystagmus slow phase eye velocity was measured with a ruler. There was no mention of videonystagmography or the various forms of BPPV or their treatments and nothing about the advances in eye movement neurophysiology in the last 35 years. A new book was long past due.

So along comes this young fella, Devin McCaslin (Master's degree in Audiology from Wayne State University, PhD in Hearing Science from The Ohio State University, currently Director of the Vestibular and Balance Program at the Mayo Clinic in Rochester, Minnesota). Dr. McCaslin published *Electronystagmography/Videonystagmography (ENG/VNG)* in 2012 and it was quite a book—well reviewed, widely read by clinicians, and widely adopted by instructors of ENG/VNG courses.

I can think of three reasons why Dr. McCaslin's book was so good:

1. Dr. McCaslin is an experienced clinician. He has spent many years doing ENG/VNG and continues to see patients despite many other demands upon his time. At one point in my own career, I decided I needed to spend my precious time writing and teaching, so I stopped seeing patients. That was a mistake. I quickly got out of touch and ended up mostly parroting hearsay. Soon I began seeing patients again and thereafter became a better writer and teacher. Dr. McCaslin hasn't made that mistake. He writes from firsthand experience in the clinic. You can tell.

2. Dr. McCaslin is a serious scholar. He reads and winnows basic research on the neurophysiology of eye movements, and as a consequence, is able to tell us the causes (insofar as they are known) of the abnormalities we see in the clinic. This information alone is worth the price of the book.

3. Dr. McCaslin is a lucid writer. To be a lucid writer, you must of course be a lucid thinker,

but that's not enough. First drafts are always terrible (at least mine always were). So you have to lay down the hours, painstakingly going over every sentence again and again until the words on the page say exactly what you mean. Dr. McCaslin does that.

Now we have before us the second edition of Dr. McCaslin's book, and it's even better than the first. Same firsthand clinical experience, same serious scholarship, same lucid writing, but now there's updated and expanded information on eye movement neurophysiology and a new set of illustrations. Also new is a whole chapter listing common (and some not so common) dizziness-causing disorders. Dr. McCaslin has outdone himself here. For each disorder, he provides historical background, pathophysiology, clinical presentation, laboratory findings, and treatment. He also provides several useful appendices—a dizziness questionnaire, suggested alerting tasks to be used during caloric testing, a table listing reliability and localizing value of various ENG/VNG findings, and best of all, a delightful brochure for children describing the ENG/VNG procedure. (With minor modification, I think this would also work for adults.)

Who is this book for? It should be required reading for all clinicians who perform ENG/VNG and for all students who aspire to do so. It should also be read by referring physicians. ENG/VNG test results alone rarely yield a diagnosis, but they often provide useful information to physicians who understand their implications and relate them to other medical data available for diagnosis. One need not look elsewhere to find cogent descriptions of ENG/VNG results and their implications. They're in this book. I learned a lot. You will too.

Charles W. Stockwell, PhD
July, 2019

Preface

The ENG/VNG examination is comprised of a number of tests that each evaluates a different aspect of the balance system. Findings are then used to assist the physician or therapist in the diagnosis and treatment of the dizzy patient. The first edition of this text, and now the second edition, is written with the purpose of providing a resource "handbook" that provides practical descriptions of the tests for the practicing clinician, as well as for the graduate student first learning about the ENG/VNG examination. In order to achieve this goal, the book is written from the perspective of a clinician with the intent of providing a text that can be used in the clinical environment.

What's new in the second edition? Based on feedback from readers of the first edition, a significant amount of information has been added to select chapters. Chapter 1 has been extensively expanded by providing a deeper level of detail to the practical anatomy and physiology of the ocular motor system. This chapter also incorporates new illustrations to supplement the additional text. In Chapter 3, new material has been added regarding recently developed questionnaires that can be utilized for assisting with the case history, as well as the addition of tests that can be used to assist the clinician at the bedside. Chapter 4 has added new information with the addition of more examples and descriptions of commonly encountered ocular motor disorders and their underlying pathophysiological mechanisms. In Chapter 5, an entire set of new illustrations are provided to better guide the clinician in the testing and treatment of benign paroxysmal positional vertigo. The ter-minology associated with positioning vertigo has changed since the initial edition of this text and this chapter reflects those changes. A new chapter has been added entitled Common Vestibular Disorders: Clinical Presentation. The purpose of this chapter is to provide the clinician with a basic understanding of the pathophysiology of the most commonly encountered disorders, the most frequent laboratory test findings, and currently accepted treatments for these disorders. When appropriate, Bárány Society Diagnostic criteria for the disorders are presented. Finally, 10 illustrative cases with accompanying eye movement videos have been added and can be accessed using the PluralPlus companion website. These cases are intended to be used in conjunction with the descriptions of a number of the disorders described in the text.

The ENG/VNG examination is a technically challenging set of tests where the correct interpretation by the clinician is critical to the patient's diagnosis and management. When performed and interpreted correctly, the ENG/VNG provides unique information for those managing dizzy patients and can expedite treatment. Alternatively, when test findings are misinterpreted or over-interpreted, the result can be delays in treatment or worse, inappropriate procedures being recommended. This book is written with the purpose of providing the clinician doing ENG/VNG with a readily accessible source for test protocols, interpretation of the various subtests, and the background information to make recommendations regarding the source of patients' dizziness.

Acknowledgments

This book is a product of my professional experiences with those that I have had the opportunity to work with over the years. My great friend and collaborator Gary P. Jacobson, PhD, first provided the spark that drove my interest in this area, and then he continued to guide my learning throughout the years. He is one of the early pioneers in the area of balance and continues to be a tireless advocate for our profession in this area of study.

Although this book has my name on the cover, it is ultimately my collaborations with others in the profession and what I have learned from them throughout the years that is embedded in the content. I must thank Drs. Bob Burkard, Neil Shepard, and Paul Kileny for their friendship, kindness, support, and guidance throughout the years.

It was my mother, Laurie LaFleur, who first exposed me to this field and showed me how rewarding a profession could be. Her sound guidance throughout the years and "lead by example" approach to how to persevere, no matter how dire the situation, has been invaluable in every aspect of my life. These skills are particularly useful when writing a book.

Finally, I must thank my wife, Heather, and children, Molly and Declan, for their support and love during this project and throughout my career.

Videos

This text comes with supplementary case videos on a PluralPlus companion website. See the inside front cover for instructions on how to access the website.

Case 1: Downbeat Gaze Nystagmus (1 video)

Case 2: Bidirectional Gaze-Evoked Nystagmus (2 videos)

Case 3: Hypermetric Saccades (1 video)

Case 4: Infantile Nystagmus (2 videos)

Case 5: Ocular Flutter (1 video)

Case 6: Slow Saccades (2 videos)

Case 7: Spontaneous Vestibular Nystagmus (4 videos)

Case 8: Posterior Canal Benign Paroxysmal Positional Vertigo (1 video)

Case 9: Square Wave Jerks (1 video)

Case 10: Geotropic Horizontal Canal Benign Paroxysmal Positional Vertigo (2 videos)

1

Neural Control of Eye Movements

INTRODUCTION

One of the ways that an examiner can obtain information about a patient who complains of dizziness is to observe the patient's eye movements in response to different stimuli. In some instances, the observation of the eyes can be more sensitive than magnetic resonance imaging in localizing and identifying impairments that can result in balance disturbances. An examiner who is knowledgeable about the neurology of eye movements is afforded the ability to distinguish between impairments involving the central nervous system and the peripheral vestibular system.

HIERARCHY OF THE OCULOMOTOR SYSTEM

The neural control of human eye movements is organized in such a way as to allow an individual to explore their world in an effective way. When an object of visual interest is identified, three factors must be in play in order to observe it in detail (Schor, 2003): first, where the target is located; second, whether the target is moving or stationary; and third, whether the observer is moving or stationary. Each of these considerations must be

taken into account because of the physiological limitations of the retina. The retina is composed of two types of photoreceptor cells known as rods and cones. Cones are concentrated primarily in and around the fovea, making it the part of the eye that has the highest spatial sensitivity and the part responsible for visual acuity (Figure 1–1). In this regard, when an observer wants to see a visual target with any detail, the oculomotor system (OMS) must align the two foveae so that the target falls on them. A single type of eye movement is inadequate

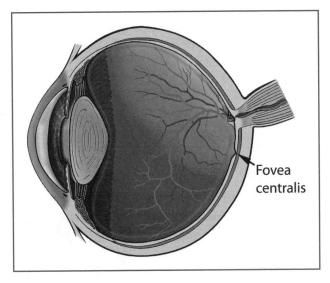

FIGURE 1–1. A diagram of the eye illustrates the location of the fovea.

1

to keep targets of interest on the foveae in all situations and is the reason why multiple eye movement systems exist. Depending on the task required to observe a target, different eye movement systems, with separate and independent neural pathways are recruited. Each of these systems employ different brain structures to process the information about the target, which ultimately converges in the "final common pathway."

Physiologists have organized the OMS into a hierarchy where each component has a different level of processing. Many authors organize the OMS into three components: (1) motor system, (2) premotor system, and (3) type of eye movement system. The motor system (i.e., the part of the system directly involved with movement of the eyes) moves the eye in the orbit and consists of the oculomotor nerves and the extraocular eye muscles. The premotor system organizes the neural input coming from higher centers (e.g., cerebral cortex and midbrain) and relays these commands to the motor system. The premotor system is located in the brainstem. Together, the motor and premotor systems comprise what has been termed the "final common pathway." Four primary control systems provide input to the final common pathway; these include the saccade, pursuit, optokinetic, and vestibular systems.

These systems all work together to enable an observer to clearly perceive objects of interest and explore the surrounding environment. First, the saccade system enables an observer to quickly bring a visual target identified in the peripheral field of vision system onto the fovea. The pursuit system is recruited when a target is moving slowly and the observer wishes to track it. The optokinetic and vestibular systems work together to keep the fovea centered on a target when the head is moving. The following section discusses the actions and neural generators of each of these functional classes of eye movements.

THE FINAL COMMON PATHWAY OF THE OCULOMOTOR SYSTEM

In order for the clinician to be able to make judgments about whether an eye movement is normal or abnormal, he or she needs to have a basic knowledge about the structure and function of the six eye muscles. Through a complex series of contractions and relaxations of six extraocular muscles (EOM), the globe can move in three axes: horizontal (i.e., z-axis), vertical (i.e., y-axis) and torsional (i.e., x-axis) (Figure 1–2). The various rotations of the eye in these three directional planes are, by convention, described as ductions, versions, and vergences.

Sherrington (1947) described the final common pathway component of the OMS as being composed of the ocular motor nerves and the extraocular muscles (EOMs). When the eye is directed straight ahead, it is referred to as being in the primary position. There are six EOMs that control the movement of each eye; these include the medial rectus, lateral rectus, superior rectus, inferior rectus, superior oblique, and inferior oblique (Figure 1–3). Each EOM has a primary action that refers to its rotational effect on the eye in the primary position. There are also secondary and tertiary actions that the muscle has on the eye (Figure 1–4). The EOMs are housed within the bone of the orbit. For each eye, these six muscles each have an opposing counterpart comprising three pairs. Each muscle in a pair moves the eye in the same plane, but in the opposite direction. The pairs are the medial rectus and lateral rectus, superior rectus and inferior rectus, and the superior and inferior oblique. If the eye is to be moved, the opposing counterpart (i.e., antagonist muscle) must be relaxed, and the muscle pulling the eye in the direction of interest (i.e., agonist muscle) must be contracted. That is, the agonist muscle will pull the eye in the direction of the target, and the antagonist muscle moves the eye away from the object of interest.

The arrangement of the EOMs enables the eye to be moved in the horizontal plane (back and forth) and the vertical plane (up and down). A third type of movement is torsional. This is a rotation of the eye around the line of sight (an imaginary line that connects the eye with the target). Sherrington's law of reciprocal innervation refers to the process that when an agonist muscle is contracted, a simultaneous equivalent relaxation must take place in the corresponding antagonist muscle. This process is mediated primarily through neural structures in the brainstem.

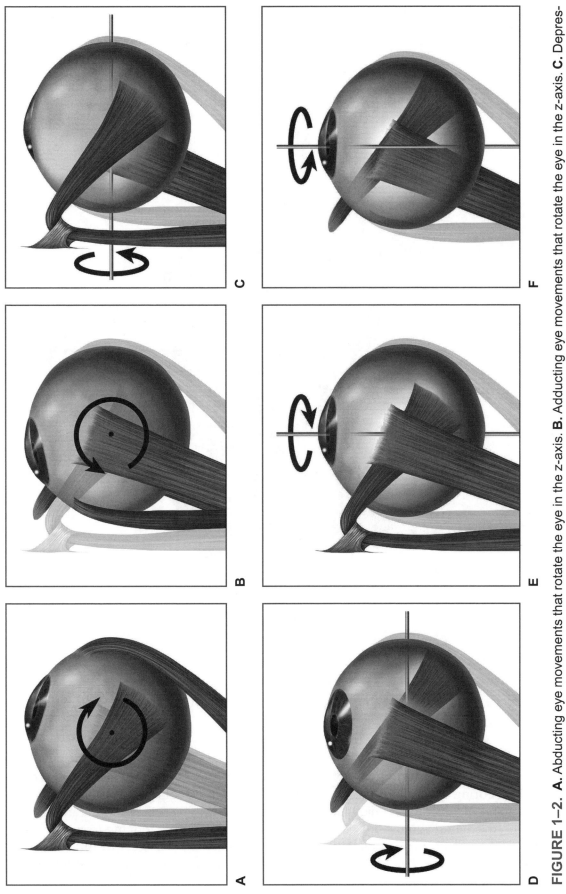

FIGURE 1–2. A. Abducting eye movements that rotate the eye in the z-axis. **B.** Adducting eye movements that rotate the eye in the z-axis. **C.** Depressor eye movements that rotate the eye in the y-axis. **D.** Elevator eye movements that rotate the eye in the y-axis. **E.** Lateral rotational eye movements that rotate the eye in the x-axis. **F.** Medial rotational eye movements that rotate the eye in the x-axis. (By Eye_movements_abductors.jpg: Patrick J. Lynch, medical illustrator derivative work: Anka Friedrich [talk]—Eye_movements_abductors.jpg [A], Eye_movements_adductors.jpg [B], Eye_movements_Depressor.jpg [C], Eye_movements_elevators.jpg [D], Eye_movements_lateral_rotators.jpg [E], Eye_movements_media_rotators.jpg [F], CC BY 2.5, https://commons.wikimedia.org/w/index.php?curid=7493751)

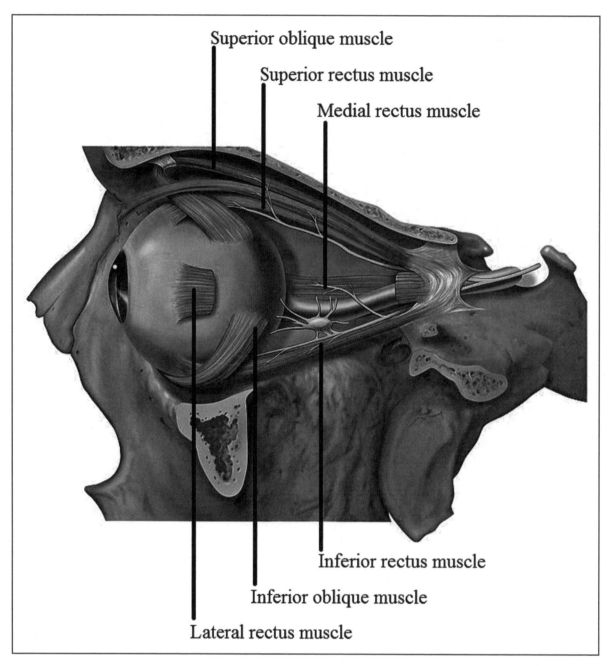

FIGURE 1–3. The six extraocular muscles of the eye. (Courtesy of Patrick Lynch, Yale University School of Medicine)

Herings law of equal innervation refers to the two eyes being yoked during an eye movement. Specifically, the law states that during a conjugate movement of the eyes, the paired agonist muscles and antagonist muscles must receive equivalent neural input so that both eyes move together.

When patient's OMS is being evaluated clinically, the eye movements are all referenced to the primary position, which is when the eyes are in their natural resting state looking forward. When patients deviate their gaze eccentrically (i.e., right, left, up, or down) the eye movement is referred to as a secondary position. When an observer gazes up and to the right or down and to the left, these are considered tertiary positions (see Figure 1–4). These types of actions of the EOMs allow for movement of the eyes in three directional planes: horizontal, vertical, and torsional (Table 1–1). In the real world, the majority of eye movements are complex requiring various levels of activation and inhibition of all the EOMs. A comprehensive overview of this topic is given by Leigh and Zee (2006).

Cranial Nerves and Nuclei of the Oculomotor System

The EOMs are innervated by oculomotor neurons (OMNs) located on each side of the midline of the brain (Figure 1–5). These cranial nuclei receive eye movement information from the premotor center and relay it through projections to innervate the EOMs (Figure 1–6). The cell bodies of these nerves form the three oculomotor nuclei: the third nucleus (oculomotor), the fourth nucleus (trochlear), and the sixth nucleus (abducens nucleus).

Oculomotor Nerve (Cranial Nerve III)

The oculomotor nuclei are located in the dorsal midbrain near the floor of the third ventricle. From the periaqueductal gray matter of the midbrain, the nerve passes through the medial longitudinal fasciculus (MLF) and emerges from the cerebral peduncle and forms the oculomotor nerve trunk. The nerve then travels through the subarachnoid space, over the petroclinoid

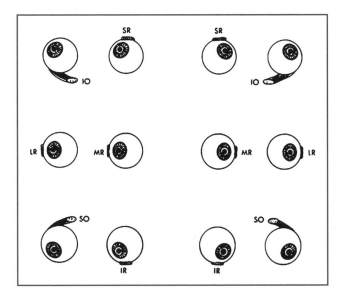

FIGURE 1–4. The different gaze positions and the primary agonist muscles that move the eye into position. MR = medial rectus; LR = lateral rectus; SR = superior rectus; IR = inferior rectus; SO = superior oblique; IO = inferior oblique. (From Barber & Stockwell, 1976)

Table 1–1. Primary, Secondary, and Tertiary Eye Movements Controlled by Extraocular Muscle

Extraocular Muscle	Primary Action	Secondary Action	Tertiary Action
Medial rectus	Moves eye inward		
Lateral rectus	Moves eye outward		
Superior rectus	Moves eye upward	Rotates top of eye toward nose	Adduction
Inferior rectus	Moves eye downward	Rotates top of eye away from nose	Adduction
Superior oblique	Rotates top of eye toward nose	Moves eye downward	Abduction
Inferior oblique	Rotates top of eye away from nose	Moves eye upward	Abduction

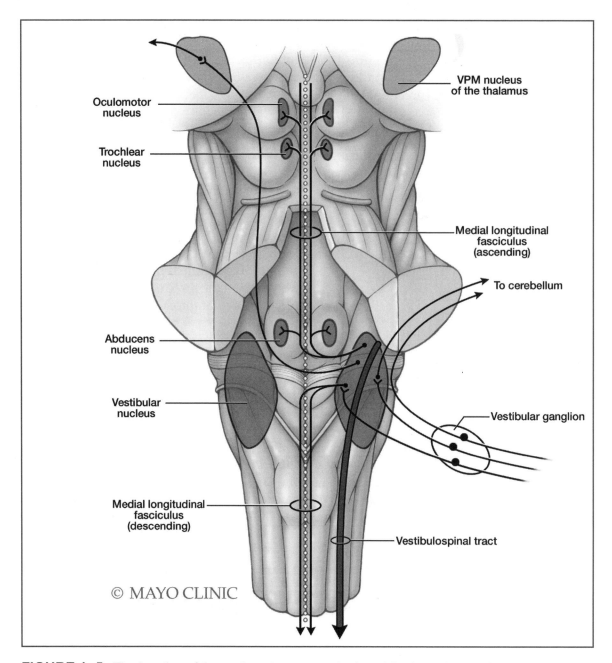

Oculomotor nucleus

Trochlear nucleus

Abducens nucleus

Vestibular nucleus

Medial longitudinal fasciculus (descending)

VPM nucleus of the thalamus

Medial longitudinal fasciculus (ascending)

To cerebellum

Vestibular ganglion

Vestibulospinal tract

© MAYO CLINIC

FIGURE 1–5. The location of the oculomotor neurons in the midbrain and pons. (Used with permission of Mayo Foundation for Medical Education and Research. All rights reserved.)

ligament where it enters the cavernous sinus. From this point, it travels along the lateral wall of the sinus, divides into the superior and inferior division, and enters the orbit within the annulus of Zinn. Once the two divisions enter the orbit, the superior division innervates the levator palpebrae muscles and superior rectus. The inferior version innervates the medial and inferior rectus, inferior oblique muscles, and the ciliary body and iris sphincter. There are a number of causes that can cause or put an individual at risk for developing a third nerve palsy. This includes aneurysms, diabetes, hypertension, trauma, and migraine. Third nerve palsies are also observed in children that may suffer a trauma at birth or neonatal hypoxia.

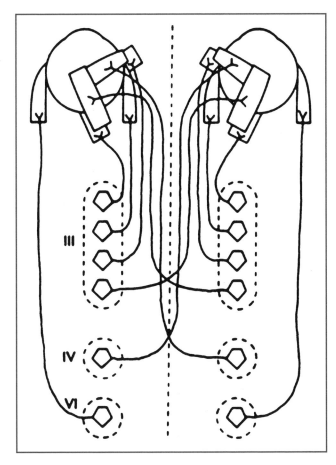

FIGURE 1–6. The extraocular muscles and their innervation by the oculomotor neurons. (From Barber & Stockwell, 1980)

Clinical Manifestations of Oculomotor Nerve Palsy:

1. Ptosis (due to involvement of the levator palpebrae muscle)
2. Dilated pupil
3. Loss of accommodation (ability of the eye to change its focus from distant to near objects
4. Limited adduction, depression, and elevation

Trochlear Nerve (Cranial Nerve IV)

The trochlear nuclei are found near the dorsal surface of the midbrain ventral and lateral to the aqueduct of Sylvius, and are located at the level of the inferior colliculus (Leigh & Zee, 2006). The fascicle then crosses the midline of the fourth ventricle and then curves around the lateral surface of the pons where it approaches the prepontine cistern, penetrates the dural, and enters the cavernous sinus. Once inside the cavernous sinus, the nerve crosses the oculomotor nerves and enters the orbit through the superior orbital fissure and innervates the contralateral superior oblique muscle. Often associated with a head injury, but can often be idiopathic and congenital.

Clinical Manifestations of Trochlear Nerve Palsy:

1. Diplopia with symptoms worse on downward gaze (patient will report difficulty navigating stairs)
2. May exhibit facial asymmetry
3. Patient will often tilt head to the contralateral side to reduce symptoms of diplopia.

Abducens Nerve (Cranial Nerve VI)

The abducens nuclei are located in the dorsal pons on the floor of the fourth ventricle and project to the ipsilateral lateral rectus muscles. There are three primary populations of neurons that compose the sixth nerve: (1) projections to the floccularnodular lobe (i.e., cerebellum), (2) motor neurons that innervate the ipsilateral lateral rectus muscles; and (3) internuclear neurons that send projections to the contralateral medial recuts subnucleus of the oculomotor nucleus. From the abducens nucleus, the nerve passes through the pons and runs along the ventral surface of the pons through the subarachnoid space. It then enters the dura mater, and travels through the inferior petrosal sinus and around the intravcavernous carotid artery. The nerve then projects through the orbit, travels through the annulus of Zinn, and terminates on the ipsilateral lateral rectus. Abducens nerve palsies are often associated with an aneurysm, trauma, or space occupying lesions around the tentorium.

Clinical Manifestations of Abducens Nerve Palsy:

1. Impaired eye abduction
2. Slight eye adduction in primary gaze
3. Horizontal diplopia when gazing toward the impaired eye
4. Impaired saccades, pursuit, and VOR

Table 1–2 provides a summary of the EOMs and their respective innervation by the OMNs.

The OMNs control the velocity and position of the eye by continually adjusting the neural input to the EOMs. Constant neural activity is fed to the EOMs by the premotor system, keeping them in a constant state of contraction, which holds the eye steady in the orbit. In instances where the eye must be moved in a certain direction, motor neurons connected to the agonist muscles increase their neural drive to the agonist muscle (contracting it), while simultaneously decreasing their firing rate to the antagonist muscles and relaxing the opposing muscle.

Figure 1–7 shows how the neural drive from the OMNs moves the eye in the horizontal plane. In this illustration, the observer has detected a target that is 30° to the right, yet the eyes are oriented forward. In order to move the eye to the right, the EOMs responsible for moving the eye right in the horizontal plane must be contracted and their antagonists must be relaxed. The primary agonist muscles for this rightward movement of the eyes are the right lateral rectus and left medial

Table 1–2. Cranial Nerve Innervation of Extraocular Muscles

Extraocular Muscle	Cranial Nerve Innervation
Medial rectus	Cranial nerve III (oculomotor)
Lateral rectus	Cranial nerve VI (abducens)
Superior rectus	Cranial nerve III (oculomotor)
Inferior rectus	Cranial nerve III (oculomotor)
Superior oblique	Cranial nerve IV (trochlear)
Inferior oblique	Cranial nerve III (oculomotor)

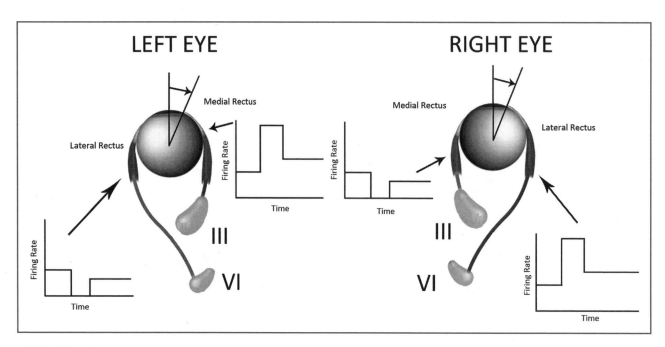

FIGURE 1–7. The relationship between changes in firing rate in the oculomotor neurons and the change in eye position for a rightward eye movement. (Adapted from Barber & Stockwell, 1976)

rectus. In order to contract the lateral rectus and medial rectus, the abducens and oculomotor neurons increase their firing rates, respectively. The antagonist muscles are the left lateral rectus and right medial rectus, and the respective abducens and oculomotor neurons decrease their firing rate to these muscles causing them to relax and allow the eyeball to be moved to the right.

THE FUNCTIONAL CLASSES OF EYE MOVEMENTS

The human oculomotor network is comprised of a complex set of neural circuits that coordinate six different types of eye movements. The gaze-holding, optokinetic, and vestibulo-ocular reflex serve to keep the foveae fixated on a target of interest. The eye movement systems that move the fovea to a target of interest are vergence, smooth pursuit, and saccades. In order to initiate these eye movements and address the visual task, the premotor system receives and organizes the neural input arriving higher centers (e.g., cortex and midbrain) and organizes it into a specific set of commands to generate the most appropriate eye movement(s) for the situation. The premotor system has been described as being located in the brainstem tegmentum, and its role in eye movements is to provide the appropriate neural drive to the three oculomotor brainstem nuclei (i.e., oculomotor, trochlear, and abducens nuclei) (Barber & Stockwell, 1980) (Table 1–3). To completely describe the human premotor system is beyond the scope of this book; however, an extensive review of this system is given by Glaser (1999). The functional classes of human eye movements are summarized in Table 1–4 and are discussed in detail in the following section.

Eye Movements That Move the Fovea Onto a Target

There are three types of eye movements that the oculomotor system uses to direct the fovea to a target. These include vergence, saccades, and smooth pursuit.

Table 1–3. Overview of the Primary Premotor Structures, Their Functions, and Associated Eye Movements.

Premotor Structure	Function	Associated Eye Movement
Medial longitudinal fasiculus	Central conduit to the motor nuclei for coordinated and synchronized eye movements	Involved in all classes of eye movements
Superior colliculus	Generates quick eye movements for orienting to visual or auditory stimuli	Saccades
Superior and lateral vestibular nuclei	Plays a major role in the generation of the VOR and optokinetic nystagmus	VOR and optokinetic
Lateral vestibular nucleus	Fixes images with head stable and environment moving	Optokinetic
Pontine excitatory burst neurons	Generates ballistic eye movements for acquisition of a visual target	Saccade
Medial vestibular nucleus	Stabilizes images during head movement and stabilizes environment	VOR
Repositus hypoglossal (PPH)	Holds a target on the fovea	Together with the MVN it participates in horizontal gaze-holding

VOR vestibulo-ocular reflex; *MVN* medial vestibular nuclei.

Table 1–4. Functional Classes of Eye Movements

Class of Eye Movement	Function
Hold Images on Retina	
Vestibular (VOR)	Maintains image on the retina during brief movements of the head
Optokinetic	Maintains image on the retina during sustained head movements
Visual Fixation	Maintains image on the fovea when the head is not moving
Moves the Fovea to a Target of Interest	
Vergence	Moves the eyes in an opposite direction so that a single target is maintained simultaneously on both foveae
Smooth pursuit system	Maintains the image of a moving target on the fovea
Saccades	Brings a target of interest onto the fovea rapidly

Version and Vergence

When the eyes are tracking a target and change directions from left to right with no change in the distance of the target, the eye movement is referred to as a version. Versions are conjugate eye movements. Vergence refers to a type of eye movement that moves the globes in a disconjugate manner (divergence or convergence) so that the observer sees a single image located at different distances. Specifically, gaze direction remains unchanged, but the distance of the target will change. This class of eye movement is somewhat different than pursuit or saccades because the movements are disjunctive. For example, when an object is close to the face, the eyes must rotate inward or converge. Alternatively, when an object is far away, the eyes must rotate outward in order to allow the observer to see one image (Figure 1–8).

Velocity and latency are the two primary characteristics that are evaluated when examining vergence. With regards to velocity, there is fast and slow vergence. Slow vergence eye movements are recruited when an object of interest is either moving away or toward the observer slowly. Conversely, fast vergence eye movements are generated when the observer quickly switches from a target that is near to one that is off in the distance. The latency of vergence movements refers to the time it takes to focus on a target. The vergence eye movement system is relatively slow in comparison to other eye movements. The latency of vergence ranges from 80 to 200 msec depending on the situation. It has been suggested that one reason for this prolonged latency is related to the time it takes for the lens of the eye to changes shape. The primary trigger for the vergence system to be recruited is retinal image blur, which is a situation where the object of interest is either too far away or too close to view in detail. Another reason is retinal disparity, which refers to the observer seeing to different images and the eyes must adjust to bring both foveae on the target and fuse the image.

Neural Mechanism

The neural mechanisms that initiate and control the vergence system have not yet been completely mapped. However, there are three primary centers that are known to control vergence eye movements. These include the cerebrum, brainstem, and the cerebellum. In the cerebrum, there are contributions from the frontal eye fields in the frontal lobe, the parietal lobe, striate cortex, middle temporal, and medial superior temporal areas. The brainstem structures responsible for vergence include the medial nucleus reticularis

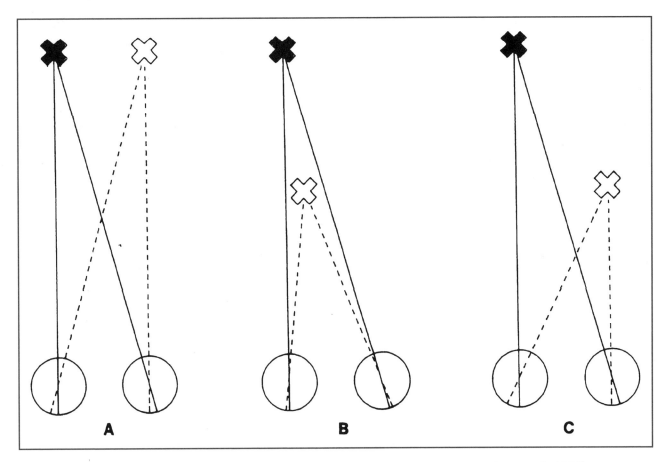

FIGURE 1–8. A. Version, **B.** Vergence, **C.** Version and Vergence. (From Barber & Stockwell, 1976)

tegmenti pontis, supra-oculomotor area, ocular motor nucleus, and abducens nucleus. The dorsal vermis, nucleus, interpositus, and flocculus are parts of the cerebellum that are known contributors to vergence.

Saccades

When a target is detected on the edge of the visual field, the OMS can quickly move the eyes conjugately and bring the image of interest onto the foveae. This type of eye movement is known as a saccade and is the type of eye movement we use to shift our gaze to interesting targets and explore our visual environment (Robinson, 1964). The saccadic control system is responsible for generating extremely fast and accurate conjugate eye movements that place the foveae in new positions. The saccade is the fastest type of eye movement and its speed is dependent on the distance the eye must travel to acquire the target (faster for objects far

away and slower for objects that are close). The speed of these eye movements is not controlled by the observer but rather by the distance of the eye excursion. That is, a higher velocity can be obtained the farther the eye has to travel to the target. Saccades can be either reflexive or voluntary and occur in the absence of a visual stimulus (i.e., in the dark or with vision denied).

The calculation by the nervous system of what the amplitude of a voluntary saccade needs to be (i.e., how big the saccade has to be to acquire the target) involves what has been termed "retinal positional error" (RPE) (Heywood & Churcher, 1981). RPE describes the disparity between where the target is in space compared with where the retina is. A more specific way of describing this may be "foveae positional error" because it is the fovea that must be aligned with the target. When the target is identified, the entire process (i.e., premotor and motor contributions) of saccade generation takes, on average, less than 350 ms. The latency (i.e., how long before the eye begins to move once a target appears) averages approximately 150 to 250 ms, and most saccades last less than 100 ms (Rucker, 2010). As previously stated, the saccade system is capable of moving the eye extremely fast. This type of eye movement can range from approximately 100° to 700° per second during excursions of 0.5 to 50 degrees. During this eye movement, the observer is essentially "blind" because the retina is incapable of resolving images when the eye is moving at speeds this high. These fast eye movements reduce the amount of time that vision is blurred.

Neural Mechanism

In order to accomplish this precise ballistic eye movement, the system makes use of cortical, brainstem, and cerebellar circuitry (i.e., the neural integrator) to calculate where the foveae of the retinas should go in order to fixate on an object of interest. A saccadic eye movement consists of what has been termed "pulse-step" innervation and has three distinct stages. First, the target of interest must be identified and its location calculated. When discussing voluntary horizontal saccades, the cerebral cortex exerts control over these fast eye movements. The cortex is responsible for processing when to initiate the saccade and to relay the commands to lower centers to bring the object of interest onto the fovea (Figure 1–9).

Cerebral Contributions to Saccades

The cortex has several areas that play a role in the generation of voluntary saccades. A subregion

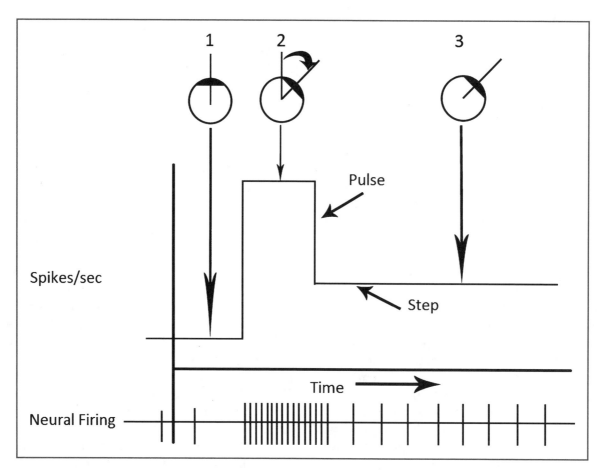

FIGURE 1–9. Relationship between the discharge rate and eye movement. 1. Eye is in primary position; 2. Eye is quickly moved to the right; 3. Eye is maintained in deviated position. (Adapted from Leigh & Zee, 2006).

of the frontal eye field (FEF), supplementary eye fields (SEF), dorsolateral prefrontal cortex, and parietal eye field (PEF) work together to encode the amplitude and direction of the saccade needed to bring the eyes onto the target. The FEF and PEF both directly relay information regarding the target of interest to a visuomotor integration center called the superior colliculus (SC) located on the dorsal aspect of the midbrain (Leigh & Zee, 2006). These cortical centers also send indirect projections to the superior colliculus via the caudate nucleus and substantia nigra pars reticulata, which are located in the midbrain. This converging information arriving at the SC is then passed on to specialized centers in the brainstem (i.e., paramedian pontine reticular formation (PPRF) and the medial longitudinal fasciculus (MLF).

Cerebellar Contributions to Saccades

The cerebellum acts to ensure the size of the saccade is appropriate based on what has been relayed from the higher centers. The frontal eye fields, by way of the caudal nucleus reticularis tegmenti pontis and superior colliculus, project saccadic information to the dorsal "oculomotor" vermis (lobules VI and VI) Purkinje cells and fastigial nucleus. The deep cerebellar fastigial nucleus sends input to the saccadic burst generator (e.g., burst and omnipause neurons) located in the brainstem via the uncinated fasciculus (Figure 1–10). The flocculonodular lobe and paraflocculus receive vestibular inputs and send projections to the medial and superior vestibular nuclei (i.e., PPRF) and play a key role in

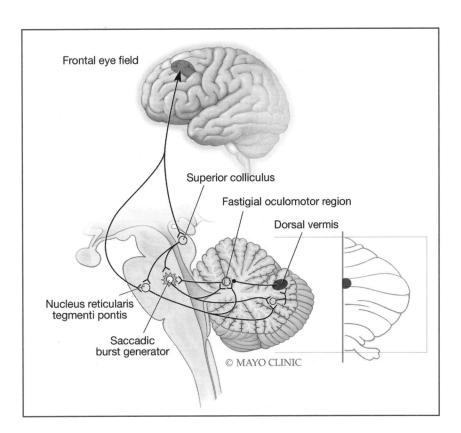

FIGURE 1–10. Role of the dorsal and fastigial oculomotor region in the control of saccades. The dorsal vermis by way of the fastigial oculomotor region modulates saccade direction and amplitude. The fastigial nucleus projects to the saccadic burst generator. The nucleus reticularis tegmenti pontis relays information from the frontal eye fields and superior colliculus to the cerebellar structures involved in the generation of saccades. (Used with permission of Mayo Foundation for Medical Education and Research. All rights reserved.)

the coordination and adaptation of the pulse command that drives the motor neurons that move the eye from point "A" to point "B" for horizontal saccades (Figure 1–11).

Brainstem Contribution to Horizontal Saccades

Beginning with the FEFs, projections carrying information about the saccade are routed through the cerebellum and the SC where they converge on PPRF. The PPRF is located in the pons and is also referred to as the paraabducens nucleus. This brainstem structure is part of the pontine reticular formation and contains three primary classes of neurons. They are referred to as excitatory burst neurons (EBN), inhibitory burst neurons (IBN) and omnipause neurons. Together they three types of neurons located in the brainstem effectively work together to generate the neural process known as "pulse-step" (Sylvestre & Cullen, 1999). EBNs are responsible for initiating the premotor command (i.e., eye velocity). This high frequency burst of neural activity is sent to the agonist motor neurons of the eye and is often referred to as the "pulse" of the saccade. The EBNs or "pulse generator" relay this information to the abducens nucleus motor neurons and internuclear neurons via the MLF to contract the ipsilateral lateral rectus and the contralateral medial rectus muscles respectively (Figure 1–12). A corresponding inhibition of the antagonist muscles is coordinated by the second type of burst neurons referred to as inhibitory. Inhibitory burst neurons (IBN) are located in the nucleus paragigantocellularis dorsalis in the PPRF. This process, known as the "pulse," overcomes the viscous drag of the eye and quickly and accurately moves the eyes in a yoked fashion to the target of interest. A third type of neuron referred to as omnipause inhibit the above-described excitatory burst neurons, when smooth eye movements are required or the eyes need to remain fixed on a target. That is, they control the activation of unwanted saccades and facilitate the generation of appropriate saccades. When a saccade command is received at the level of the brainstem, these omnipause neurons reduce their firing rate. This has the consequence of releasing the burst neurons from inhibition and enabling them to generate the high-frequency burst of neural activity needed to activate the motor neurons and move the eye. Once the position of the eye matches the desired eye position that was communicated from the higher centers, the omnipause neurons assume their tonic resting rate the saccade stops.

The second stage of a saccade consists of a continued neural discharge that holds the eyes on the target and is known as the "step" response. The "step" generator is distributed throughout the medulla and brainstem and is responsible for translating the eye velocity command into an eye positon command for the ocular motor neurons. This mathematical calculation by the medial ves-

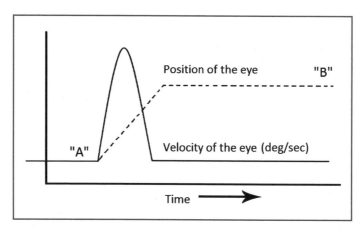

FIGURE 1–11. Relationship between the velocity of the eye and the position of the eye during a saccadic eye movement.

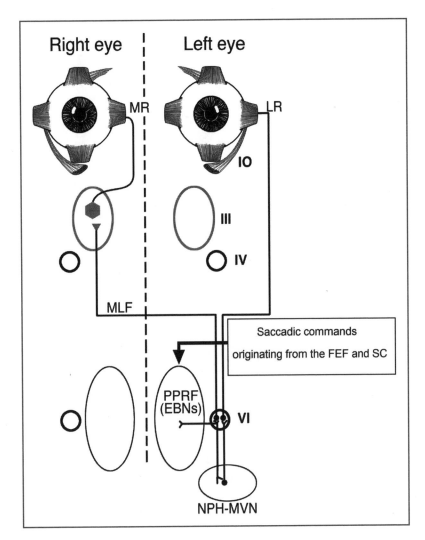

FIGURE 1–12. Illustration of the pathway in the brainstem for the generation of horizontal saccades. PPRF = paramedian pontine reticular formation; EBNs = excitatory burst neurons; MLF = medial longitudinal fasciculus; III = third nucleus; IV = fourth nucleus; VI = sixth nucleus; NPH = nucleus prepositus hypoglossi; MVN = medial vestibular nucleus; MR = medial rectus; and LR = lateral rectus. (Adapted from Wong, AMF, *Eye Movement Disorders*, 2008)

tibular nucleus (MVN) and nucleus prepositus hypoglossi (NPH) is referred to in the literature as the neural integrator. The neural integrators purpose is to hold gaze steady on the target of interest following the rapid eye movement that initially acquired the target. Together, this neural process of generating a saccade and holding the eye steady on the target is known as the "pulse-step" (Sylvestre & Cullen, 1999). A recording of a random saccade test is shown in Figure 1–13.

Smooth Pursuit System

The pursuit system is a voluntary oculomotor control system that enables an observer to hold the foveae on a target that is moving slowly (<70° per second). The primary purpose of this system is to keep slow moving images stabilized on the foveae when the target is moving and the head is stable. Creatures that have foveae are capable of generating smooth pursuit eye movements, whereas

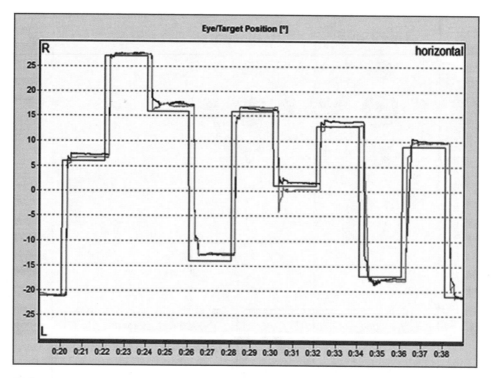

FIGURE 1–13. A recording of a normal random saccade paradigm and the associated eye movements. (Interacoustics version; Interacoustics, Assens, Denmark)

those that do not are incapable of producing this type or eye movement. A target is required in order to recruit the pursuit system to track a target. It can be visual, auditory, proprioceptive, or tactile. Typically, a target is initially acquired quickly (approximately 100 ms) using the saccade system. If the target of interest is moving, the pursuit system is engaged to hold the visual target stable on the retina. The way the pursuit system holds the target on the retina is by continually sampling where the target is in relation to the fovea and adjusting for the amount that the target "slips" off the retina. The pursuit system is limited with regard to how fast it can track a target. When target velocities exceed 60° per second, the pursuit system is no longer able to match the eye velocity to the target velocity, and the target is no longer maintained on the fovea. In this case, the target must be reacquired using the saccade system. Interestingly, the pursuit system seems to be driven almost entirely by a moving visual stimulus. Although one can produce saccades in the absence of visual stimuli, this is not true for pursuit.

Neural Mechanism for Horizontal Pursuit Eye Movements

The neural pathways responsible for generating smooth pursuit eye movements are complex and, to date, have not yet been completely described. Smooth tracking of eye movements is accomplished using a combination of cortical, cerebellar, and brainstem centers. In order to track a visual target, a series of events must be accomplished, which involve processing by each of the aforementioned centers. First, motion-sensitive cells known as M-cells (i.e., magnocellular) in the retina detect that an object is moving. These cells send signals about target velocity and direction through the magnocellular layers located in the lateral geniculate nucleus (LGN) of the thalamus to the primary visual cortex of striate cortex (area V1). Area V1 has specialized cells that further refine the information about the particular direction of the target. From area V1, information about the visual target is relayed to the extrastriate areas V2, V3, as well as the middle temporal visual area (MT or V5) that further encodes the velocity and direction of the moving target. The encoded information about the target is then distributed from the MT to the medial superior temporal (MST) area and from there to specialized subregions of the visual motor region of the frontal cortex referred to as the frontal and supplemental eye fields. There are also simultaneous projections from the MT and MST to several other specialized areas. These include the lateral intraparietal area (LIP) located in the posterior parietal cortex, the dorsolateral pontine nuclei (DLPN) which is located in the pons and the nucleus of the optic tract (NOT). It is noteworthy that the NOT only participates in the generation of horizontal pursuit eye movements. The updated and processed information regarding the moving target all converges on the DLPN and is then projected to the cerebellum. Cerebellar structures that are integral to processing the information about target velocity and direction are the flocculus/paraflocculus, vermis, and fastigial nucleus. Projections from these cerebellar structures are received by the medial vestibular nucleus (MVN) in the brainstem and then relays through the final common pathway. Specifically, the MVN sends projections across the midline of the brainstem to the contralateral abducens nucleus (VI). From the abducens nucleus, the information regarding the target is sent both back across the midline to innervate the contralateral medial rectus and the lateral rectus on the same side where the velocity of the eye is matched to the velocity of the target (Figure 1–14). A recording of a pursuit test is shown in Figure 1–15.

EYE MOVEMENTS THAT KEEP THE FOVEA FIXED ON A TARGET

There are three types of eye movements that the oculomotor system uses to keep the fovea stable on a target. These include gaze-holding, optokinetic, and vestibulo-ocular reflex (VOR). The VOR is discussed in-depth in Chapter 2.

Gaze-Holding: "The Neural Integrator"

Gaze-holding describes the function of holding the foveae motionless on a target in the primary position or eccentric (deviated) position. When gaze is directed away from midline, the brain must program a tonic neural command of sufficient size to cause sustained contraction of the paired agonist extraocular muscles and a reciprocal command to decrease electrical tone delivered to the paired antagonist muscles. This is necessary to counteract the visuo-elastic restoring forces of the orbit that tend to pull back the eye to the primary position. This eye-position signal is generated by a gaze-holding network [i.e., the neural integrator (NI)].

Neural Mechanism

The NI is a distributed function (i.e., distributed among several structures in the brainstem) and is highly dependent on an intact vestibulocerebellum (flocculus, ventral paraflocculus, nodulus, and uvula) (Leigh & Zee, 2006). The flocculonodular lobe is located near the paraflocculus and both in close proximity to the VIII cranial nerve. These two regions of the cerebellum receive neural input from the labyrinth; dorsolateral pontine nuclei (DPN); nucleus prepositus hypoglossi (NPH); nucleus reticularis tegmenti pontis (NRTP); mesencephalic reticular formation; vestibular nuclei; and middle superior temporal area (MST) (Figure 1–16). These two regions of the vestibulocerebellum are critical to gaze-holding and vestibulo-ocular reflex cancellation. When patients with impairments in the NI are asked to hold their eyes on a target in an eccentric position, they often demonstrate a slow drift of their eyes off the target followed by a quick corrective saccade of the eye back onto the target (Figure 1–17). When gazing at a target in an eccentric position, the NI is continuously updating the neural command to extraocular muscles to ensure that the eyes stay on the target; however, impairment in this gaze-holding system results in a reduced step response and thus a centripetal drift of the eyes off the target. A corrective saccade directed away from the primary position is generated by the OMS to reacquire the target. This phenomenon has been termed gaze-evoked nystagmus, and it manifests as a jerk nystagmus that is characterized by a low amplitude and high frequency.

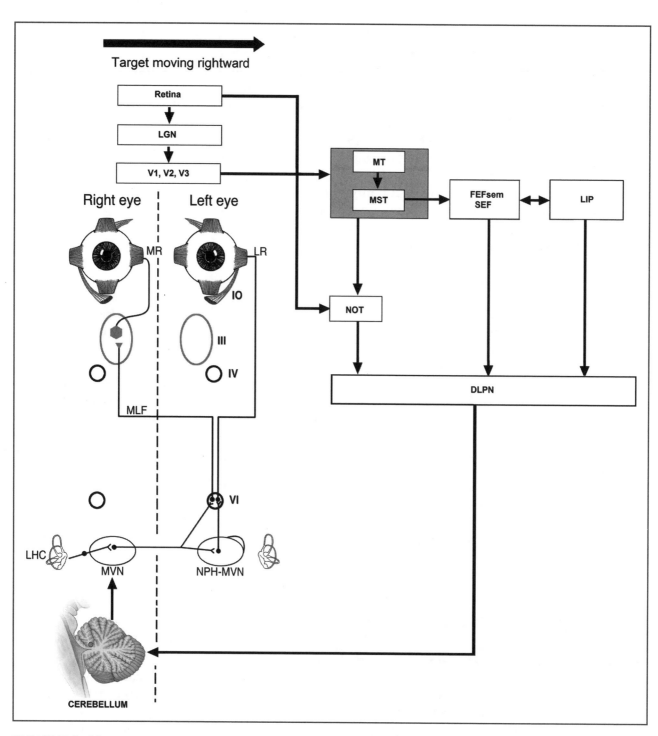

FIGURE 1–14. Pathway for horizontal pursuit. LGN = lateral geniculate nucleus; V1 = striate cortex; V2, V3 = extrastriate cortex; MT = middle temporal visual area; MST = medial superior temporal visual area; MST = medial superior temporal visual area; FEFsem = pursuit subregion of the frontal eye field; SEF = supplemental eye field; LIP = lateral intraparietal area; NOT = nucleus of the optic tract; DLPN = dorsolateral pontine nuclei; MVN = medial vestibular nucleus; LHC = left horizontal canal; NPH = nucleus prepositus hypoglossi; MLF = medial longitudinal fasiculus, LHC = left horizontal canal, MR = medial rectus, and LR = lateral rectus. (Adapted from Wong, AMF, *Eye Movement Disorders*, 2008)

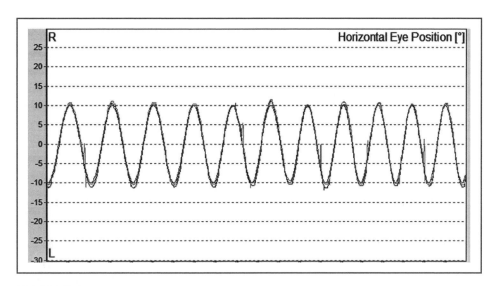

FIGURE 1–15. A recording of the eye movements in response to a pursuit stimulus. (Interacoustics version; Interacoustics, Assens, Denmark)

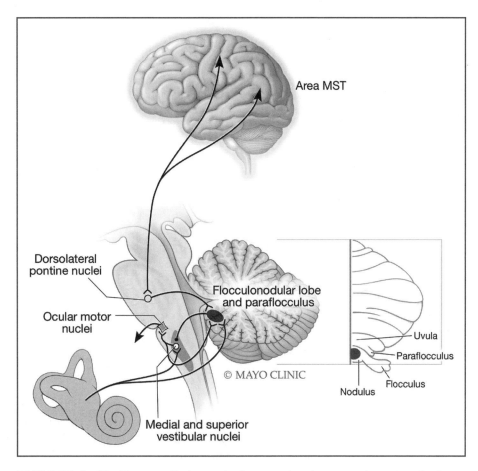

FIGURE 1–16. The vestibulocerebellum as it relates to the control of eye movements. (Used with permission of Mayo Foundation for Medical Education and Research. All rights reserved.)

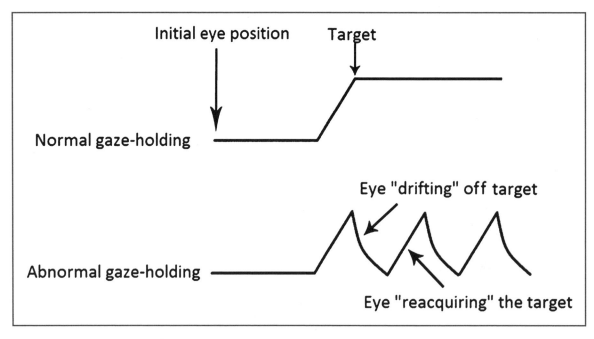

FIGURE 1–17. A comparison of normal gaze-holding and abnormal gaze-holding and the associated eye movement.

OPTOKINETIC SYSTEM

The optokinetic (OKN) system is a reflexive functional class of eye movement that works in concert with the vestibular system to stabilize a moving visual environment on the retina when the head is stationary. It is activated by movement of the visual field around an observer or when the visual scene in front of the observer is large. When the reflex is generated, the observer will have the illusionary sensation that they are moving in the opposite direction as the visual field. This has been termed circularvection. The OKN subsystem generates a response that is complementary to the one that is provided by the vestibular labyrinths (Leigh & Zee, 2006). That is, the canal system in the peripheral vestibular system is best suited to transducing high-frequency head movements (angular), whereas the OKN system provides the ability to keep an image steady using low frequency sustained movement. Together, the responses from the OKN system and the vestibular system generate a slow compensatory eye movement that is proportional to the velocity of the head movement. When the head velocity is slow, the compensatory input is driven primarily by the OKN system; however, when the head is moved at a frequency above approximately 1 Hz, the input is provided primarily by the peripheral vestibular system. Stimuli moving to the right are slowly followed by both eyes. Once the eyes reach a certain position in the orbit, they are quickly reset in the opposite direction, at which point the stimuli are reacquired and tracked again. This slow tracking movement, (which has the same velocity as the head movement) followed by the quick resetting of the eye in the opposite direction has been termed optokinetic nystagmus (Figure 1–18).

Neural Mechanism

In order to generate compensatory eye movements that are appropriate for observing the moving visual stimulus, the OKN system processes the visual input using two different pathways. OKN eye movement is initiated at the retina, which contains ganglionic cells that respond exclusively to motion in certain directions and orientations. Motion-generated signals sent from the retina

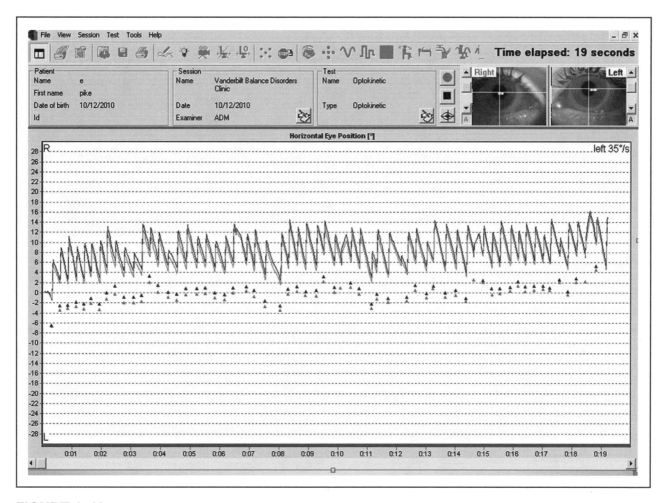

FIGURE 1–18. A recording of the eye movements in response to a full-field optokinetic stimulus consisting of stripes. (Interacoustics version; Interacoustics, Assens, Denmark)

pass through the optic nerve at which point the signal diverges and inputs are sent to the cortex (via lateral geniculate nucleus) and brainstem.

The brainstem pathway receives the OKN signals from the optic nerve. At a certain point they decussate at the optic chiasm and are projected to specialized nuclei in the brainstem [i.e., nucleus of the optic tract (NOT)] that code motion. Specifically, the NOT is composed of cells with receptive fields sensitive to moving stimuli. Once the NOT has received the input from the contra-lateral eyes, it relays the signals to the vestibular nuclei. The vestibular nuclei project this electrical code to the OMNs that drive eye movement to track the moving stimulus. The cortical pathway receives and processes the target information, which is routed via the lateral geniculate nucleus to the MST, where information regarding ipsilateral motion is coded. This visual input, which has been processed by the cortex, is relayed to the NOT and then to the premotor system to move the eye accordingly.

2

Anatomy and Physiology of the Vestibular System

INTRODUCTION

The vestibular system is composed of a set of five electrical generators, or end organs, on each side that accomplish three primary tasks. First, it works to stabilize the visual environment when the visual surround is moving or the observer is moving. The labyrinth of the inner ear transduces linear and angular accelerations of the head and routes that information through the VIIIth nerve to the vestibular nuclei in the brainstem. The vestibular nuclei send projections to the ocular motor nuclei, which synapse on ocular motor neurons that contract and relax the extraocular muscles to accommodate the vestibulo-ocular reflex (VOR). Second, it acts to provide information to the central nervous system for controlling skeletal muscle tone for adjusting posture. The neural code that is generated by the peripheral vestibular system regarding head movement is also sent to the cervical spinal motor neurons commonly referred to as the vestibulo-colic reflex. Projections also continue on to lower spinal motor neurons to drive what has been termed the vestibulo-spinal reflex (VSR).

Third, it provides the central nervous system with spatial information regarding linear and angular movements. The vestibular input collected during head movements is also relayed to cortical centers where the organisms' perception regarding movement and orientation is processed. Secondary functions of the vestibular system are varied. For instance, it provides information to the autonomic nervous system and has a role in regulating hemodynamic reflexes to keep the brain perfused with blood. One of the key abilities it has is the ability to adapt the vestibular reflexes following injury to the peripheral system or when there has been a significant change in vision. This action is accomplished through the vestibular systems direct communication with the cerebellum and is discussed in-depth in Chapter 3.

Understanding the vestibular reflex pathways allows the clinician to understand and make sense of symptoms described by the patients and the associated deficits of the balance system. A thorough understanding of the anatomy and physiology of the vestibular system is required in order to correctly interpret the associated eye movements and postural changes that occur following an insult to the vestibular system.

THE SENSORY TRANSDUCTION OF THE PERIPHERAL VESTIBULAR SYSTEM

The peripheral vestibular system is an elegant network of membranous sacs (i.e., membranous labyrinth) and contains the inertial sensors that transduce angular and linear acceleration. These inner ear structures are located in the petrous portion of the temporal bone within a bony labyrinth (Figure 2–1). The membranous labyrinth is suspended within the bony labyrinth by connective tissue and contains the three semicircular canals (SCC) on each side, and two orthogonal otolith organs. The organs have two types of fluid that are separated by a membrane. Perilymph has an ionic composition similar to cerebrospinal fluid that is high in [Na+] = 140 mEq/l and low in [K+] = 10 mEq/l. Endolymph has a chemical composition that is similar to intracellular fluid and [K+] = 144 mEq/l and [Na+] = 5 mEq/l (Fife, 2009). The cells in the stria vascularis of the cochlea are able to convert perilymph into endolymph. Endolymph is moved through the system and absorbed by the darks cells of the cristae and maculae (Figure 2–2). The three SCCs on each side are termed the horizontal (lateral), superior (anterior), and posterior. The canals are orthogonal to each other and have a partner on the other side of the head that creates a 3D coordinate system for sensing rotation. The otolith organs housed in the vestibule are responsible for sensing linear acceleration and deceleration in the horizontal and vertical plane.

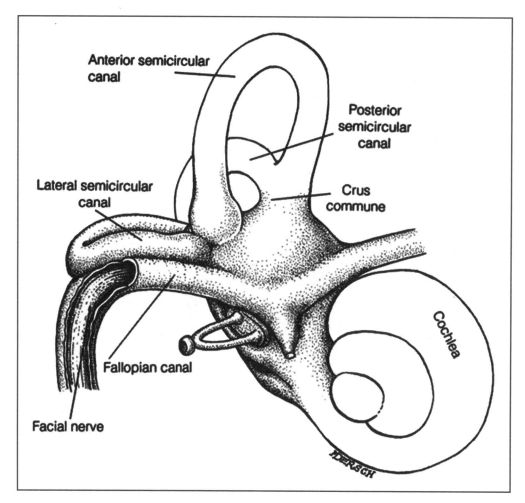

FIGURE 2–1. The anatomy of the bony labyrinth. (Illustration by Mary Dersch from Pender, 1992, with permission of Daniel Pender)

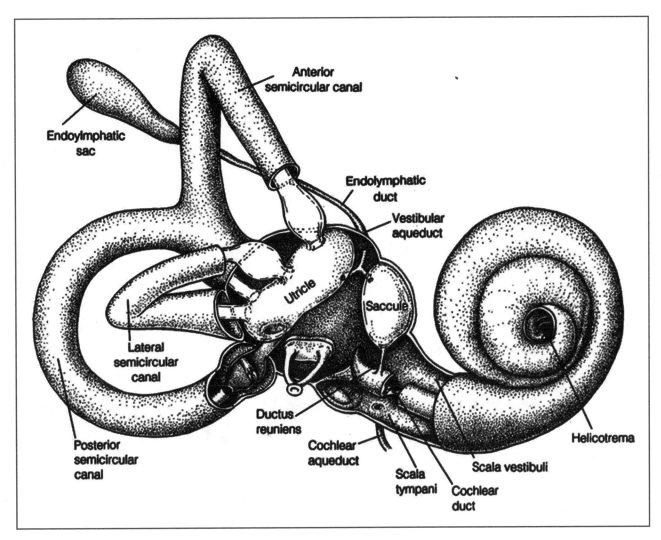

FIGURE 2–2. The anatomy of the membranous labyrinth. (Illustration by Mary Dersch from Pender, 1992, with permission of Daniel Pender)

The two organs are orthogonal to each other and referred to as the utricle and saccule. Each canal has an enlarged end called an ampulla that contains a sensory organ. The otoliths organs act as inertial accelerometers and each have a sensory organ known as the maculae. Anatomically, the semicircular canals (SCCs) and otolith organs are, at the same time, both similar and different. Each organ has a mass that is connected to stereocilia that project from the tops of specialized hair cells. It is the effect of inertia during acceleration or deceleration on the mass that results in a movement of the cilia and electrical transduction at the base of the hair cells.

VESTIBULAR HAIR CELLS

There are two primary types of hair cells in the vestibular system; these are the cylindrical type II and the flask-shaped type I hair cells. Type I hair cells are surrounded at the base by a large afferent nerve ending called a *calyx* or *chalice*. The neural efferent connections synapse on the calyx rather than the cell body. In contrast to the type I cells, type II hair cells are cylindrical and have afferent and efferent nerve terminals connecting directly to the base of the cell. Although there are distinct morphological differences in the two types of cells, they both convert mechanical energy into a neural code that provides the brain with information about orientation and acceleration of the head. There are three primary components to both types of cells; the stereocilia, the cell body, and the afferent and efferent nerve endings. Both types of hair cells have approximately 70 stereocilia that progressively increase in height and converge on one long filament referred to as a *kinocilium*. The stereocilia form a gradient from shortest to tallest terminating on a single longer and thicker kinocilium. Both Type and I and II hair cells have a high tonic resting rate. That is, in the absence of any stimulus, they generate a spontaneous firing rate in the nerve of about 70 to 90 spikes per second (Goldberg & Fernandez, 1971a). As previously stated, vestibular hair cells are sensitive to mechanical force and the stereocilia of each cell are linked to one another by a protein strand called *tip links*. Research has shown that when a parallel force is applied to the top of the stereocilia, the tip links open cation channels in the stereocilia. The stereocilia of vestibular hair cells are directionally polarized meaning that when the hairs are deflected toward the kinocilium, ions from the K+ rich endolymph are able to enter the gates. This has the net effect of increasing (making more positive) the cell membranes resting potential (i.e., depolarize it). This increase in the cell membranes voltage in turn triggers the activation of voltage-sensitive calcium channels located at the bottom of the hair cell. The activation of the calcium channels allows calcium to flow into the cell and trigger the release of excitatory neurotransmitters (e.g., glutamate), which leads to an increase in the firing rate in the vestibular nerves. An equivalent force in the opposite direction (away from the kinocilium) decreases the resting potential of the cell (i.e., hyperpolarize) and decreases the firing rate in the nerve. When a force perpendicular (straight down) to the hair cells is applied, there is little or no change in the resting potential of the cells (Hudspeth & Corey, 1977; Hudspeth, 1982). These changes in firing rate in the afferent fibers as a result of changes in the hair cell voltage are relayed to secondary neurons of the vestibular nuclei located in the brainstem (Figure 2–3).

SEMICIRCULAR CANAL ANATOMY AND PHYSIOLOGY

The three SCCs are arranged orthogonally (at right angles) to each other, enabling the system to detect

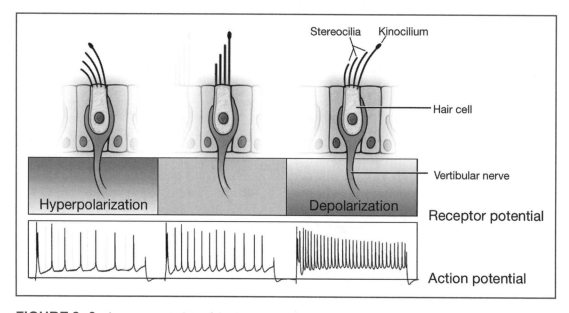

FIGURE 2–3. A representation of the hair cells and the firing of primary vestibular afferent neurons for different directions of deflection. (Used with permission of Mayo Foundation for Medical Education and Research. All rights reserved.)

the direction and amplitude of a head movement in any direction. When a person is upright, the lateral canals are positioned 30 degrees superior from the horizontal plane. The two vertical SCCs are oriented at 45° in the sagittal plane and the horizontal canals are tilted upward approximately 30°. Each SCC canal has a partner on the opposite side that is coplanar and detects movement in the same plane (Figure 2–4). The orientation and pairings of the SCCs are a key component in facilitating the eye movements that are associated with the vestibulo-ocular reflex (VOR). When one member of the pair is stimulated (i.e., excited) by a head movement in the plane of stimulation for that canal, the partner is inhibited. For instance, when the head is moved quickly to the right in the horizontal plane, the right horizontal SCC is excited and its counterpart the left horizontal SCC is inhibited. The pairings for the vertical canals are the right anterior and left posterior (RALP) and the left anterior and right posterior (LARP) canals.

Each SCC is attached to the vestibule and has an enlarged end called the ampulla (Lysakowski, 2005). The ampulla houses each canal's sensory epithelium (i.e., crista ampullaris). The crista ampullaris is shaped like a dome and is composed of several parts. One component of the crista ampullaris is the cupula. The cupula is a gelatinous mass that extends from the base of the ampulla to the roof and effectively seals off the two sides of the ampulla (Figure 2–5) (McLaren & Hillman, 1979). Embedded in the base of the cupula are the approximately 7,000 stereocilia of the type I and type II receptor hair cells. In the cupula, type I hair cells are centered on the top of the cristae in the SCCs and near the striola on the utricle and saccule. Type II hair cells are focused around the sides of the crista and on the lateral edges of the otoliths organs. The approximately 7,000 hair cells in each of the crista are polarized in the same direction (Berthoz, 1996). When the head is moved in the plane of a particular SCC, inertia and the viscosity of the endolymph causes the fluid to lag behind the head movement (i.e., the semicircular canal and hair cells). This has the effect of moving the endolymph in the opposite direction of the SCC which in turn creates a force that pushes on the crista ampullaris in the SCC that is in the plane of the acceleration. The result is a deflection of the hair cell bundle toward the kinocilium resulting in a decrease in hair cell membrane voltage and an increase in firing rate of the afferent fibers. Deflection of the stereocilia bundle away from the kinocilium results in a decrease in neural afferent firing rate (Figure 2–6). The stereocilia in the vertical canals (anterior and posterior) are polarized toward the canal side of the ampulla. That is, the taller ends of the stereocilia

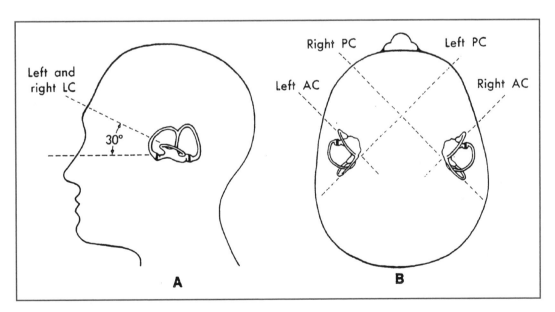

FIGURE 2–4. Spatial orientation of the SCCs. LC = lateral canal; AC = anterior canal; PC = posterior canal. (From Barber & Stockwell, 1980 with permission from Charles Stockwell)

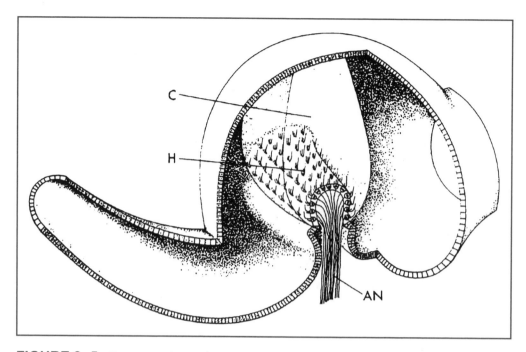

FIGURE 2–5. Cross-sectional view of the ampulla of a semicircular canal. C = cupula, H = hair cells, AN = afferent nerves (From Stockwell and Barber, 1980 with permission from Charles Stockwell)

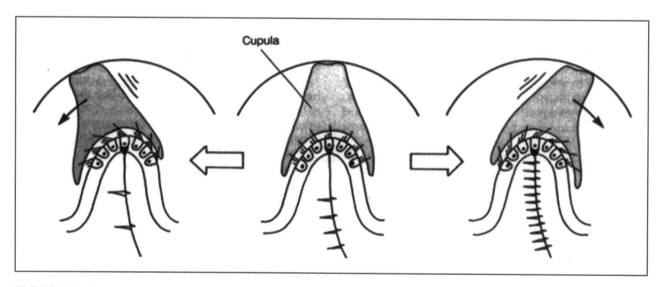

FIGURE 2–6. Cupular deflection in one direction results in an increase in firing in the nerve and a decrease in the opposite direction. (Illustration by Mary Dersch from Pender, 1992, with permission of Daniel Pender)

bundles are directed away from the utricle. Movement of the endolymph away from the ampula and utricle is referred to as ampullofugal and in this instance is excitatory. The stereocilia in the horizontal canals are oriented toward the utricu-lar side of the ampulla. This arrangement creates a difference in the directional sensitivity of the vertical and horizontal canals (Figure 2–7). In the horizontal canals, movement of endolymph toward the ampulla (ampullopetal) generates an

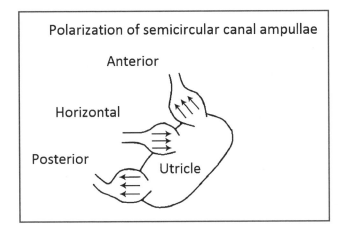

FIGURE 2–7. Polarization patterns of the hair cells in the SCCs. The *arrows* indicate the directions in which the stereocilia are oriented.

increase in firing rate in the nerve, whereas in the vertical canals the opposite is true (endolymph flow toward the ampulla results in a decrease-firing rate in the nerve). The distribution of the hair cells in the cristae is complex (Brichta & Goldberg, 1996). Type I hair cells produce an irregular firing pattern and are found to be clustered in the center of the crista (Goldberg & Fernandez, 1971a, 1971b). Goldberg, Highstein, Moschovakis, and Fernandez (1987) suggest that this arrangement of the type I hair cells in the crista may be responsible for producing quick bursts of neural activity that adjust the head when the canals are stimulated. In contrast, type II neurons are found to be located on the periphery of the crista and have been suggested to be primarily responsible for driving the eye movement of the vestibulo-ocular reflex (VOR) (Goldberg et al., 1987). The cupula and the endolymph surrounding it have essentially the same specific gravity making the cristae insensitive to gravity. When the head is still, the cupula is suspended in the endolymph in a neutrally buoyant position and the vestibular afferents fire at their tonic resting rate; however, when the head is moved in an angular fashion, the endolymph lags behind the canal walls. When this happens the cupula acts as a partition in the ampullar cavity and the endolymph presses on the cupula and bends it in the opposite direction of the head movement. When the hair cells embedded in the base of each of the cupula are deflected,

ion channels in the tips of the stereocilia open or close (depending on the direction of the head movement) and allow more or less endolymph into the cell, as compared with when the system is at rest. More endolymph entering the cell raises the resting potential and increases the amount of activation that occurs at the synapses between the cell and the nerve (increasing the firing rate in the nerve). This excitatory action is known as an ampullopetal response. Less endolymph entering the cell lowers the resting potential and decreases the activation of the synapses between the cell and the nerve (decreasing the firing rate in the nerve). This inhibitory action is termed an ampullofugal response. These changes in the vestibular nerve firing rate drive the compensatory eye movements of the VOR and are discussed later.

OTOLITH ORGAN ANATOMY AND PHYSIOLOGY

Although the ENG/VNG examination does not assess the two otolith organs, a basic understanding of them is necessary for any clinician assessing balance function. The saccule and utricle have a specialized sensory epithelium that enables them to act as biacclerometers and sense persistent tilt and low-frequency linear acceleration. They are positioned in the otic capsule in such a way that they respond to movements in the horizontal and vertical planes. The utricular macule is oriented in the horizontal plane in the elliptical recess of the vestibule near the anterior opening of the horizontal SCC. It is tilted down and back approximately 25 to 30 degrees (Schwarz & Tomlinson, 2005). The utricle is two times larger than the saccule and is loosely attached to the skull (Jaeger & Haslwanter, 2004; Rosenhall, 1973; Uzun-Coruhlu, Curthoys, & Jones, 2007; Wright, Hubbard, & Clark, 1979). The macule of the saccule is oriented primarily in the vertical plane and is located on the medial wall of the vestibule in the spherical recess inferior to the utricle and directly beneath the stapes in the sagittal plane (Figure 2–8). This proximity to the middle ear space makes the saccule sensitive to high-intensity air-conducted stimuli (ACS). It is noteworthy that in several animal species utilize the saccule as a hearing receptor (Popper & Fay, 1973). Each otolith has a sensory epithelium called a maculae that rests on a gelatinous membrane (i.e., otolithic membrane). The macula utriculi and sacculi are one of the two types of sensory epithelia in the vestibular system (the other is the semicircular canals). Small (i.e., 5 to 7 μm) calcium carbonate crystals (Ca(CO3)

referred to as "otoconia or otoliths" with a specific gravity of 2.71 g/mL are embedded in a gelatinous matrix known as the otolithic membrane (Figure 2–9) (Ross, Donovan, & Chee, 1985). The crystals are dense compared with the surrounding endolymph and therefore have a higher specific gravity (i.e., they are heavier) (Money et al., 1971).

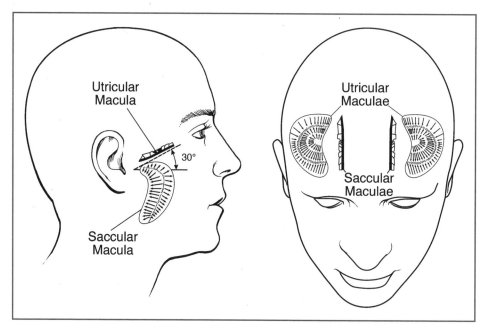

FIGURE 2–8. Orientation of the maculae of the utricle and saccule. The *arrows* indicate the direction in which the stereocilia are oriented.

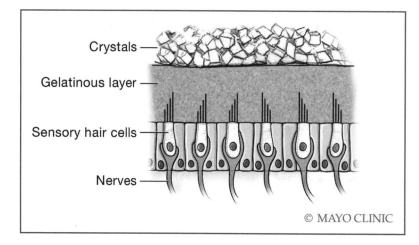

FIGURE 2–9. Otolith organ is shown. (Used with permission of Mayo Foundation for Medical Education and Research. All rights reserved.)

The macules are composed of several components that enable them to effectively transduce and code linear acceleration. First, the otoconia are embedded in a gelatinous matrix known as the otolithic membrane. The otolithic membrane of the utricle is loosely attached to the skull and it transduces head movement in primarily the horizontal plane. The otolithic membrane of the saccule is more firmly attached and processes the constant pull of gravity as well as vertical head translations (Fettiplace & Fuchs, 1999). The cilia projecting from the hair cells in both maculae are embedded into the bottom of each otolithic membrane. It has been estimated that humans have approximately 18,000 receptors in each saccule and 33,000 receptors in each utricle (Lopez et al., 2005). In this way, the maculae act as bio-accelerometers that are sensitive to linear motion. Much like the crista ampullaris in the SCCs, the stimulus for activating vestibular hair cell transduction is deflection of the hair stereocilia with respect to the cell bodies embedded in the neuroepithelium of the macula or crista. Given that the otolithic membranes of the saccule and utricle are heavier than the endolymph, a shift or tilt of the head displaces them, so they align with the earth's vertical gravity vector (Fernández & Goldberg, 1976). Furthermore, when the head is translated quickly, the free-floating nature of the otolithic membranes causes them to lag behind resulting in a deflection of the hair cells in the direction opposite that of the head movement (Figure 2–10).

In contrast to the cristae, the polarization patterns of the hair cells in the maculae are more complex. Each macula has a line running through it which is composed of very small otoconia. This anatomical line is known as a striola and it acts to divide the maculae into two parts. In the saccular macula the hair cells are oriented in opposing directions around the striola. In the utricular macula, the hair cells are oriented toward the striola. This pattern of polarization enables an organism to sense linear head motion in nearly any direction.

The saccule has two systems that it employs to enhance its response sensitivity to tilt and linear acceleration. First, like the SCCs, commissural fibers exist between the two saccules. When saccular afferents are stimulated they receive ipsilateral excitation and contralateral inhibition via the commissural fibers; however, it has been reported that only 10% of second-order neurons excited by ipsilateral saccular afferent stimulation receive commissural inhibition (Uchino, 2001). This suggests that during linear acceleration (deceleration) the saccule is less dependent on the contralateral end organ to produce an electrical asymmetry (for detecting motion) than are SCCs. The second mechanism employed by the saccule to increase its sensitivity has been termed "cross-striolar inhibition" (Uchino, 2001). The mechanism of excitation and inhibition in the saccule is related to the geometric arrangement of the hair cells around the striola. When a linear acceleration occurs, some

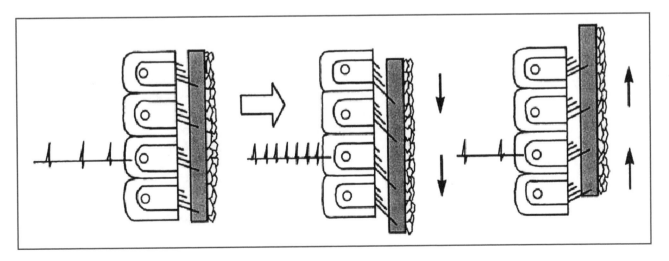

FIGURE 2–10. Mechanism of macule hair cell activation.

hair cells are depolarized while others on the side opposite the striola are hyperpolarized; thus, each saccule is independently capable of producing an electrical asymmetry necessary for the detection of motion. The majority of the vestibular neurons that are modulated by cross-striolar inhibition have axonal projections to the spinal cord (Sato, Ohkawa, Uchino, & Wilson, 1997); therefore, if one saccule is impaired by disease, information from the intact saccule will still be available to the central vestibular system to adjust posture and eye movements. The SCC system does not benefit from this redundancy and thus may help to explain why patients with canal impairments suffer poorer postural stability than their counterparts with unilaterally impaired saccules.

PRIMARY VESTIBULAR AFFERENT PROJECTIONS

Each of the end organs in the peripheral vestibular system sends their dendrites to the cell bodies located in Scarpa's ganglion (SG). SG is the origin of the two branches of the vestibular nerve that are located in the internal auditory canal. One division is termed the superior (anterior) vestibular nerve and it innervates the horizontal and anterior cristae, utricle, and a small portion of the saccule macule. The inferior (posterior) vestibular nerve innervates the posterior SCC and the inferior division of the saccule macule. The inferior and superior vestibular nerves run together as a bundle into the lateral medulla (Figure 2–11). The two vestibular branches of the vestibular nerve are composed of approximately 25,000 single nerve fibers that have a firing rate between 10 and 100 spikes/second (Ishiyama, Lopez, Ishiyama, & Tang, 2004; Ishiyama et al., 2005). According to Rasmussen (1940), the number of afferent nerve fibers is evenly distributed between the otolith organs and the SCCs. The primary excitatory neurotransmitter of the vestibular afferents is glutamate (Straka, Biesdorf, & Dieringer, 2000). There are three primary types of vestibular afferents. They include dimorphic, calyceal, and bouton. Calyceal afferents synapse on Type I hair cells and have chalice-shaped synapses. Bouton affer-

ent fibers synapse on multiple Type II hair cells. Dimorphic afferents have calyceal synapses and innervate both Type I and Type II hair cells. There is a distinct difference in the spatial distribution of these three types of afferents throughout the vestibular system. Type I hair cells located in the middle of the cristae (i.e., central zone) and both striolas of the otoliths are innervated by calyceal afferents. The bouton type afferents innervate the lateral areas (i.e., peripheral zone) of the crista and the extrastriolar zone of the maculae. The dimorphic fibers are distributed across all regions in both the cristae and the maculae.

There are two primary classes of vestibular nerve afferents that are differentiated by their response characteristics. *Regular* afferent fibers have a spontaneous firing rate of approximately 50 to 100 spikes per second and have what is termed a tonic response pattern. Tonic refers to the fact that the firing rate will either increase or decrease around the baseline firing rate in manner that closely matches the stimulation of the hair cells in the vestibular organs (i.e., linear for the otoliths and rotary for the SCCs). The anatomical characteristics of regular afferents are that they, in most instances, have thin or medium sized axons and are located in the peripheral zones of both the otolith and cristae. The other type of vestibular afferent is known in the literature as *irregular*. These fibers are characterized by medium and thick axons and are centered in the central zones of the vestibular end organs. They are referred to as irregular because their firing response characteristics are variable. That is their baseline spontaneous firing rate is more variable than regular afferents and they are very sensitive to stimuli acting on the vestibular system.

It has been suggested that the different classes of afferents and their varied firing rates may be related to their position in each vestibular neuroepithelium in order to serve different functions. For example, regular afferents are connected to the peripheral areas of the crista and the macula (i.e., extrastriolar zone). Conversely, the irregular afferents project from the central zone of the crista and are centered on the striola of the macula. This distribution of afferents with different firing characteristics offers insight into the roles of each. It has been suggested that (Goldberg, 2000) afferents

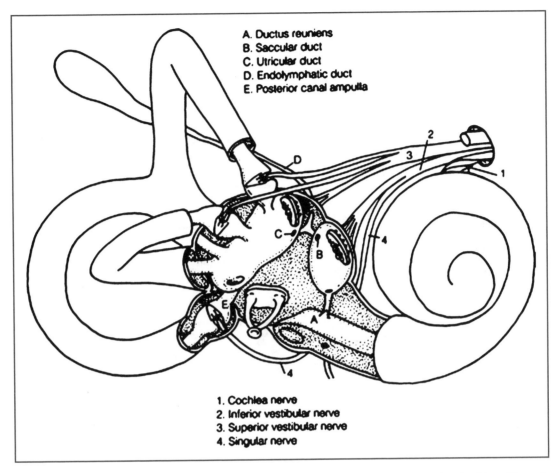

A. Ductus reuniens
B. Saccular duct
C. Utricular duct
D. Endolymphatic duct
E. Posterior canal ampulla

1. Cochlea nerve
2. Inferior vestibular nerve
3. Superior vestibular nerve
4. Singular nerve

FIGURE 2–11. Afferent nerve fibers from the vestibular receptors. (Illustration by Mary Dersch from Pender, 1992, with permission of Daniel Pender)

with regular firing rates may code head velocity and phase information that is sensed by the semicircular canals. In order for the VOR to generated the appropriate eye movements for low-frequency head movement regular afferents have been shown to be activated. Irregular afferents with their high gains may be more sensitive to acceleration.

The vestibular labyrinth also has efferent innervation. There are approximately 500 efferent neurons that synapse on Type II hairs cells as well as the axons of the vestibular afferent discussed above. When the efferents firing rates is increased, there is a corresponding increase in firing in the irregular vestibular afferents. It has been suggested that these efferent nerve fibers work to supplement the vestibular compensation process and rebalance firing rates between the two end organs in situations where one is impaired.

Blood Supply to the Peripheral Vestibular System

The primary source of blood supply to the membranous labyrinth is the labyrinthine artery which, in most instances, originates from the anteroinferior cerebellar artery (Figure 2–12) (Mazzoni, 1969). When the labyrinthine artery enters the temporal bone, it feeds structures within the internal auditory canal. Upon entering the inner ear, the labyrinthine artery bifurcates into two divisions: the common cochlear artery and the anterior vestibular artery. The common cochlear artery further divides in the main cochlear artery and the posterior cochlear vestibular artery. The main cochlear artery irrigates the spiral ganglion. The posterior vestibular artery supplies the ampulla of the posterior canal and the infe-

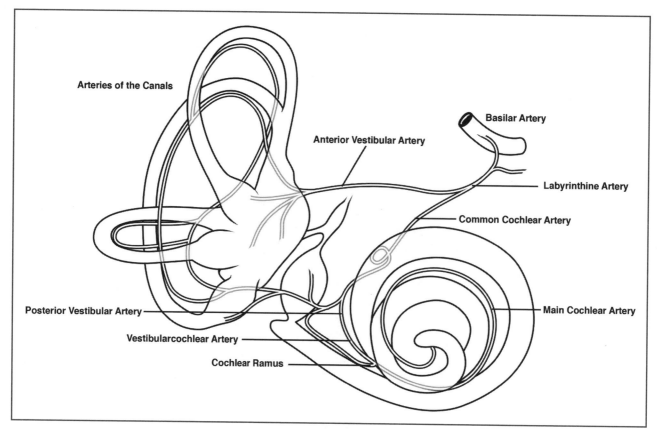

FIGURE 2–12. Arterial supply to the inner ear.

rior portion of the saccule. The anterior vestibular artery supplies the utricle, the ampulla of the horizontal and superior canals, and a small part of the saccule. These arteries do not have collateral anastomotic connections that can continue to supply the end organs in cases of ischemic events. The selective supply of the vestibular end organs by different arteries can lead to various patterns of pathology during quantitative testing.

ANATOMY OF THE CENTRAL VESTIBULAR SYSTEM

Primary vestibular afferents divide into an ascending and descending branch as they enter the brainstem and project to second-order neurons in the vestibular nuclei (VN) (i.e., the vestibular equivalent of the cochlear nuclei). The ascending branch terminates on cells in the cerebellum or rostral portion of the VN. The descending branch sends projections to the caudal portion of the VN. The VN are located on the floor of the fourth ventricle in the pons and serve as the primary distribution center for neural activity generated by the peripheral vestibular system. The neural activity received by the VN from the canal and otolith organs ascends ipsilaterally and contralaterally, mainly via the medial longitudinal fascicle, to the midbrain tegmentum with the interstitial nucleus of Cajal. Connections also exist between the VN and the descending spinal cord pathways (i.e., the lateral and medial vestibulospinal pathways, and the reticulospinal pathway) that are responsible for posture and gait (Figure 2–13). There are four anatomical divisions of the VN. The superior vestibular nucleus is located on the floor of the fourth ventricle and re-

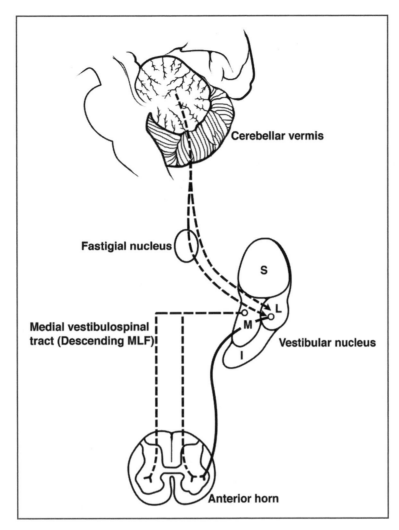

FIGURE 2–13. Vestibulocerebellar and vestibulospinal projections. (Adapted from Baloh, 1998b)

ceived the majority of the input from the SCCs. The medial vestibular nucleus is the largest of the four centers and is located caudal to the superior vestibular nucleus. It receives projections from the SCCs as well as sends projections down through the vestibulospinal tract. The inferior vestibular nuclei are located caudally to the lateral nuclei. They receive input from the cerebellum, adjacent vestibular nuclei, and the spinal cord. The lateral vestibular nuclei (i.e., Deiters' nucleus) receive afferent peripheral vestibular input from the utricles and vestibulocerebellum. These connections between the vestibulocerebellum and the VN via the fastigial nucleus are

"what make it possible for patients to recover function following impairment (i.e., improve the dynamic properties of the VOR and vestibulospinal reflex) to a single end organ (Ito, 1993). The lateral vestibular nuclei also send projections down through the ipsilateral lateral vestibulospinal pathway.

There are direct connections between the cerebellum, the VN, and the vestibular nerve. Inputs from the VN and vestibular afferents project through the juxtarestiform body of the inferior cerebellar peduncle to the vestibular cerebellum. The vestibulocerebellum is a key driver of balance function and is composed of the flocculus, para-

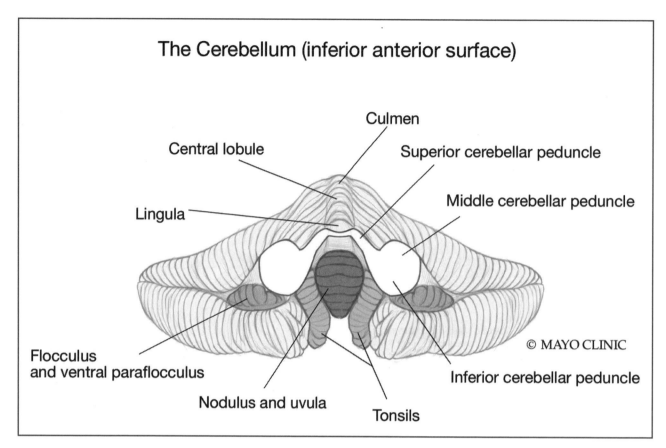

The Cerebellum (inferior anterior surface)

Culmen

Central lobule

Superior cerebellar peduncle

Middle cerebellar peduncle

Lingula

Flocculus
and ventral paraflocculus

Inferior cerebellar peduncle

© MAYO CLINIC

Nodulus and uvula

Tonsils

FIGURE 2–14. An illustration showing the inferior anterior surface of the cerebellum. Visible in the drawing are the three cerebellar peduncles that relay information to and from the cerebellum as well as the structures that compose the vestibulocerebellum (i.e., flocculus, ventral paraflocculus, nodulus, and uvula). The superior cerebellar peduncle arises from the cranial part of the anterior cerebellar notch and is a major fiber bundle that sends efferent information out of the structure. The middle cerebellar peduncle (brachium pontis) is larger than the superior and inferior peduncles and is made up almost exclusively of the axons from the second neurons on the corticopontocerebellar pathway. The inferior cerebellar peduncle is a thick bundle of white fibers that acts to connect the cerebellum with the spinal cord and medulla. It arises from the dorsolateral aspect of the superior half of the medulla oblongata. (Used with permission of Mayo Foundation for Medical Educationand Research. All rights reserved.)

flocculus, nodulus, and uvula (Figure 2–14 and Table 2–1).

There are also strong connections between the VN, the reticular activating system, and the autonomic nervous system. These systems contribute to the secondary reactions, such as pallor, sweating, nausea, and vomiting, that occur when an individual suffers from a loss of function in one of the end organs (Figure 2–15). The vestibulcortical pathway includes broadly distribute projections involving at least three deccusations in the brainstem for ascending vestibular information: one between the vestibular nuclei, one in the pons, and one in the rostral midbrain tegmentum. The vestibulocortical pathway includes projections from the superior and lateral VN, through the thalamus (Figure 2–16), to the multisensory vestibular cortex areas known as the parieto-insular vestibular cortex (PIVC) and the medial superior temporal area (MST) of the visual cortex. There are at least two transcallosal crossings connecting the PIVC or the MST that are thought to bind ves-

Table 2–1. Inputs, Projections and Eye Movement Abnormalities of the Vestibulocerebellum

Vestibulocerebellar Structure	Inputs	Projections	Observed Findings When Lesioned
Flocculus	Vestibular Nucleus Vestibular nerve Nucleus prepositus hypoglossi (NPH) Inferior olivary nucleus Paramedian tracts Nucleus reticularis tegmenti pontis Mesencephalic reticular formation	Ipsilateral superior and medial vestibular nuclei	Downbeat nystagmus (enhances laterally) Impaired smooth pursuit Impaired VOR cancellation (during caloric and during rotational testing) Postsaccadic drift Impaired VOR compensation
Paraflocculus	Contralateral pontine nuclei		
Nodulus and Uvula	Medial and inferior vestibular nuclei, vestibular nerve, NPH Inferior olivary nucleus	Vestibular nuclei	Impaired velocity storage (i.e., periodic alternation nystagmus) Downbeat nystagmus (primary position and observed during positional testing)

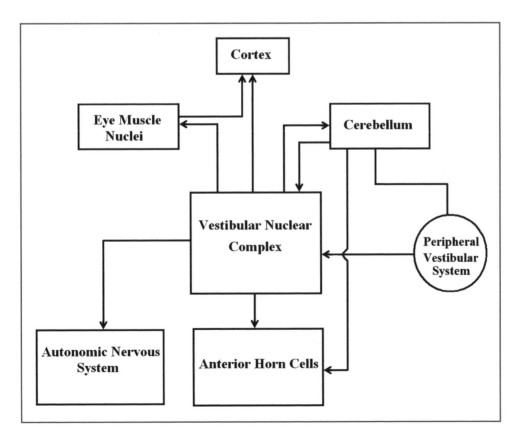

FIGURE 2–15. The vestibular nuclei and their connections. (From Musiek, Baran, Shinn, & Jones, 2012)

tibular, proprioceptive, and visual sensory input into one percept of spatial orientation as well as contribute to the perception of motion (Berthoz, 1996) (Figure 2–17).

Semicircular Canal and Ocular Pairings

One of the key principles of vestibular physiology is referred to as Ewald's first law. This refers to the fact that stimulation of a SCC will generate a corresponding eye movement in the plane of the SCC. This principle was further developed by scientists Flourens and Mach. The SCCs are circular tubes oriented orthogonally to each other with a hole in the center and a cupula located at one end which can be deflected when subjected to the movement of the fluid. Each canal is sensitive to movement in the plane perpendicular to the center of the hole. The SCCs and eyes are linked

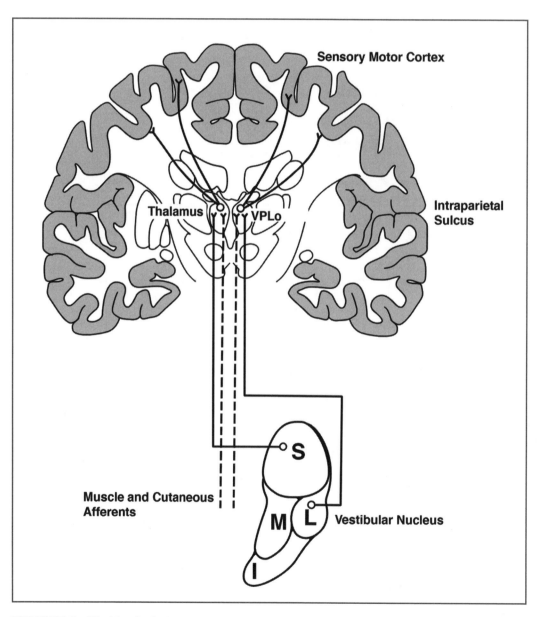

FIGURE 2–16. Vestibulothalamocortical pathways.

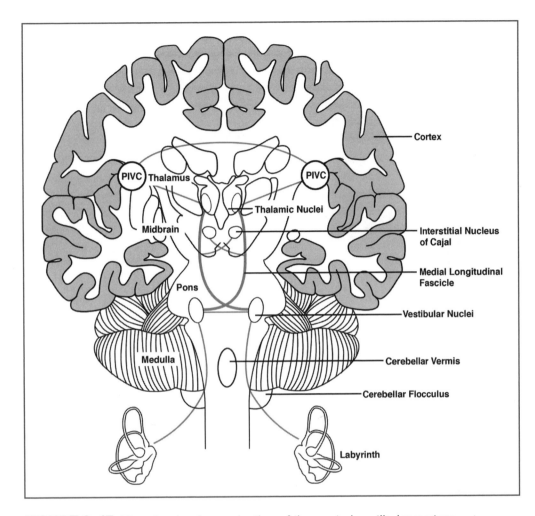

FIGURE 2–17. The structural organization of the central vestibular system.

through a series of pathways that extend from the peripheral vestibular system to the EOMs by way of the brainstem. Afferent projections from the ampullas of the canals project to the VN which then connect to the motor neurons of the EOMs. When the SCCs are accelerated in their plane of stimulation, the eyes are moved in approximately the same plane (Ewald's law) (Figure 2–18). This phenomenon is facilitated by the fact that each EOM receives both excitatory and inhibitory input from the canal system (Ito, Nisimaru, & Yamamoto, 1977). Furthermore, afferent input from each canal is sent to one muscle attached to the ipsilateral eye and one muscle attached to the contralateral eye. As described previously, each SCC canal has a partner on the opposite side that is coplanar and detects movement in the same plane (e.g., RALP and LARP) (Figure 2–19). In other words, any angular acceleration that increases neural firing rate in one canal also causes a corresponding decrease in the firing rate in its partner on the opposite side. This type of arrangement is known in engineering terms as a push-pull organization and provides the coordinate system for the VOR and vestibulocolic reflex (VCR). Given that each canal sends projections to the opposing eye muscles of its partner, the eyes move in the opposite direction of the head movement. This direct relationship between the SCCs and the eyes reduced the amount of central neural processing that must be performed in order to keep they eyes on a target during a head movement.

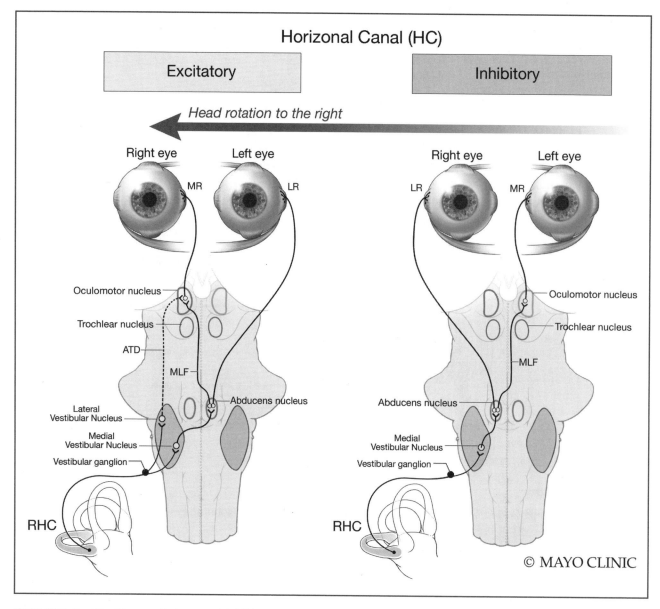

FIGURE 2–18. The excitatory and inhibitory connections between the horizontal semicircular canals and the extraocular eye muscles in response to a head movement to the right. MR = medial rectus; LR = lateral rectus. (Used with permission of Mayo Foundation for Medical Education and Research. All rights reserved.)

An example of how this system works would be when the head is moved in the RALP plane. In this case, when the head is moved in a manner that stimulates the anterior canal, there is an increase in neural activity above the baseline rate that is routed to the ipsilateral superior rectus and contralateral inferior oblique, and muscle tone is increased (the muscles are contracted). Simultaneously, the left inferior canal is moved in such a way as to reduce the firing rate in the nerve (ampullofugal) and the ipsilateral inferior oblique and contralateral superior rectus are inhibited resulting in a decrease in muscle tone in these muscles. A summary of the excitatory and inhibitory connections from each canal is presented in Table 2–2. These slow reflexive movements of the eyes that occur with stimulation of the peripheral vestibular system during head movement are one component of the VOR.

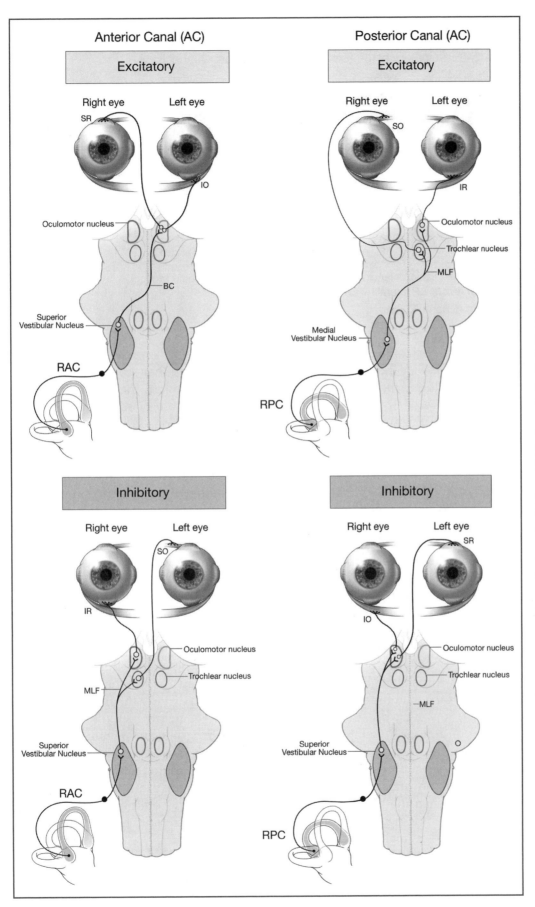

FIGURE 2–19.
The excitatory and inhibitory connections between the anterior and posterior semicircular canals and the extraocular eye muscles. SR = superior rectus; IR = inferior rectus; SO = superior oblique; IO = inferior oblique; RAC = right anterior canal; RPC = right posterior canal; MLF = medial longitudinal fasciculus. (Used with permission of Mayo Foundation for Medical Education and Research. All rights reserved.)

Table 2–2. Summary of the Excitatory and Inhibitory Connections in Three Canals

Semicircular Canal	Extraocular Muscles Excited	Extraocular Muscles Inhibited
Posterior (inferior)	Ipsilateral (SO) Contralateral (IR)	Ipsilateral (IO) Contralateral (SR)
Anterior (superior)	Ipsilateral (SR) Contralateral (IO)	Ipsilateral (IR) Contralateral (SO)
Horizontal (lateral)	Ipsilateral (MR) Contralateral (LR)	Ipsilateral (LR) Contralateral (MR)

SO superior oblique; *IO* inferior oblique; *IR* inferior rectus; *SR* superior rectus; *MR* medial rectus; *LR* lateral rectus.

Adapted from Barin (2009).

The connections between the horizontal SCCs are of particular interest because these are the canals that are most commonly assessed during the ENG/VNG examination. The horizontal VOR is the primary reflex that is measured during the caloric portion of the ENG/VNG examination. It is a neural circuit that has only a few synapses, allowing for an extremely short latency (i.e., 7 ms) and is evoked with movement of the head or body. The purpose of the VOR is to enable clear vision in dynamic situations by moving the eyes in an equal and opposite direction of the head movement. This type of action keeps the fovea on the object of interest allowing for clear vision during dynamic situations.

When the head is stationary, the tonic firing rate in the primary vestibular afferents on both sides is essentially equal, and the eyes do not move. It is angular acceleration and deceleration of the head that is the stimulus that activates the VOR. When an individual turns their head quickly to the left, the skull (and the membranous labyrinths) moves to the left; however, because of the inertial properties of endolymph, it lags behind. A good explanation of this phenomenon is Newton's law of inertia: "An object at rest will remain at rest unless acted on by an unbalanced force." In the case of the VOR, when the head is stationary, the endolymph is not moving. When the head is moved, the endolymph is inclined to remain at rest due to inertia, and so it lags behind the head movement. Given that the ampulla is sealed by the cupula, the endolymph cannot pass through it. This causes a corresponding increase

in pressure that occurs on one side of each cupula (opposite sides) causing them to bend. In the case of the head turn to the left, the left lateral canal is the leading ear for the head movement, and the right end organ is housed in the lagging ear. A head turn to the left causes endolymph to flow to the right and consequently deflects the cupula to the right (toward the utricle). Given that the stereocilia are embedded in the bottom of the cupula, they are also deflected. The deflection of the stereocilia stretch the tip links located on the ends of the filaments and mechanically opens cationic channels. Membranes toward the utricle opens the ion channels in their tips and allows endolymph to flow into the cell. As endolymph, (which is high in K+), enters the cell, the resting potential increases, resulting in an increase in activity at the synaptic junction at the base of the cell increasing firing in the nerve. Conversely, the cupula in the right ear is deflected away from the utricle (inhibitory or utriculofugal) driving the firing rate in the right vestibular nerve below its tonic resting rate.

The changes in baseline firing rate in the superior vestibular nerves caused by the acceleration of the head to the left are routed to the medial vestibular nuclei (MVN). In the example presented, the superior vestibular nerve on the left side is firing at a rate higher than its tonic resting rate which increases the level of activity in the left MVN. A simultaneous decrease in firing rate occurs in the right MVN. The left MVN projects the increased level of neural activity to both ipsilateral and contralateral secondary vestibular neurons.

Specifically, the left MVN sends projections to the left oculomotor nucleus (III) and sends decussating projections to the right abducens nucleus (VI). On the right side, a similar but opposite chain of events occurs. The right MVN relays the decrease in neural activity to the right oculomotor nucleus and also across the midline to the left abduces nucleus. The abducens and oculomotor nuclei send motor projections to the effector organs of the horizontal VOR (i.e., extraocular muscles). In our example of a head turn to the left, the right abducens nucleus and left oculomotor nucleus route the increased neural input received from the medial VN to the motor neurons of the right lateral rectus muscles and left medial rectus extraocular muscles. This pattern of input received by the EOMs initiates a contraction (i.e., shortening) of these two muscles resulting in the eye being pulled slowly to the right. This conjugate movement of the eyes to the right should be proportional to the size or magnitude of the head turn (Figure 2–20).

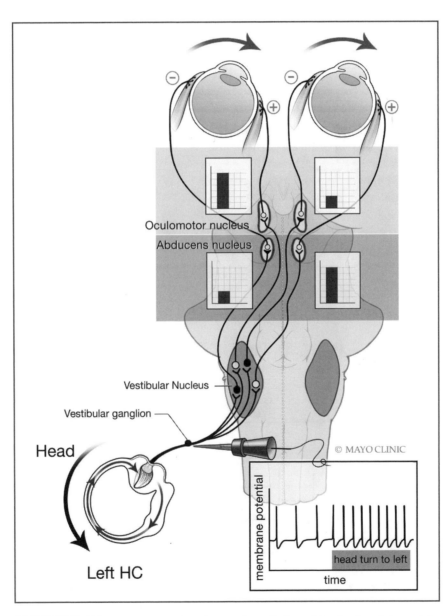

FIGURE 2–20. Direct neural pathway of excitation of the horizontal semicircular canal–ocular reflex during rotation of the head to the left. (Adapted from Carey and Della Santina, Principles of Applied Vestibular Physiology, 2004)

There is also a corresponding decrease in neural drive to the antagonist extraocular muscles (i.e., right lateral rectus and left medial rectus). The decrease in neural activity received by the left medial VN from the peripheral system is relayed to the left oculomotor nuclei and right abducens resulting in a relaxation of the left medial rectus and right lateral rectus muscles. These coor-dinated eye movements would not be possible without the medial longitudinal fasciculus (MLF). The MLF is the brainstem pathway that coordi-nates the outputs of the VN to the oculomotor and abducens nuclei. This pathway makes it pos-sible for these compensatory eye movements to be conjugate (i.e., for the visual axes to be parallel) (Figure 2–21).

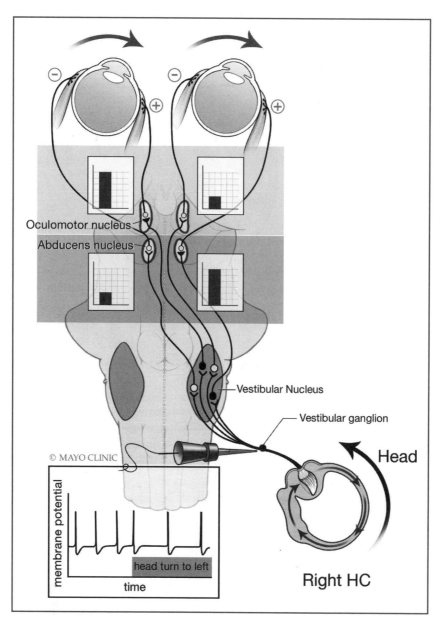

FIGURE 2–21. Direct neural pathway of inhibition of the horizontal semi-circular canal–ocular reflex during rotation of the head to the left. (Adapted from Carey and Della Santina, Principles of Applied Vestibular Physiology, 2004)

In instances when an individual is subjected to a continuous rotation, the eyes are driven by the vestibular system to their lateral extremes in the orbits. When the eyes reach this critical point in the orbits, they must be reset to their original position and begin the deviation again or stop moving. If the eyes stop moving during the head movement, then the environment blurs due to the poor resolving capabilities of the retina. At this point, the eyes are able to be reset by specialized neurons in a distributed group of cells called the paramedian pontine reticular formation (PPRF). The PPRF briefly interrupts the flow of electrical activity from the vestibular periphery which allows the oculomotor system to initiate a saccade to send the eyes back to midline. The PPRF cells then go through a refractory cycle where input from the vestibular system is permitted once again to drive the eyes laterally. Again, this drive from the vestibular periphery is interrupted by neurons in the PPRF, and continues in this manner. This repetitive eye movement is called nystagmus.

VESTIBULAR NYSTAGMUS GENERATED BY HEAD MOVEMENT

Nystagmus refers to an involuntary eye movement where there is a slow eye movement away from the target. Although there are many forms of nystagmus, the one that is associated with the VOR is known as *peripheral vestibular nystagmus*. This type of nystagmus represents a normal response by the vestibular system to head acceleration or can be present in the case of peripheral vestibular system impairment. The reaction consists of producing a compensatory eye movement that is equal to, and opposite, the head movement followed by a quick movement of the eye in the opposite direction. Vestibular nystagmus generated by stimulation of the SCCs through angular acceleration/and or impairment consists of two primary components. The first component is a slow deviation of the eyes in the direction opposite the head turn. This is known as the "slow phase." The slow phase is generated by the vestibular system and is the response of the VOR to acceleration. This is the component that is measured during quantitative assessment (caloric and rotary chair testing) of the horizontal canals. The slow phase is followed by a second faster component called the "fast phase" (Figure 2–22). Without a corrective movement of the eye in the opposite direction, the eye would reach the limits of the orbit and the VOR would stop functioning. The fast component of the VOR is not generated by the vestibular system, but rather by a pulse generator associated with the saccade system (PPRF). The PPRF is a distributed group of cells that are located near the abducens nuclei and have been shown to be active immediately prior to a fast phase being generated (Curthoys, 2002). It has been suggested that the PPRF monitors the ongoing VOR, and when the eye reaches a certain position in the orbit, burst neurons fire and quickly move the eye in the opposite direction. For angular accelerations, fast-phase nystagmus components have been shown to be larger than the slow-phase components. This would effectively put the eye in a position to acquire targets that are arriving (Baloh & Honrubia, 1990). An extensive review of the generation of the quick phase of vestibular nystagmus is presented in an article by Curthoys (2002).

It is possible for patients to have selective impairments in the PPRF that disrupt the ability to generate fast phases. Figure 2–23 compares the saccades of a neurologically intact patient with a patient who has a defect in the PPRF system. The impaired patient is incapable of producing the ballistic eye movements required for the generation of saccades. The patient was identified as having a saccade defect during the ENG/VNG test and

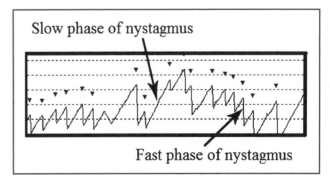

FIGURE 2–22. Nystagmus as recorded and displayed by an Interacoustics VNG system. (Interacoustics, Assens, Denmark)

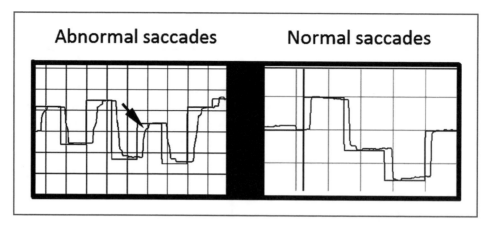

FIGURE 2–23. Saccades in a patient with a diagnosed "saccade defect" compared with saccades in a neurologically intact patient.

was subsequently diagnosed by a neurologist as having a global saccadic palsy secondary to "progressive supranuclear palsy."

How Nystagmus Is Quantified

Although it may seem counterintuitive, by convention, nystagmus is described by the direction of its fast phase. For instance, nystagmus with a fast phase to the right and a slow phase to the left would be said to be "right-beating." When the VOR is invoked during a movement of the head, the nystagmus typically beats in the direction of the head turn. There are several variables that can be used to quantify nystagmus; these include velocity, amplitude, latency, and duration (Jacobson & Newman, 1993). In order to accurately measure nystagmus, the clinician must have an understanding of how the eye movements are being plotted during the recording. Specifically, the majority of commercial eye movement recorders plot eye movement (x-axis) as a function of time (y-axis). Most computerized systems allow the examiner to adjust the time scale, whereas the calibration procedure determines the scale for the eye movement. The slow-phase velocity (SPV) of nystagmus is the most commonly used variable to quantify nystagmus and represents the amplitude of the response over a period of time (Figure 2–24). The SPV of nystagmus represents the distance that

the eye moves during the slow phase divided by how long the eyes took to make the excursion. To measure the slow phase of a beat of nystagmus, most computerized systems incorporate a line that can be aligned with the slow phase and provide a measure of the slope. By convention, most systems use a time base of 1 s. The latency of the nystagmus, whether provoked by the caloric irrigation or another subtest during the examination, is the time it takes the response to occur once a test has been initiated. A measure of the frequency of the nystagmus can be obtained by counting the number of beats that occur during a specific time period.

THE VOR DURING SUSTAINED MOVEMENT

The VOR works to maintain clear vision during head movements, and each head movement has a frequency; however, the vestibular system is not equally sensitive to all frequencies due to endolymph-cupular dynamics. The SCCs are less sensitive to angular accelerations below 0.05 Hz and above 3 Hz (Baloh & Honrubia, 2001). Furthermore, because the cupula is insensitive to gravity (the cupula and the endolymph have the same specific gravity), the vestibular system is poor at transducing sustained constant-velocity move-

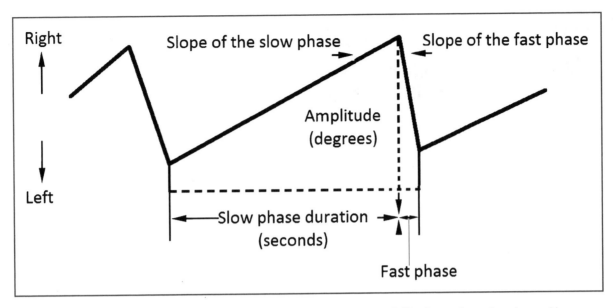

FIGURE 2–24. The variables of nystagmus that can be measured. (Redrawn from Jacobson, Newman, and Kartush, 1993)

ments. Specifically, during a constant-velocity rotation, fluid motion approximates the speed of the canals and the cupula drifts back to its neutral position, and peripheral drive to the central nervous system ceases (Goldberg & Fernandez, 1971a). In order to compensate for the fact that the VOR is poor at transducing low-frequency accelerations and sustained constant-velocity rotations, the vestibular system has a central nervous system function that enhances its sensitivity during these dynamic situations. When the time constant (time taken for a response to decay to 37% of its initial value) of the VOR is measured in response to a sustained rotational stimulus, the nystagmus persists approximately three times longer than the "drive" from the periphery (Raphan, Matsuo, & Cohen, 1979). This extension of the VOR response past the point where there is no longer any neural drive coming from the peripheral end organs has been termed "velocity storage" (VS). VS is mediated by a distributed system of neural structures which are collectively termed the "neural integrator" (NI) (Leigh & Zee, 2006). These structures include the VN, commissural fibers connecting the VN, and the connections between VN and the cerebellum.

The NI facilitates the process of VS in two primary ways. First, the NI collects and stores electrical activity arriving from the primary vestibular afferents. In this way it acts as a capacitor (i.e., a circuit that stores a charge). Second, the NI gates the outflow of electrical activity that it has collected. The amount of neural activity that the NI releases from its "storage bank" is dependent on the type of movement being encountered and whether or not the peripheral vestibular system is impaired. The primary purpose of VS is to extend the time constant of the VOR one order of magnitude beyond what the canal responses produce during low-frequency or constant-velocity rotations. The centrally mediated prolongation of the nystagmus after the canal responses have ceased providing input effectively extends the low-frequency response of the vestibular system; however, it has been reported that in cases of peripheral vestibular system impairment, the VS mechanism opens the valve and significantly increases the outflow. The VS mechanism is implicated in several tests used to assess the vestibular system (e.g., headshake and rotational testing). In fact, it has been reported that patients with impairments in the VS mechanism may contribute to balance impairments in unsteady, fall-prone patients. (Jacobson & McCaslin, 2004).

PERIPHERAL VESTIBULAR IMPAIRMENT AND CENTRAL NERVOUS SYSTEM COMPENSATION

When a person with two healthy peripheral vestibular systems suddenly loses function in one of them, they manifest a distinct pattern of symptoms. First, the patient complains of "true" vertigo defined as the entire environment rotating around the patient or the patient turning inside the environment. They may also describe experiencing nausea and vomiting secondary to involvement of the vestibulo-autonomic system. Second, if the patient's vestibular impairment is acute, they manifest a primarily linear horizontal nystagmus with the quick phase directed away from the impaired ear. This nystagmus typically enhances when the patient is unable to fixate (e.g., when the nystagmus is observed using video goggles and vision is denied.) Third, the patient demonstrates postural impairments, such as falling to the affected side, or they may complain that they experience difficulty walking straight or are very unstable in environments that are poorly lit. Fourth, patients will report a sense of spatial disorientation that is related to an interruption in vestibular neural activity that is projected to the vestibular cortex. Interestingly, in neurologically intact individuals these symptoms begin to subside within a week. After the vertigo has stopped, patients may still complain of feeling strange when making quick head movements, but typically within less than a month they are able to resume their pre-attack lifestyle. This ability for the vestibular system to recover following an insult to the peripheral end organ or vestibular nerves has been termed "vestibular compensation" or "vestibular adaptation." It is vital for the clinicians administering VNG examinations to understand the neural basis of the phenomenon and its effect on the various subtests of the VNG.

Effect of Unilateral Vestibular Lesions

In order to understand what happens in the case of a peripheral vestibular system impairment, one must have an understanding of what happens in an intact system. Figure 2–25 shows that when a person turns their head to the left, there is an increase in tonic neural activity on the left side (i.e., in the direction of the head turn) and a corresponding decrease in activity on the right side (i.e., the side contralateral to the head turn). This type of head turn produces an asymmetry in the neural drive from the peripheral vestibular system. This peripherally generated asymmetrical neural drive is relayed through the oculomotor neurons to the extraocular muscles. The pattern of neural activity received by the motor system produces the aforementioned slow eye movement in the opposite direction of the head turn that is proportional to the velocity of the head movement. Once the eye reaches a specific point in the orbit, the vestibular input is blocked briefly allowing the oculomotor system to reset the eye in the direction of the head movement (i.e., nystagmus).

Damage to one of the peripheral vestibular end organs or vestibular nerves can occur for several reasons. For example, there may be a disease process that injures the hair cells in the labyrinth or destroys neurons in the nerve. An illustration of what happens physiologically when a person incurs a loss of function of one of their peripheral vestibular systems is presented in Figure 2–26. As can be seen from the figure, there is a significant decrease in the tonic activity from the right peripheral system routed to the vestibular nuclei. This asymmetry in tonic neural activity generates an electrical "code" that the brain falsely interprets as a head turn. In fact, during the acute phase following a loss of peripheral vestibular function, the patient perceives that they are turning toward the healthy ear. It is this false perception of rotation generated by the loss of peripheral vestibular function that has been termed vertigo. In addition to the perception of rotary motion, patients may also experience vegetative symptoms. The tonic neural asymmetry results in a sensory "mismatch" between information that the vestibular system is providing (i.e., patient is turning) compared with other supporting senses (e.g., somesthetic system and vision) that the patient is, in fact, sitting still. The patient experiences autonomic system symptoms of pallor, sweating, nausea, and vomiting.

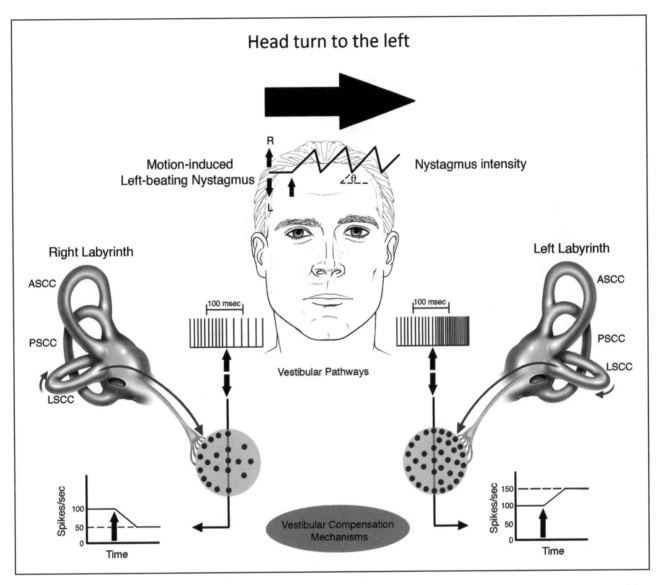

FIGURE 2–25. The change in primary afferent firing rate and resulting eye movement following rotation of the head to the left. The circle represents the vestibular nuclei and the number of dots the level of neural activity. ASCC anterior semicircular canal; PSCC posterior semicircular canal; LSCC lateral semicircular canal. (Adapted from Barin & Durrant, 2000)

The perception of vertigo is a product of the aberrant nystagmus (i.e., spontaneous vestibular nystagmus) generated by the asymmetry registered at the vestibular nuclei. In a normally functioning vestibular system, when the head is moved the VOR drives the eyes in an equal and opposite direction. This stabilizes the environment and the perception of movement is mitigated; however, in the case of a loss of vestibular function on one side, the head is static, but nystagmus is generated

due to the tonic neural asymmetry. Because the eyes are moving (i.e., spontaneous nystagmus) in the absence of any head movement, the perception of the patient is that of rotation. The nystagmus generated by the loss of function in the peripheral vestibular system is primarily (although not entirely) horizontally linear and is a direct result of the loss of neural tonic input from the impaired side. The reason that the nystagmus is not purely horizontal is that the input from the two vertical

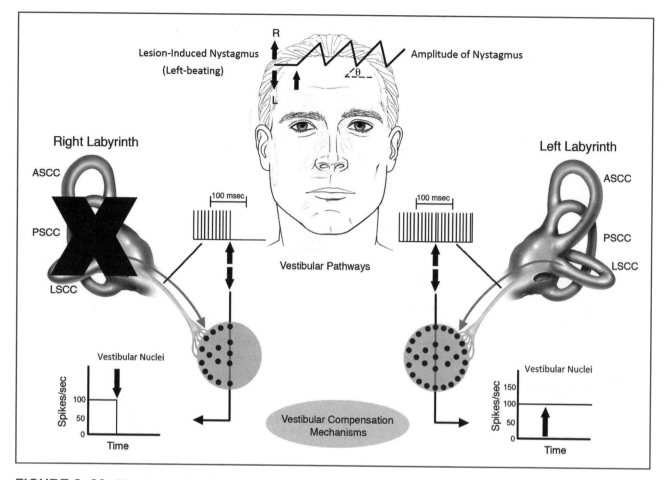

FIGURE 2–26. The change in primary afferent firing rate and resulting eye movement following an acute loss of peripheral vestibular function on the right side. ASCC anterior semicircular canal; PSCC posterior semicircular canal; LSCC lateral semicircular canal. (Adapted from Barin & Durrant, 2000)

canals (i.e., posterior and anterior) cancels out incompletely leaving a small residual torsional component. Acutely, the slow component of the nystagmus is directed toward the impaired ear; however, due to compensation mechanisms, the direction of the nystagmus is not always a reliable indicator of the impaired ear.

Neural Basis of Vestibular Compensation

The vestibular system has an elegant adaptive mechanism that is activated during an acute loss of vestibular input from one side. In situations where there is an extended asymmetry in the neural firing rate due to impairment of the peripheral system, central vestibular system structures are first recruited to eliminate the asymmetry. Then they begin the process of restoring the dynamic function of the VOR. This process is termed "vestibular compensation" and consists of two primary stages. The first stage consists of eliminating symptoms such as spontaneous nystagmus and skew deviation by rebalancing the tonic neural activity in the vestibular nuclei. This stage has been referred to in the literature as "static compensation." The second stage is much more subtle, takes longer, and has been termed "dynamic compensation." Dynamic compensation involves a central recalibration of the response properties of the VOR (i.e., timing and gain) in order to restore the compensatory actions of the VOR to preimpairment levels. A patient's stage of compensation can have dramatic effects on the results of the various VNG subtests, and thus an understanding of the underlying mechanisms of compensation is important for all clinicians. The following two sections outline the processes that occur during static and dynamic compensation in a simplified manner.

Static Compensation

The process of static compensation occurs almost immediately following unilateral vestibular deafferentation (uVD). This process consists of compensation mechanisms restoring the static balance in tonic neural activity between the vestibular systems. In other words, the asymmetry between the vestibular end organs is eliminated and there is no spontaneous vestibular nystagmus when the patient is not moving. As was discussed previously, each vestibular nerve routes a large amount of neural activity into the vestibular nuclei (VN) (e.g., 1,000,000 spikes per second). Following uVD, one of the VN ceases to receive this input resulting in an asymmetrical tonic neural resting rate between the two sides. The difference in neural input between the two VNs triggers the VOR into action thereby producing an aberrant nystagmus known as "spontaneous vestibular nystagmus" (SVN). Acutely, the fast phase of the nystagmus beats away the impaired ear. As soon as hours after uVD occurs, a phenomenon known in the literature as "cerebellar clamping" is initiated (Figure 2–27).

Midline cerebellar structures quickly respond to the imbalance in the tonic resting rates between the two VNs and increase the tonic inhibition in the contralesional VN. This increase in inhibition acts to decrease the tonic resting rate of the VN

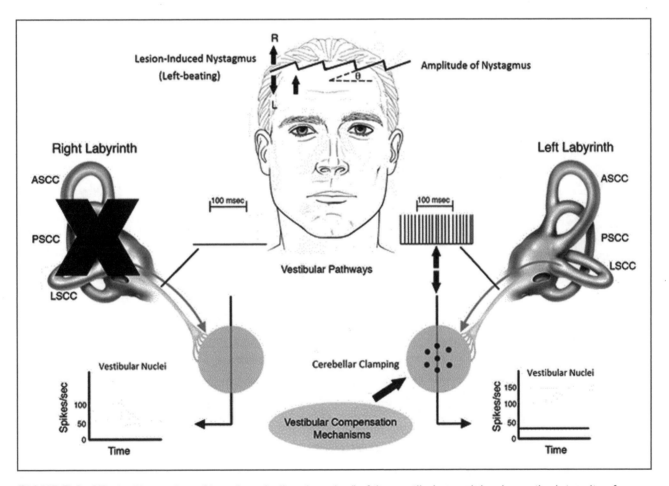

FIGURE 2–27. An illustration of how "cerebellar clamping" of the vestibular nuclei reduces the intensity of spontaneous vestibular nystagmus. ASCC anterior semicircular canal; PSCC posterior semicircular canal; LSCC lateral semicircular canal. (Adapted from Barin & Durrant, 2000)

on the intact side, and as a consequence of this, the asymmetry between the two VNs is reduced (or clamped). The process not only reduces the amplitude of the SVN (decrease in the severity of the vertigo), but also the severity of the symptoms generated by the autonomic nervous system, such as nausea and pallor. At this point the neural tonic resting rate of both VN is reduced compared with levels before the insult. In fact, if a patient is tested using caloric or rotational stimuli, they often manifest findings consistent with a bilateral peripheral vestibular impairment. The process of cerebellar clamping is more complex than presented here, and a more detailed account of the process is given by Curthoys and Halmagyi (1996). Once the activity to the contralesional VN has been "clamped," the next stage in the process of static compen-

sation begins. In order to regain normal performance of the VOR, the neural resting rates of both VN need to be brought back to their original levels. First, the level of clamping must be reduced on the intact side. In order to accomplish that task, the midline cerebellum decreases the level of neural drive sent through its direct inhibitory connections to the VN. This effectively increases the level of neural tonic firing rate (i.e., reduces inhibition) in the contralesional VN and releases it from its "clamped" state (Figure 2–28).

Second, the tonic resting rate must be restored on the impaired side. Reports have shown that as soon as 52 hours following uVD, the neural resting rate in the ipsilesional VN can be equivalent to rates that preceded the insult (Curthoys & Halmagyi, 1996). This increase in the tonic firing rate

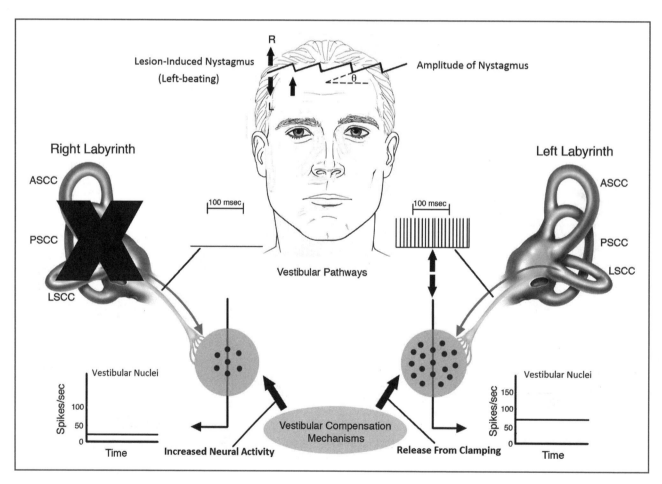

FIGURE 2–28. An illustration of how the cerebellum releases the "clamping" on the intact side and increases neural activity at the level of the vestibular nuclei on the impaired side. ASCC anterior semicircular canal; PSCC posterior semicircular canal; LSCC lateral semicircular canal. (Adapted from Barin & Durrant, 2000)

in the ipsilesional VN has been suggested to have several different origins with the primary one being a release of inhibition mediated by the midline cerebellum (Jacobson, Pearlstein, Henderson, Calder, & Rock, 1998). The process of static compensation is completed when the neural resting rates in the two VN are equilibrated (Figure 2–29).

Dynamic Compensation

Following the process of static compensation, the dynamic response properties of the VOR remain impaired. Specifically, compensation mechanisms modify the properties of the central vestibular system to account for the fact that the impaired organ does not produce the appropriate neural drive during head movements. The tonic resting rate of the two VNs is equal at this stage; however, in the case of head movements there is little or no increase in neural input from the ipsilesional peripheral system. The VOR response is at this point only receiving drive from one labyrinth and cannot provide accurate compensatory eye movements during dynamic situations. The process of dynamic compensation consists of central structures adjusting the vestibular systems neural output to accurately drive the VOR with only one labyrinth (Figure 2–30).

Two of the primary facilitators of dynamic compensation are visual input (Leigh & Zee, 2006) and the midline cerebellum (Beraneck, McKee, Aleisa, & Cullen, 2008). Although research has shown that together these two systems play a critical role in the recovery of VOR function after

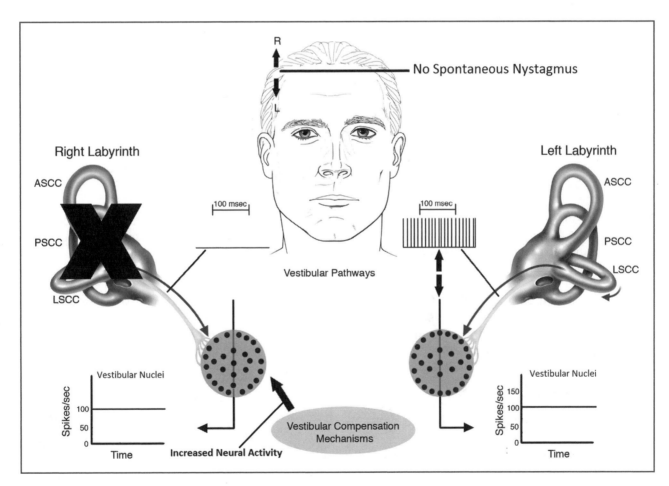

FIGURE 2–29. The level of activity at the peripheral vestibular afferents and vestibular nuclei following static compensation. Note that there is no longer any spontaneous vestibular nystagmus. ASCC anterior semicircular canal; PSCC posterior semicircular canal; LSCC lateral semicircular canal. (Adapted from Barin & Durrant, 2000)

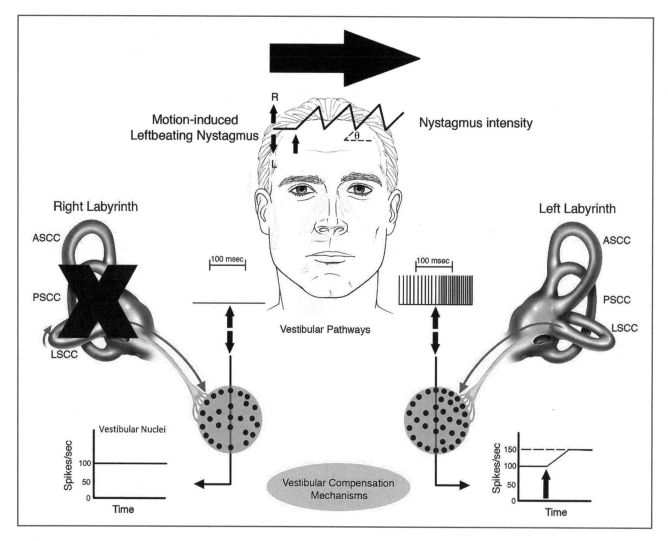

FIGURE 2–30. The change in primary afferent firing rate and resulting eye movement following rotation of the head to the left after the patient has achieved dynamic compensation. ASCC anterior semicircular canal; PSCC posterior semicircular canal; LSCC lateral semicircular canal. (Adapted from Barin & Durrant, 2000)

uVD, there are other contributors (e.g., commissural fibers between the VN and spinal input). The ability of this process to completely restore dynamic function is also dependent on the severity of the impairment. In complete or severe uVDs, there are often permanent decrements in VOR performance. In such cases, the compensation process makes sacrifices in the response characteristics of the VOR in order to maximize performance in frequencies critical for functioning. For example, the neural integrator decreases the amount of neural activity held by the velocity storage mechanism (low frequency) and allocates it to frequencies encountered during ambulation (high frequency). These adjustments to the central vestibular system that occur during dynamic compensation following uVD often result in permanent abnormalities in the VOR at high accelerations and sensitivity to low-frequency stimuli (Barin & Durrant, 2000; Leigh & Zee, 2006).

IMPAIRED CENTRAL NERVOUS SYSTEM COMPENSATION

The clinician seeing patients with dizziness will inevitably evaluate some that either poorly compensate or do not compensate at all. It is often the case that these are patients that have been evaluated and diagnosed with a peripheral end-organ impairment by a physician and then enrolled in a vestibular rehabilitation program. However, they show little or no reduction in their symptoms after months or even years of therapy. This population of patients that present with impaired compensation can often be frustrated with their lack of progress in therapy. One factor to consider in patients who have poorly compensated is whether the peripheral impairment is fluctuating (e.g., Ménière's disease). Fluctuating peripheral vestibular function (i.e., irritative lesions) creates a challenge for the central nervous system because the input to central vestibular structures is variable. The compensation mechanisms are continually active because they are trying to equilibrate a system that is dynamic. There are certain signs that the clinician can identify during an exam that may confirm an irritative vestibular impairment. One such sign is a phenomenon known as recovery nystagmus (RN) is observed. This form of spontaneous nystagmus has also been referred to as "Bechterew's" nystagmus and is characterized by the fast-phase beating toward the ipsilesional ear (Jacobson et al., 1998 ; Leigh & Zee, 2006). Clinically, RN can be difficult to interpret because in cases where the impaired ear is clearly identified, the nystagmus appears to be beating in a paradoxical direction (fast phase toward the impaired ear). When a lesion affecting one inner ear of balance is stable, compensation mechanisms are highly effective; however, in cases where the function of the impaired vestibular system fluctuates, central compensation mechanisms need to adjust accordingly. An example of this would be when a patient has active Ménière's disease. Acutely, following an attack, the patient demonstrates a spontaneous nystagmus where the fast phase beats toward the intact ear. The presence of the persistent neural asymmetry between the two end organs triggers central nervous system compensation mechanisms to become active and the asymmetry is reduced by cerebellar clamping (Figure 2–31). RN is most commonly observed during the "clamping" phase of compensation or when the level of neural activity at the VN is reduced bilaterally. At this stage in the compensation process, if there is a recovery of function on the impaired side, it will create another tonic neural asymmetry, only this time in the opposite direction. Given that the

level of tonic activity in the vestibular nucleus on the intact side has been reduced, a recovery of function in the previously impaired ear raises the tonic neural output of the impaired ear over that of the healthy ear. This set of circumstances generates a spontaneous nystagmus where the fast phase beats toward the impaired but recovering ear. If the recovery of the ear is stable, the patient should statically compensate and the RN will disappear. It is critical that the clinician understand the circumstances and characteristics of RN so as to avoid any misinterpretation during ENG/VNG examination. Because of the unstable nature of some disease processes and the dynamic nature of central nervous system compensation, the clinician cannot always rely on the direction of the nystagmus to identify the impaired ear. A comprehensive review of RN is given by Jacobson et al. (1998).

Another issue to consider in patients who demonstrate an inability to adequately compensate are those who have a vestibular system that is functional but generates an erroneous output. Patient with disorders affecting the central nervous system, such as cerebellar degeneration, concussion, severe vascular disease (e.g., brainstem leukoaraiosis), or demyelinating disorders (e.g., multiple sclerosis) are often challenged with fully compensating following a peripheral vestibular insult. This is has been suggested to be due to the inability of the central compensation mechanism to properly integrate the sensory input from vision, proprioception, and the vestibular system. Correct integration of these three sensory systems enables the central vestibular system to detect when the peripheral vestibular system is deficient. When there is impairment somewhere along the central vestibular pathways, it may be impossible for the system to detect that the peripheral vestibular system is deficient, and accordingly, the rebalancing of the tonic neural activity in the vestibular system to accommodate the loss may be inadequate.

Patients who have suffered a vestibular crisis may adopt a sedentary lifestyle which has been shown to prolong the time it takes to compensate. This is due to the disorientation caused by the spontaneous vestibular nystagmus, unsteadiness from abnormal vestibulospinal input, and provocative sensations that accompany head movement (e.g., retinal slip). In an attempt to not exacerbate

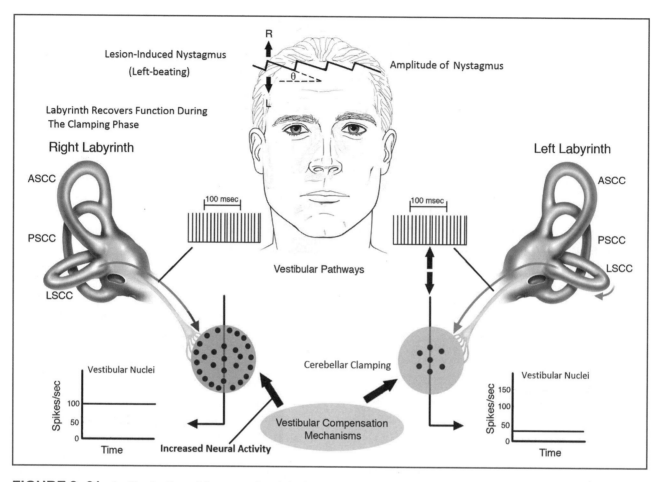

FIGURE 2–31. An illustration of the neural activity in the peripheral nerves and vestibular nuclei following recovery of function to the impaired labyrinth. Note that the nystagmus beats in the opposite direction from the previous examples (i.e., recovery nystagmus). ASCC anterior semicircular canal; PSCC posterior semicircular canal; LSCC lateral semicircular canal. (Adapted from Barin & Durrant, 2000)

their symptoms, patients may limit mobility and head movement and inadvertently rob the central compensation system of the sensory input it needs to adapt to the injury.

Long-term use of vestibular suppressant medications (e.g., meclizine) can disrupt central vestibular system compensation. These drugs are often prescribed to ameliorate the symptoms of vertigo during the early stages of an acute vestibular crisis. However, it is often the case that patients will continue to take these medications long past the acute phase of the vertiginous event. Vestibular suppressants mask the vestibular asymmetry. This creates as situation where the central nervous system centers responsible for adjusting the tonic neural activity at the level of the brainstem (e.g.,

midline cerebellum) to compensate for the asymmetry are not recruited.

LAWS OF COMPENSATION

Vestibular compensation is most effective when the following conditions are met:

1. Patients are not taking vestibular suppressants.
2. Patients must be active (a basic tenant of vestibular rehabilitation therapy).
3. Patients have intact vestibular pathways.
4. Patients have vision.

3

Pretest Procedures for VNG

INTRODUCTION

When the clinician first greets the patient in the waiting room, the examination has officially begun. The examiner should introduce himself or herself and always ask the patient if there is someone that they would like to accompany them during the testing. This is an important question because many patients with vertigo have a misunderstanding or distorted perception of what is going to happen during the VNG test. Having a family member or friend with them during the examination can greatly reduce the patient's level of anxiety and increase the quality of the data collected. At this stage of the interview, the examiner should note if the patient is in a wheelchair, hearing impaired, or visually impaired. In cases where a patient is severely hearing impaired, he or she should be made aware that it is okay to wear hearing aids or activate their cochlear implant. If a patient is severely visually impaired, the clinician needs to determine if calibration is possible. If the patient is blind, caloric testing can still be completed using a default calibration; however, only statements about whether or not the patient has vestibular function can be made. Given that the system will essentially be uncalibrated for the patient, conventional quantitative measures derived from the caloric testing cannot be employed (e.g., unilateral weakness and directional preponderance). The clinician should also be vigilant to the presence of "blind nystagmus" in patients with severe visual impairments. Prior to doing any testing, a thorough case history, otoscopic examination, and gross eye movement evaluation should be conducted.

CASE HISTORY

Agarwal and colleagues (2009) estimate that 24 to 60 million people experience symptoms of vestibular impairment during their lifetime. It has been estimated that dizziness is the presenting complaint in 2.5% of patients who are evaluated by primary care physicians each year (Sloane, 1989). If this is true, then primary care physicians evaluate over 8 million dizzy/vertiginous/unsteady patients per year. It is estimated that 26% of the 8 million dizzy patients are unable to work because of dizziness, and this results in a financial impact of $2.25 billion (assuming that the dizziness results in $30,000 per person in economic damage from medical claims, health insurance, and disability payments). Dizziness and vertigo also represented 2% to 3% of all emergency department consultations from 1995 to 2004 (Kerber, Meurer, West, & Fendrick, 2008). This amounted to 26 million visits to emergency departments in the United States for dizziness during that time span. Additionally, it probably is not surprising that when patients are evaluated in the emergency department or the primary care setting, the final diagnoses are more often general medical diagnoses (e.g., hypertension, elevated blood glucose, and coronary artery disease) compared with the final diagnoses when the same patients are evaluated by ear specialists. Case history taking in the assessment of the dizzy/unsteady patient can be a frustrating experience for both the clinician and the patient. The clinician must attempt to acquire from the patient salient pieces of information in a short period of time. The clinician must synthesize this information as it is being acquired so that the examination of the patient (e.g., the choice of examinations) can be tailored to the patient's complaints. The case history also enables the clinician to generate hypotheses about the source of the patient's complaints (i.e., the differential diagnosis), which are either supported or not supported by the results of objective tests (e.g., neuroimaging, electroneurodiagnostic tests). Often, patients complicate the history-taking process by recounting what they feel is valuable information that, in fact, contributes little to the differential diagnosis. Patients may feel that they have been ignored if they are not given sufficient time to provide the clinician with information. Despite these shortcomings, many clinicians believe that a well-conducted case history is the most important part of dizziness assessment (e.g., Baloh & Honrubia, 2001). Dizziness is similar to other medical problems in that a thorough case history (qualitative information), paired with laboratory testing (quantitative testing), can help confirm the underlying etiology of the impairment; thus, it is crucial that adequate time for the case history be allotted during the examination. Prior to the interview, the examiner should have reviewed the patient's past medical history. This enables the examiner to determine if there are any predisposing factors that may be contributing to the condition of the patient. The formal case history is typically conducted at the beginning of the assessment, but it can also begin prior to the appointment. Patients may be sent structured questionnaires to their home so that the forms can be filled out with the help of a significant other and with no time limitation. (An example of a dizziness case history form is included in Appendix A.) In this regard, patients can begin to organize the occurrences and triggers of their dizziness, which will facilitate the interview with the examiner; however, a face-to-face systematic interview is often most useful because it affords the patient to describe the symptoms in his or her own words. This can often help the interviewer categorize the nature of the complaints or sensations and direct the interview in a meaningful way. At the time of the appointment, it should be determined if the patient would like any accompanying family members or friends to be present during the testing. This helps to put the patient at ease, and also occasionally, the person accompanying the patient can provide additional information regarding the dizziness. When taking a case history, the clinician should be seated directly across from the patient and ask questions that allow for interpretation. Although there is a standard set of questions that are related to dizziness, the patient should be encouraged to provide a description of the symptoms in their own words. It is important that the questions help the clinician to better understand the nature of the patient's sensations, as well as engage the patient in a historical account of when the dizziness started and what the status of it is at the time of the interview.

The following section presents questions that are often used to categorize information obtained from patients suffering from dizziness. Counseling materials from Mayo Clinic, as well as a case history form developed by the Mayo Clinic Neuro-vestibular Team (MINT), can be found in Appendices A, B, and C.

Key Questions

The key questions to ask are given below.

Question 1: Can you describe the sensations that you are experiencing?

Question 2: How long does the dizziness last?

Question 3: Can you make the dizziness happen?

Question 4: Are there any other symptoms that accompany the dizziness?

Question 5: Do you have any other medical conditions?

Question 6: What medications are you taking?

Question 1: Can You Describe the Sensations that You Are Experiencing?

A good way to start the interview is to ask the patient to describe their symptoms. "Dizziness" is an imprecise term that patients often use to describe a number of different symptoms they are experiencing. For example, the symptoms the patient describes may be a feeling of floating or being lightheaded. The patient may also complain of vertigo, which is defined as "the sensation of motion when no motion is occurring relative to earth's gravity" (American Academy of Otolaryngology–HNS, 1995). The first step in a case history is to ask the patient to describe in their own words the sensations they are experiencing. It is common for the patient with dizziness to have more than one symptom. For instance, a patient may complain of a sensation of rotary motion accompanied by severe imbalance. The clinician should follow up with questions regarding what the impact of the sensations is on the patient's everyday activities and whether they change over time (e.g., "worse when I get up in the morning"). Occasionally patients have difficulty describing the symptoms and the examiner can direct the interview with questions such as "Are you unsteady?" or "Do the sensations feel like they are in your head?" During this initial part of the case history, the clinician should be guiding the questioning and patient descriptions of what they are experiencing in a way that differentiates symptoms of vertigo from those of nonvertigo. According to Baloh and Honrubia (1990), less than 50% of patients who present with dizziness have true vertigo (Tables 3–1 and 3–2).

Question 2: How Long Does the Dizziness Last?

Following a description of the symptoms, the examiner should begin determining the time

Table 3–1. Symptoms and Sensations Related to Vertigo

Symptoms
The illusion of movement that usually is rotational (e.g., spinning) but can also be linear displacement (e.g., linear movement, tilt)
Sensations
"I feel like the room is spinning." (subjective vertigo)   "The room is spinning around me." (objective vertigo)   "I feel like I am shifting or falling." (subjective vertigo)

Table 3–2. Symptoms and Sensations Not Related to Vertigo

Symptoms
Panic attacks, persistent sensation of rocking in the absence of any movement, hyperventilation, motion sickness
Imbalance or unsteadiness while ambulating or standing
Lightheadedness or presyncope
Sensations
"When I sit and think about my problems I get dizzy."   "I have trouble focusing my eyes."   "I feel lightheaded."

course of the sensations. For example, is the patient experiencing dizziness that is episodic, or is it constant? If it is episodic, then the clinician should ascertain how often the episodes occur (e.g., every day or once a month) and how long they last (e.g., seconds or hours). Is the patient free of symptoms between the spells? When conducting a case history with a patient experiencing episodic dizziness it is important to have them describe the characteristics of the initial symptom(s) (first attack) and their last attack. Understanding the characteristics of the first and last bouts of dizziness enable the clinician to make a determination as to whether spells are related or if they are independent of one another. In the latter case, a specific history may need to be taken and developed for each of the complaints. An example of this would be a patient who initially experienced a spontaneous attack of rotational vertigo and nausea that lasted for a day and then complained of dizziness only when lying down or sitting up in bed. In patients with persistent dizziness, the clinician should question the patient as to when the initial symptoms became evident and whether the dizziness seems to be getting progressively worse, resolving, or staying the same. Table 3–3 is an adaption from Bennett (2008) that pairs common disorders and their time course.

Question 3: Can You Make the Dizziness Happen?

Determining if there is anything a patient can do to provoke the symptoms, or whether they are spontaneous is another key question in understanding the nature of the dizziness. The inquiry into what the circumstances are when the dizziness occurs should follow the description by the patient about the symptoms and their duration. For example, can the patient bring on the dizziness by performing a certain head movement? If a patient stands up and feels lightheaded, it may indicate a form of presyncope or positioning vertigo. Alternatively, a patient may have had an attack of vertigo that lasted anywhere from a day to a month and he or she continues to be very unstable during everyday activities. One method of helping to further discern the cause of dizziness is to pair the time course of the dizziness (Question 2) with circumstances that provoke it (Bennett, 2008). This can help the examiner begin to classify the possible origin of the sensations that the patient is experiencing (Table 3–4).

Question 4: Are There Any Symptoms that Accompany the Dizziness?

Due to the proximity of the hearing and balance organs to one another, it is important that the clinician inquire about any otological symptoms that are concomitant with the dizziness. Patients who have disorders affecting the inner ear may present with tinnitus, hearing loss, and pain or pressure. Alternatively, patients may also have associated symptoms that are neurological. Impairments in the brain or central nervous system commonly manifest symptoms of dizziness. Disorders such as neoplasms, multiple sclerosis, cerebellar degenerations, and migraine can all result in severe sensations of dizziness. Visual disturbances can have either a central or peripheral origin. In order to differentiate between a central and peripheral visual impairment, the patient should be questioned as to whether they have double vision (diplopia), whether the visual disturbance becomes worse with head movement (i.e., VOR related), and whether there is any complete loss of vision. One of the most common forms of dizziness that occurs with neurological symptoms is migrainous vertigo. In fact, Isaacson and Rubin (1999) have reported that approximately one-third of the migraine population complains of associated vertigo. Tables 3–5 and 3–6 present otological and non-otological symptoms that can accompany dizziness, along with the potential causes.

Table 3–3. Common Disorders and Their Time Course

Short Duration	Intermediate Duration	Long Duration
BPPV Benign Paroxysmal Positional Vertigo	Migraine	Head injury (trauma)
Superior canal dehiscence	Metabolic disorders	Vestibular neuritis
Vascular insufficiency	Ménière disease	Stroke
Medication effects	Syphilis	Medication effects
Chiari malformation	Panic attacks	Labyrinthitis
	Transient ischemic accident	

Table 3–4. Characteristics of Vertigo and Potential Origin

Vertigo of Short Duration	Potential Origin
Change in the position of head or head and body	BPPV Benign Paroxysmal Positional Vertigo
Loud sounds or exertion	Superior canal dehiscence
Standing up or sitting up quickly	Orthostatic hypotension

Vertigo of Intermediate or Long Duration	Potential Origin
Stress	Anxiety and/or depression
Headache	Migraine or space-occupying lesions
Diet	Ménière disease
Upper respiratory infection	Vestibular neuritis/labyrinthitis
Head trauma	Concussion/blast exposure

Table 3–5. Otological Symptoms of Dizziness

Dizziness with Associated Otological Symptoms	Potential Causes
Tinnitus (non-pulsatile/pulsatile)	Ménière disease
Hearing loss (conductive/sensory, neural/mixed)	Acoustic neuroma
	Vestibular schwannoma
Fullness (pressure/popping)	Perilymph fistula
Otalgia	Labyrinthitis
Otorrhea	Cholesteotoma
	Stroke (anterior inferior cerebellar artery)
	Otitis externa
	Otitis media

Table 3–6. Neurological Symptoms of Dizziness

Dizziness with Associated Neurological Symptoms	Potential Causes
Headaches	Stroke
Weakness (paralysis/numbness)	Migraine
	Multiple sclerosis
Facial palsy	Vertebrobasilar insufficiency
Loss of consciousness	
Photophobia/phonophobia	Viral infection (Ramsay Hunt syndrome)
Dysphagia/dysphonia/dysarthria	Tumors
Changes in vision	
Ataxia	

Question 5: Do You Have Any Other Medical Conditions?

The patient's current medical status and medical history are important components in the case history because there are medical conditions that

are known to contribute to dizziness. Prior to the face-to-face interview, the clinician should have reviewed the patient's medical history and noted any conditions that may indirectly or directly affect the vestibular system or contribute to sensations of dizziness. Any surgeries, otological or otherwise, should be documented and further examined. As with the associated symptoms, the patient can be questioned regarding any medical conditions that are otological or nonotological. For example, a patient who has a history of ear disease (e.g., cholesteatoma) may have had numerous surgeries, and based on the symptoms a causal relationship may be established. A patient who has heart disease (e.g., coronary artery disease) may likely complain of lightheadedness. In patients who are anxious or depressed, a relationship may exist between the dizziness and the situation that results in a patient having a panic attack. Finally, patients should be questioned regarding their family's history of neurological and/or otological disease. For example, questions inquiring whether there are any family members with migraine or multiple sclerosis can be helpful because many of the disorders that cause dizziness can be genetically transmitted. Table 3–7 shows common medical conditions and the symptoms of dizziness that they produce.

Question 6: What Medications Are You Taking?

The majority of patients seen for balance function testing are using medications to either treat dizziness or another medical condition. The examiner should have the patient bring a list of all prescription and over-the-counter medications (including nutritional supplements). It is the responsibility of the clinician to understand the symptoms and side effects that these medications have on dizziness and how these agents contribute to a patient's complaints. It is also important that the examiner be aware of the effect of medication on quantitative vestibular testing. Some medications affect the peripheral vestibular system, whereas others act on the central nervous system. Patients taking drugs that affect the nervous system may produce findings that are similar to those of patients with a cerebellar impairment, oculomotor impairment, or a decrease in peripheral vestibular system function. Patients suffering from an acute attack of vertigo are often prescribed antivertigo medications (meclizine or Valium). These medications act to reduce the symptoms of dizziness, as well as prevent nausea and vomiting. To reduce the patient's

Table 3–7. Types of Dizziness and Related Medical Conditions

Medical Condition	Type of Dizziness
Cardiovascular	Syncope (orthostatic hypotension)
Migraine	Motion intolerance/vertigo
Multiple sclerosis	Ataxia, lightheadedness, vertigo
Autoimmune disease	Ataxia, oscillopsia, lightheadedness
Chronic subjective dizziness	Rocking sensation, lightheadedness
Viral infections (nervous system)	Ataxia/vertigo
Stroke	Vertigo, short-duration unsteadiness

symptoms of vertigo, the actions of these medications work to target the neurotransmitters acetylcholine, histamine, and gamma-aminobutyric acid (GABA) at the level of the vestibular nerve and nuclei (Baloh, 1998b; Foster & Baloh, 1996). The antinausea mechanisms of the medications block the input to the medullary vomiting region and reduce the symptoms (Timmerman, 1994). The nature of these medications is such that they sedate the central nervous system and can thus produce abnormalities during oculomotor testing, static positional testing, and caloric testing. A summary of common medications and their effects is presented in Table 3–8.

THE DIZZINESS SYMPTOM PROFILE (DSP)

Although the formal evaluation of the patient with dizziness typically begins with the case history, it can often be a lengthy process to extract the salient pieces of information. The clinician uses the case history to develop hypotheses regarding the origin of the patient's symptoms and correlate these with the results of laboratory tests (e.g., neuro-

Table 3–8. Common Medications, Their Mechanisms, and Adverse Effects

Common Medications	Mechanism	Adverse Effect
Alcohol (e.g., Tennessee Moonshine)	Enhancement of GABA receptor function (global sedation of central nervous system)	Brainstem–cerebellar signs, positional nystagmus
Anticonvulsants (e.g., Dilantin[a], Tegretol[b])	Inhibit voltage-dependent sodium and calcium channels (thought to inhibit neuronal firing); enhancement of GABA receptor function	Brainstem–cerebellar signs, sedation
Antidepressants/anxiety benzodiazepines (e.g., Valium[c], Xanax[a])	Enhancement of GABA receptor function (global sedation of central nervous system including vestibular nerve and nuclei)	Brainstem–cerebellar signs, sedation, may inhibit central nervous system compensation, ataxia
Antivertigo/nausea antihistamines (e.g., meclizine)	Block dopamine (primarily inhibitory neurotransmitter) thereby increasing excitation at the level of the brainstem	Sedation, may inhibit central nervous system compensation
Aminoglycosides (e.g., vancomycin, streptomycin, gentamicin)	Act as protein synthesis inhibitors (disrupts bacteria growth)	Ototoxcity, neurotoxcity, vestibulotoxicity
Chemotherapeutics (e.g., cisplatin, carboplatin)	Act as alkylating agents (inhibit cancer cells from growing)	Ototoxcity, neurotoxcity, vestibulotoxicity
Antihypertensives (e.g., Lasix[d], atenolol)	Diuretics diminish sodium reabsorption	Presyncope, orthostatic hypotension

GABA = gamma-aminobutyric acid.
[a]Pizfer, New York, NY; [b]Novartis Pharmaceuticals, East Hanover, NJ; [c]Roche Laboratories, Nutley, NJ; [d]Sanofi Aventis, Bridewater, NJ.

imaging, vestibular laboratory tests). The challenge that is often encountered with patient with dizziness is obtaining an informative directed case history in a short period of time while not cutting the patient off. There is no doubt that a well-conducted structured case history affords clinicians the ability to provide a timely and accurate diagnosis for dizzy patients. Jacobson and colleagues (2018) have recently developed a case history device that includes the standardized diagnostic criteria of the most common dizzy disorders. This tool provides the clinician with a reduced number of possible diagnoses that can be used to help develop the differential diagnosis. Once the DSP is completed by the patient, this information can be then be used to supplement the clinicians case history and direct office examination. For example,

when the results of the DSP suggest the possibility of vestibular migraine, the clinician can follow up with more detailed questions related to headaches in order to either rule in or out the contribution of headache to the patient symptoms. This device can also assist in directing patients to the appropriate subspecialty providers (e.g., neurology, otology, or behavioral medicine) to address their symptoms. The final version of the DSP is composed of 31 items (Table 3–9). The authors report that the DSP is in agreement with the differential diagnoses of otologists for Ménière's disease (100% agreement), vestibular migraine (95% agreement), and benign paroxysmal positional vertigo (82% agreement). This device should prove useful in creation of differential diagnoses for dizzy patients that can be evaluated and managed locally.

Table 3–9. The Dizziness Symptom Profile (DSP)

Instructions: "The following pages contain statements with which you can agree or disagree. To what extent do you personally agree or disagree with thee statements in regards to your dizziness? Use the following scale: 0 = Strongly Disagree, 1 = Disagree, 2 = Not Sure, 3 = Agree, 4 = Strongly Agree"

Item	Statement	Strongly Disagree		Not Sure		Strongly Agree
1	My dizziness is intense but only lasts for seconds to minutes	0	1	2	3	4
2	I have had a single severe spell of spinning dizziness that lasted days or weeks.	0	1	2	3	4
3	I have spells where I get dizzy and also have irregular heartbeats (palpitations).	0	1	2	3	4
4	I hear my voice more loudly in one ear compared to the other.	0	1	2	3	4
5	I am unsure of my footing when I walk outside.	0	1	2	3	4
6	I get dizzy when I turn over in bed.	0	1	2	3	4
7	I get dizzy when I am in open spaces and have nothing to hold onto.	0	1	2	3	4
8	I have a roaring sound in one ear only before or during a dizziness attack.	0	1	2	3	4
9	I am depressed much of the time.	0	1	2	3	4
10	I lost hearing in one ear after an attack of spinning dizziness.	0	1	2	3	4
11	I had a big dizzy spell that lasted for days where I could not walk without falling over.	0	1	2	3	4
12	I get dizzy when I sneeze.	0	1	2	3	4
13	There are times when I get dizzy and also have a headache.	0	1	2	3	4
14	I get dizzy when I strain to lift something heavy.	0	1	2	3	4
15	I get a short-lasting, spinning dizziness that happens when I bend down to pick something up.	0	1	2	3	4
16	My hearing gets worse in one ear before or during a dizziness attack.	0	1	2	3	4
17	I had a single constant spell of spinning dizziness that lasted longer than 2–3 days.	0	1	2	3	4
18	When I get a headache I am very sensitive to sound (I try to find a quiet place to rest).	0	1	2	3	4
19	I get short-lasting, spinning dizziness that happens when I go from sitting to lying down.	0	1	2	3	4
20	I can trigger a dizzy spell by placing my head in a certain position.	0	1	2	3	4

Table 3–9. *continued*

Item	Statement	Strongly Disagree		Not Sure		Strongly Agree
21	I had a spell of spinning dizziness that lasted for days or weeks after I had a cold or flu.	0	1	2	3	4
22	I have a feeling of fullness or pressure in one ear before or during a dizziness attack.	0	1	2	3	4
23	I get headaches that hurt so badly that I am completely unable to do my daily activities.	0	1	2	3	4
24	I have spells where I get dizzy and it is difficult for me to breathe.	0	1	2	3	4
25	I have a sensation of dizziness or imbalance daily or almost daily.	0	1	2	3	4
26	My vision changes before a headache begins.	0	1	2	3	4
27	I am unsteady on my feet all the time.	0	1	2	3	4
28	I am anxious much of the time.	0	1	2	3	4
29	When I cough I get dizzy.	0	1	2	3	4
30	When I get a headache I am very sensitive to light (I try to find a dark room to rest).	0	1	2	3	4
31	I feel dizzy all of the time.	0	1	2	3	4

Subscale assignments:

Vestibular migraine (5 items): 13, 18, 23, 26, 30
Ménière's disease (5 items): 4, 8, 10, 16, 22
Unspecified unsteadiness (4 items): 5, 7, 25, 27
BPPV (5 items): 1, 6, 15, 19, 20

SCD: 12, 14, 29 (3 items)
Vestibular neuritis/labyrinthitis (4 items): 2, 11, 17, 21
CSD (5 items): 3, 9, 24, 28, 31

ASSESSMENT OF DIZZINESS HANDICAP

Conventional tests of balance function (e.g., electronystagmography) yield valuable information regarding damage (impairment) to the balance system; however, these tests provide very little information regarding the debilitating effects (handicap) that disorders of the balance system may have on an individual's functional, emotional, and/or physical aspects of life (Jacobson & Newman, 1990). In this regard, the World Health Organization (WHO) has provided definitions to differentiate between impairment and handicap. The WHO defines "impairment" as an abnormality or loss of physiological, psychological, or anatomical structure or function (WHO, 2002). Using this definition, impairment in the balance system may be dysfunction in any of the systems necessary to maintain balance (i.e., vestibular system, visual system, and/or the proprioceptive system). Abnormalities of the balance system are often able to be confirmed through quantitative balance function tests (e.g., electronystagmography). Alternatively, "handicap" is defined as a disadvantage for a given individual, resulting from an impairment that limits or prevents the fulfillment of a role that is normal" (WHO, 2002). In order for the clinician to obtain a complete picture of the patient's disability, an assessment of the patient's perceived handicap should be acquired. The challenge is that it is not uncommon for patients with a history of dizziness to be asymptomatic at the time of testing and, therefore, to have normal results on quantitative balance function tests. The clinician should be vigilant to the fact that sensations of dizziness and imbalance can lead the patient to restrict social and physical activities. Furthermore, patients experiencing dizziness may suffer from significant emotional distress that can be as debilitating as the symptoms of dizziness. It is imperative that the clinician keep in mind that each patient's response to the dizziness or imbalance is unique. In other words, the patient's reaction to the sensations varies based on their personality type, age, physical health, and/or psychosocial adjustment. Conventional balance function tests are incapable of assessing the degree of participation restriction and activity limitation caused by a balance disorder. To address this, Jacobson and Newman (1990) developed a measure known as the Dizziness Handicap Inventory (DHI).

The DHI is a 25-item questionnaire designed to assess the self-perceived handicapping effects of vestibular system disorders on patients. None of the items use the word "dizziness" but instead employs the term "problem" (Table 3–10). The DHI is grouped into three subscales: a 9-item func-

tional scale, 9-item emotional scale, and 7-item physical scale. The functional scale was developed to assess what the effect of "the problem" is on the patient's daily life. The physical scale assesses how head and body movements affect "the problem," and finally, the emotional scale evaluates what effect "the problem" has on the patient's emotional well-being. Patients respond to each question by answering "yes," "sometimes," or "no" to each item and are given a score of 4, 2, or 0, respectively. Following completion of the scale, the examiner can calculate the score for each subscale or use the total score.

The DHI is a reliable and valid measure of the patient's perception of handicap (Enloe & Shields, 1997; Jacobson & Calder, 1998; Jacobson & Newman, 1990; Jacobson, Newman, Hunter, & Balzer, 1991). The total score of the DHI has good face validity and high internal consistency (Cronbach's alpha = 0.78–0.89) and high test–retest reliability ($r = 0.97$, $df = 12$, $p < 0.0001$). Satisfactory internal consistency was noted for the functional, emotional, and physical subscales. In an effort to describe the degree to which dizziness handicaps a patient's quality of life, Jacobson and McCaslin (unpublished data) categorized the level of severity using the total score of the DHI. Specifically,

Table 3–10. Dizziness Handicap Inventory

Instructions: The purpose of this questionnaire is to identify difficulties that you may be experiencing because of your dizziness or unsteadiness. Please answer "yes," "no," or "sometimes" to each question.

Answer each question as it pertains to your dizziness problem only.

		Yes (4)	Sometimes (2)	No (0)
P1.	Does looking up increase your problem?			
E2.	Because of your problem do you feel frustrated?			
F3.	Because of your problem do you restrict your travel for business or recreation ?			
P4.	Does walking down the aisle of a supermarket increase your problem?			
F5.	Because of your problem do you have difficulty getting into or out of bed.			

Table 3–10. *continued*

	Yes (4)	Sometimes (2)	No (0)
F6. Does your problem significantly restrict your participation in social activities such as going out to dinner, going to the movies, dancing, or to parties?			
F7. Because of your problem do you have difficulty reading?			
P8. Does performing more ambitious activities like sports, dancing, household chores, such as sweeping or putting dishes away, increase your problem?			
E9. Because of your problem are you afraid to leave your home without having someone accompany you?			
E10. Because of your problem have you been embarrassed in front of others?			
P11. Do quick movements of your head increase your problem?			
F12. Because of your problem do you avoid heights?			
P13. Does turning over in bed increase your problem?			
F14. Because of your problem is it difficult for you to do strenuous housework or yardwork?			
E15. Because of your problem are you afraid people may think that you are intoxicated?			
P16. Because of your problem is it difficult for you to go for a walk by yourself?			
P17. Does walking down a sidewalk increase your problem?			
E18. Because of your problem is it difficult for you to concentrate?			
F19. Because of your problem is it difficult for you to walk around your house in the dark?			
E20. Because of your problem are you afraid to stay home alone?			
E21. Because of your problem do you feel handicapped?			
E22. Has your problem placed stress on your relationships with members of your family and friends?			
E23. Because of your problem are you depressed?			
F24. Does your problem interfere with your job or household responsibilities?			
P25. Does bending over increase your problem?			

FUNCTIONAL	EMOTIONAL	PHYSICAL	TOTAL SCORE

Source: From Jacobson and Newman (1990).

the interquartile ranges for the total DHI score were calculated using the scores from 200 consecutive patients reporting to a dizziness clinic. A score of 0–14 points was considered to represent no dizziness handicap. Total DHI scores of 15 to 26 were classified as mild handicap, and a score of 27 to 44 was considered moderate handicap. A total DHI score of 44 or greater was classified as severe dizziness handicap (Table 3–11). In a similar attempt to categorize dizziness handicap using the total DHI score, Kinney, Sandridge, and Newman (1997) reported similar scores from a sample of 51 dizzy patients.

A handicap measure referred to as the Vanderbilt Pediatric Dizziness Handicap Inventory for Patient Caregivers (DHI-PC) is another self-report measure that was based on the format of the adult version of the DHI described above (McCaslin, Jacobson, Labert, English, & Kemph 2015) (Table 3–12). This measure has been shown to be valuable for clinicians for clinicians assessing dizziness disability/handicap in the pediatric population (i.e., between the ages of 5 and 12 years of age) The device is administered as a parental proxy (parent completes the form based on their knowledge of the child's impairment). This instrument is typically used in a prepost treatment paradigm to assess changes in health-related quality of life for younger patients. The DHI-PC consists of 21 items. Short-term test–retest reliability (i.e., three week interval between test and retest) of this DHI-PC was assessed for a subset of 10 patients (caregivers, mean age 38 years, sd = 7 years, 10 female). The results indicated the short-term, test–retest reliability to be strong ($r = 0.98, p < 0.001$). The total score of the DHI-PC has good face validity and high internal consistency (Cronbach's alpha = 0.93). The interquartile ranges for the total DHI-PC score are as follows: a score of 0 to 16 points was considered to represent no dizziness handicap, scores of 16 to 26 were classified as mild handicap, and a score of 26 to 43 was considered moderate handicap. A DHI-PC score >43 points indicates the child has severe activity and participation limitation.

BEDSIDE EVALUATION OF THE OCULAR MOTOR SYSTEM

There are several reasons why the clinician should always perform an examination of the movement of the eyes before any formal testing begins. First, this brief examination provides valuable information regarding the integrity of the cranial nerves and central nervous system control of the eyes (i.e., saccades and gaze). Second, it reveals if the range of motion of the extraocular muscles (EOMs) is intact and the eye movements are conjugate (move together). Finally, a close evaluation of the eyes allows the examiner to identify the presence of any nystagmus. Having this information prior to performing the VNG enables the clinician to adapt the test protocol, if necessary, and avoid technical errors and misinterpretation of the examination. For instance, the clinician occasionally encounters patients presenting with abnormalities of the eyelid. One such abnormality is referred to as ptosis (Greek for fall). Ptosis is a drooping of one or both eyelids and is readily identified during the gross eye movement examination. Ptosis may be suggestive of impairment to the muscle that lifts the eyelid or impairment to the oculomotor nerve (cranial nerve III) which controls the muscle or involvement of the superior cervical sympathetic ganglion. Bilateral and unilateral ptosis has also been associated with genetic disorders involving the oculomotor nerve (i.e., CFEOM1, CFEOM3, and congenital ptosis) (Leigh & Zee, 2006). When recording the eye movements of a patient with unilateral ptosis a monocular recording (of the intact eye) is often indicated.

For the purpose of reporting findings during the gross eye movement examination, it is important that the clinician understand the terminology

Table 3–11. Dizziness Handicap Inventory Data

Quartile	Score	Handicap
1	0–14	None
2	15–26	Mild
3	27–44	Moderate
4	44+	Severe

Source: From Jacobson and McCaslin (unpublished data).

Table 3–12. Vanderbilt Pediatric Dizziness Handicap Inventory–Patient Caregiver (DHI-PC) (Ages 5–12 Years)

NAME: _____ DATE: _____

Instructions: The purpose of this questionnaire is to identify difficulties that your child may be experiencing because of his or her dizziness or unsteadiness. Please answer "yes," "no," or "sometimes" to each question. **Answer each question as it pertains to your child's dizziness problem only.**

	Yes (4)	Sometimes (2)	No (0)
1. Does your child s problem make him/her feel tired?			
2. Is your child s life ruled by his/her problem?			
3. Does your child s problem make it difficult for him/her to play?			
4. Because of his/her problem, does your child feel frustrated?			
5. Because of his/her problem, has your child been embarrassed in front of others?			
6. Because of his/her problem, is it difficult for your child to concentrate?			
7. Because of his/her problem, is your child tense?			
8. Do other people seem irritated with your child s problem?			
9. Because of his/her problem, does your child worry?			
10. Because of his/her problem, does your child feel angry?			
11. Because of his/her problem, does your child feel down ?			
12. Because of his/her problem, does your child feel unhappy?			
13. Because of his/her problem, does your child feel different from other children?			
14. Does your child s problem significantly restrict his/her participation in social or educational activities, such as going to dinner, meeting with friends, field trips, or to parties?			
15. Because of your child's problem, is it difficult for him/her to walk around the house in the dark?			
16. Because of his/her problem, does your child have difficulty walking up stairs?			
17. Because of his/her problem, does your child have difficulty walking one or two blocks?			
18. Because of his/her problem, does your child have difficulty riding a bike or scooter?			
19. Because of his/her problem, does your child have difficulty reading or doing schoolwork?			
20. Does your child's problem make it difficult to successfully do activities that others his/her age can do?			
21. Because of his/her problem, does your child have trouble concentrating at school?			
	TOTAL SCORE		

that accompanies the descriptions of how the eye moves. This is important to both understand descriptions of the eye movements in previous medical records but also so that when observing the eyes during the bedside examination, the movements can be described accurately using accepted terminology. The eye is capable of rotating in three axes. These include the roll axis (*x*-axis), the yaw axis (*z*-axis), and the pitch axis (*y*-axis). These eye rotations are accomplished by contraction and relaxation of the extraocular muscles described in detail in Chapter 1.

One type of movement of the eye is a duction. Ductions refer to the monocular movement of each eye. For instance, a horizontal movement of an eye away from the nose is commonly referred to an A-B-duction, and a movement of the eye toward the nose is called an A-D-duction (Figure 3–1). When referring to movements in the vertical plane, an upward movement of the eye is known as an elevation (sursumduction) and a downward movement is referred to as a depression (deorsumduction). When the upper pole of the eye is rotated toward the midsagittal plane, the movement is referred to as an incycloduction. When the upper pole of the eye rotates away from the midsagittal plane, the movement is referred to as an excycloduction.

Versions describe both eyes moving in a conjugate manner. That is, both eyeballs move in the same direction at the same time. When both eyes

rotate upward in the pitch axis, it is referred to as elevation, while looking downward in the same axis is referred to as depression. When both eyes are rotated in the yaw axis to the right, the movement is referred to as a dextroversion. Conversely, a binocular conjugate movement of both eyes to the left is known as a levoversion. Finally, the both eyes moving in the x-axis, where the upper pole of the eye rotates tot the right is known as a dextrocycloversion, whereas this same action to the left is called a levocycloversion.

The third primary type of eye movement is vergence. Vergences are simultaneous binocular movements of eyes in opposite directions (i.e., disjunctive). For example, when an object is coming toward or moving away from the viewer, this type of eye movement is employed to keep the object of interest in focus. Convergence is when both eyes simultaneously rotate in the yaw axis toward the median plane, whereas divergence is when both eyes rotate in the same axis away from the median plane. When the eyes simultaneously move in the roll axis with the upper pole of the eye rotating away from the midsagittal plane it is referred to as an incyclovergence. Excyclovergence refers to the same movement but with the upper poles of the eyes rotating away from the midsagittal plane (Figure 3–2).

There are two primary reasons that it is critical to identify when a patient does not have conjugate eye movements. First, when the clinician is preparing the patient for the ENG/VNG test, if the eyes are determined to not be conjugate, he or she needs to make sure that each eye is recorded from separately. Second, identifying disconjugate eye movements can provide insight into a patient's reported symptoms and impairment. For example, a patient with disconjugate eye movements often complains of double vision (diplopia). Diplopia is commonly observed in patients with either a mechanical problem affecting the EOMs, a lesion in the neuromuscular junction (brainstem), or a disorder affecting the cranial nerves that innervate the EOMs (oculomotor, abducens, or trochlear). An example of one such disorder is internuclear ophthalmoplegia (INO). There are varying levels of severity of INO ranging anywhere from simply slow movements of the adducting eye (the eye moving toward the nose) to total paralysis. INO can be either unilateral or bilateral and implicates

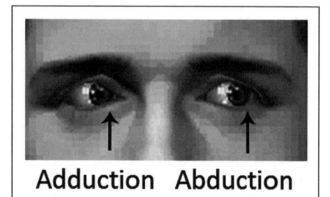

Adduction   Abduction

FIGURE 3–1. Image shows the adducting eye and abducting eye. Abduction is a horizontal movement of the eye away from the midline (*right arrow*). Adduction is a horizontal movement of the eye toward the midline (*left arrow*).

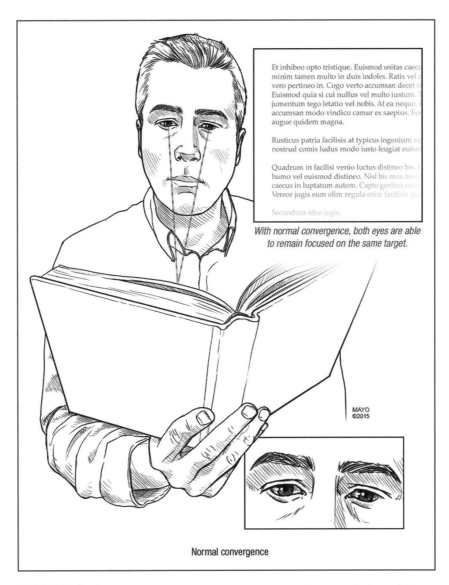

With normal convergence, both eyes are able to remain focused on the same target.

Normal convergence

FIGURE 3–2. Example of convergence. (Used with permission of Mayo Foundation for Medical Education and Research. All rights reserved.)

the medial longitudinal fasciculus (reviewed in Chapter 1). This disorder is commonly observed in patients suffering from multiple sclerosis or brainstem stroke. An INO should be identified prior to testing during the gross eye movement examination. Figure 3–3 illustrates the eye movements of a patient with an INO during the gaze examination. A thorough ocular motor examination should also include an evaluation of visual fixation while the patients fixate on a target. During this task, the clinics should instruct the patient to look at a target and then closely watch the patient's eyes to determine if there are any saccadic intrusions.

These intrusive saccades include eye movements that take the eye off the target involuntarily (e.g. square-wave jerks, opsoclonus, flutter). The examiner should also note and describe any nystagmus observed during the gross eye movement examination. Nystagmus (described in Chapter 2) can be either physiological (i.e., normal) or pathological (i.e., abnormal) (Baloh, 1998a). Physiological nystagmus can be induced several different ways. For example, it can be observed when a patient is rotated in a chair, subjected to a full-field stimulus (optokinetic), induced by a caloric stimulus into the ear canal, or stimulated when the eyes are

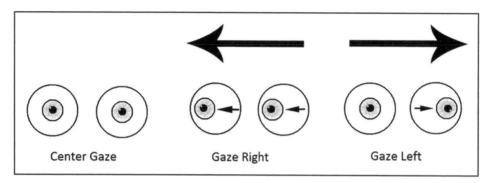

FIGURE 3–3. Illustration of the eye movements of a patient with right internuclear ophthalmoplegia. The right eye is affected, and when gaze is directed to the left, there is an impairment of adduction.

driven to extremes during lateral gaze (i.e., greater than 40°). There are also several varieties of pathological nystagmus. The three primary types are spontaneous, gaze evoked, and positional (Baloh & Kerber, 2011). When the examiner performs a gross eye movement evaluation, he or she must be able to discern normal nystagmus from abnormal nystagmus. If it is determined that a patient has pathological nystagmus, the direction (e.g., down-beating or up-beating), effect of eye position (e.g., enhancement on lateral gaze), and effect of fixation should be described. One common method of describing the effect of eye position on nystagmus has been reported by Baloh and Honrubia (1990). This method makes use of a "tic-tac-toe" plot that represents the cardinal positions of gaze Arrows are drawn longer or shorter to represent the intensity of the nystagmus. The direction of the arrow describes which way the fast phase of the nystagmus is beating.

Common Types of Aberrant Nystagmus Observed During the Gross Eye Movement Examination

Peripheral Vestibular Nystagmus

The characteristics of spontaneous nystagmus of peripheral origin are: (a) mixed horizontal-torsional nystagmus, (b) significant decrease in intensity with fixation, and (c) unidirectionality (follows Alexander's law). A summary of the features of spontaneous nystagmus are presented in Figure 3–4 using the box diagram method.

(See Chapter 2 for a detailed account of these characteristics.)

Down-Beating Nystagmus of Central Origin

The characteristics of down-beating nystagmus of central origin are (a) little or no change in intensity with fixation, and (b) enhancement on lateral gaze. A summary of the features of down-beating nystagmus are presented in Figure 3–5 using the box diagram method. (See Chapter 5 for a detailed account of these characteristics.)

Symmetrical Gaze-Evoked Nystagmus

The characteristics of symmetrical gaze-evoked nystagmus are: (a) bidirectionality (left-beating on left gaze and right-beating on right gaze), (b) little or no change in intensity with fixation, and (c) high frequency and low amplitude. A summary of the features of gaze-evoked nystagmus are presented in Figure 3–6 using the box diagram method. (See Chapter 5 for a detailed account of these characteristics.)

Congenital Nystagmus

The characteristics of congenital nystagmus are: (a) conjugate high-frequency nystagmus, and nystagmus that is variable in direction. A summary of the features of congenital nystagmus are presented in Figure 3–7 using the box diagram method.

Congenital nystagmus (CN) is observed at birth or very shortly afterward. Patients with

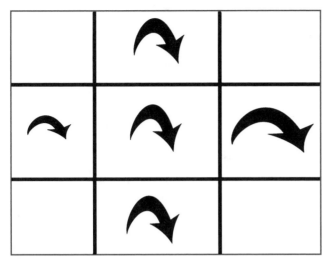

FIGURE 3–4. Example of how a left-beating peripherally generated spontaneous nystagmus that follows Alexander's law would be characterized using the method described by Baloh and Honrubia (1990).

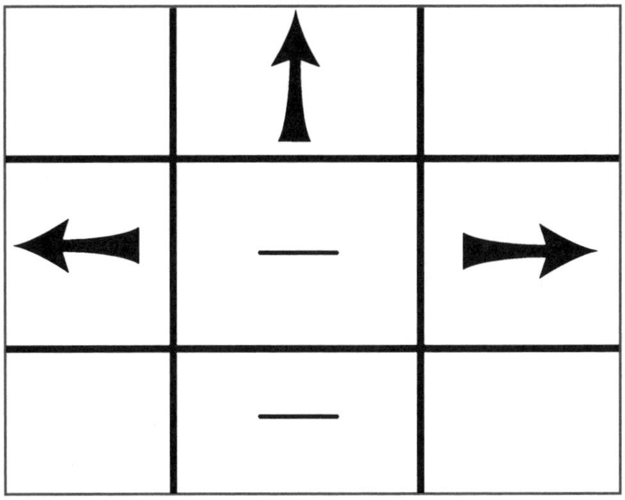

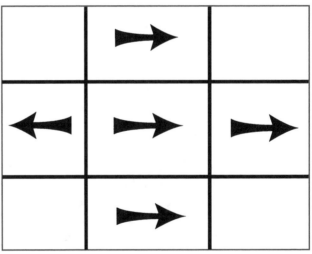

FIGURE 3–6. Example of how a bidirectional centrally generated gaze-evoked nystagmus would be characterized using the method described by Baloh and Honrubia (1990).

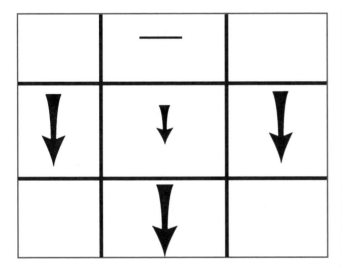

FIGURE 3–5. Example of how a down-beating centrally generated spontaneous nystagmus would be characterized using the method described by Baloh and Honrubia (1990).

FIGURE 3–7. Example of how a congenital nystagmus would be described using the method described by Baloh and Honrubia (1990). Note that on upward gaze the nystagmus continues to be horizontal.

CN may have normal vision or may be visually impaired. This type of nystagmus is important to identify early during the ENG/VNG examination for two reasons. First, CN is due to a genetic (X-linked recessive or dominant trait) or developmental brain defect that may preclude the need for further testing (Gay, Newman, Keltner, & Stroud, 1974). Second, the clinician needs to be prepared to account for these eye movements during the interpretation phase of the various ENG/VNG subtests. Figure 3–8 illustrates how congenital nystagmus manifests during various oculomotor tests. CN is characterized by a bilateral pendular nystagmus or jerk nystagmus.

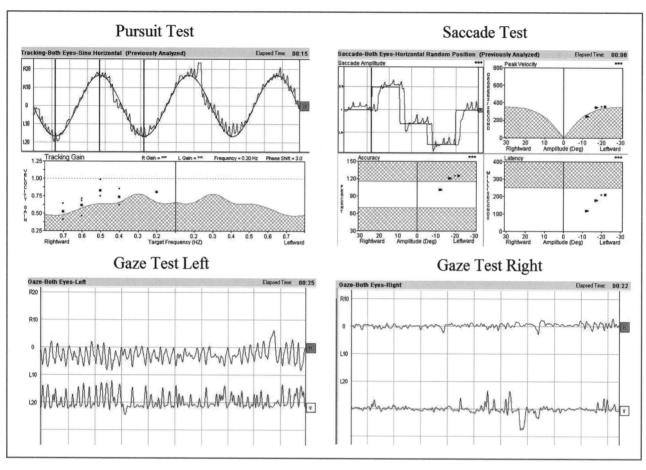

FIGURE 3–8. Example of how a congenital nystagmus manifests in various oculomotor subtests.

Finally, the examiner should attend to how well the patient is able to follow instructions and sustain appropriate effort during the examination. This provides valuable insight into how well the patient will perform during the upcoming subtests of the ENG/VNG. Reinstruction should be provided if the patient has difficulty performing the task. In order to perform the gross eye movement examination, the examiner simply needs a chair, their fingers, and a pair of Frenzel glasses or VNG goggles.

Performing the Gross Eye Movement Examination

Instructions and Preparation

Seat the patient on the examination table in a room that is well lit and free of any moving distrac-tions. Inquiry regarding the patient's visual acuity should be undertaken (e.g., glasses or prosthetic eye). A hand is placed on the patient's forehead to ensure that there will be no head movement. The patient should then be instructed to hold his or her head very still and follow the examiner's finger with his or her eyes.

Ocular Motor Exam

Ocular Range of Motion. To evaluate the range of motion of the extraocular muscles, and whether the eyes are conjugate or not, the clinician draws a large imaginary "H" in the air (Figure 3–9). The legs of the H should be approximately 25° to 30° from midline. The vertical legs of the H pattern permit assessment of the inferior/superior oblique muscles and superior/inferior rectus muscles. The horizontal arm of the H tests the lateral and medial rectus muscles. The clinician

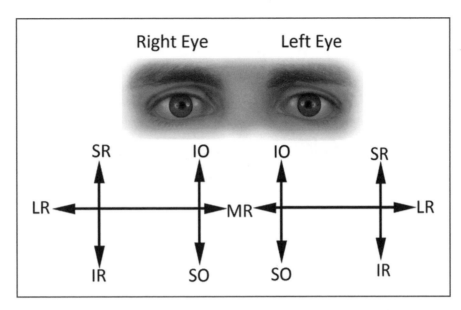

FIGURE 3–9. Movements of the extraocular muscles. LR = lateral rectus; SR = superior rectus; IR = inferior rectus; MR = medial rectus; SO = superior oblique; IO = inferior oblique; SR = superior rectus.

should determine if the patient's eye movements are conjugate (move identically).

Ocular Alignment. Patients suffering from significant ocular misalignment will often present with a primary symptom of diplopia and head tilt. Diplopia refers to the sensation of seeing two distinct objects or the same object at two different locations in space. The clinician should query the patient as to whether the diplopia is vertical or horizontal and whether it is binocular or monocular. Patients presenting with more subtle ocular misalignments may complain of brain fog, difficulty with attention, frequent headaches, and sore eyes. Ocular alignments are in most instances referred to by the resting position of the eye. A *phoria* describes a deviation of the visual axes during monocular observation of a single target (i.e., one eye is covered). While observing the target with both eyes, a patient can fuse the target and keep both eyes on the target. However, when one eye is covered the fusion is disrupted and the eye not viewing the target will return to its resting position (Figure 3–10). A tropia is a deviation of the visual axes during binocular observation of a target (Figure 3–11). This is referred to as static deviation and it occurs in all instances of a patient viewing a target (Table 3–13).

A concomitant ocular misalignment of the eyes in the vertical plane may result in significant ocular torsion and head tilt that together make up the ocular tilt reaction (OTR). Skew deviation is a vertical misalignment of the eyes that can be in response to an acute tonic neural asymmetry in the utricular-ocular reflex or an impairment in the supranuclear inputs stemming from disease in the brainstem, cerebellum. Specifically, when an ocular motor examination is performed on a patient with skew deviation, the clinician will observe a vertical misalignment of the eyes that is unrelated to impairment in the extraocular muscles (e.g., trochlear nerve palsy). Three key factors are used to identify a significant OTR; lateral head tilt, skew deviation with depression of one eye and elevation of the other, and a torsional rotation of the eyes (superior pole) toward the down ear.

Horizontal ocular-misalignment may alternate with changes in the direction of horizontal gaze. This finding is most commonly associated with cerebellar disease and the abducting eye will in most instances be the higher eye. Whenever an ocular misalignment in the horizontal plane is observed, the clinician should rule out an abducens or oculomotor nerve palsy so as to not mischaracterize the nature of the misalignment.

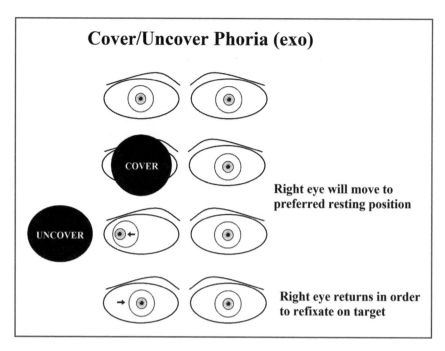

FIGURE 3–10. Cover-uncover—phoria

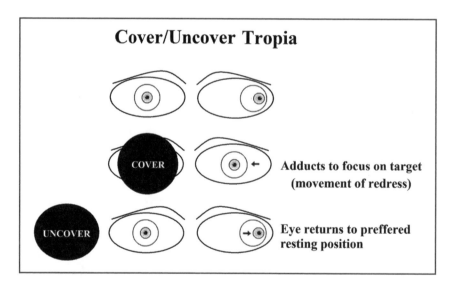

FIGURE 3–11. Cover-uncover—tropia

Table 3–13. Ocular Misalignments—Strabismus

Tropia	Deviation of visual axes during binocular viewing of a single target (Static deviation in all circumstances)
Phoria	Deviation of visual axes during monocular viewing of single target (Latent deviation)

To evaluate ocular alignment the Cover-Uncover Test (CUT) and Cover-Cross Cover Tests (CCCT) can be employed. The CUT is accomplished by having the patient focuses on a target and the clinician covers one eye. The clinician should be looking for what has been termed "movement of redress" of the uncovered eye. If the test is positive, then the tropia of the uncovered eye should be described (hypo/hyper/eso/exo). The CCCT is used to identify any movement of the occluded eye once uncovered. The CCCT and CUT are typically done together and usually referred to as the "Cover-Uncover Test." The CCCT is enables the clinician to identify phoria when the Cover test is negative (Table 3–14).

Saccades. To evaluate the saccade system, the clinician should hold up each hand in a fist approximately three feet apart. The patient is then asked to quickly divert his or her gaze to the examiner's finger when it "pops" up, without moving the head. The clinician then proceeds to quickly lift an index finger on one hand at a time alternating left to right. The latency, accuracy, and velocity of the patient's eye movements should be observed.

Smooth Pursuit. To evaluate the smooth pursuit system, the clinician should place a hand on the patient's forehead to ensure that there will be no head movement. The patient should then be instructed to keep his or her head very still and

follow the examiner's finger from side to side at approximately 2 to 4 Hz. The examiner should take care to note if the patient's eye movements are smooth and/or if they fall behind and then have to quickly catch up (saccadic pursuit).

Gaze Holding. To evaluate the gaze system the clinician should place a hand patient's forehead to ensure that there will be no head movement. The patient should then be instructed to keep their head very still and follow the examiner's finger approximately 30° up, down, right, and left. The examiner should take care to note any associated nystagmus and its characteristics (e.g., down-beating, up-beating).

VOR Suppression (i.e., Cancellation). The VOR is the critical system for keeping the eyes on an object of interest during head movement; however, there are times when it is necessary to suppress the VOR. VOR cancellation is required for tasks that involve situations where the head and the eye are rotating together (i.e., simultaneous eye-head tracking). For example, if an individual is observing a tennis match from afar, they will most likely track the ball with both the head and the eyes. If the VOR is not suppressed in this instance, vestibular nystagmus will be generated and the ability to see the ball will be interrupted. Although the primary structure that regulates VOR cancellation is the vestibulocerebellum (i.e., flocculus and

Table 3–14. Cover Test (Tropia) and Uncover Test (Phoria)

Cover Test (Tropia)	*Uncover Test (Phoria)*
The patient is instructed to focus on a stationary object.	The patient is instructed to focus on a stationary object.
Cover one of the eyes.	Cover one of the eyes and block fixation for at least 10 seconds.
The clinician looks for "movement of redress" of the eye that is not covered.	Remove the cover from the eye.
This will identify a tropia of the eye that is not covered (eso-exo-hyper-hypo).	Look for "movement of redress" of the eye that has just been "uncovered."
	Identifies phoria of the eye that is being uncovered (eso-exo-hyper-hypo)

paraflocculus) there a numerous other neural centers that play a role including the dorsal pontine nuclei and frontal eye fields. These structures also regulate regulating the smooth pursuit system. In this regard, when there are abnormalities in the VOR cancellation it is common to also have abnormalities in smooth pursuit.

The test can be easily performed by having the patient sit in an exam chair with their arms extended outward, hands together, and their thumbs pointing upwards. The patient is then instructed to keep their eyes fixed on their thumbs while the examiner rotates the patient's torso "en bloc" back and forth. It is important to ensure that the patients head stays in line with the outstretched arms. The rotation of the torso (and arms) should be approximately 30 degrees (from center—60 degrees total) with a frequency of approximately 2 Hz. A negative VOR cancellation test is little or no observable nystagmus during the rotations back and forth. A positive result during the VOR cancellation test is when there is observable nystagmus consistent throughout the rotations. During the test, the clinician should stand to the side while still being able to observe the eyes so as to avoid invoking an optokinetic response. If the patient's vision is extremely poor to the extent they cannot see their thumbs clearly, then they are not appropriate candidates for the test.

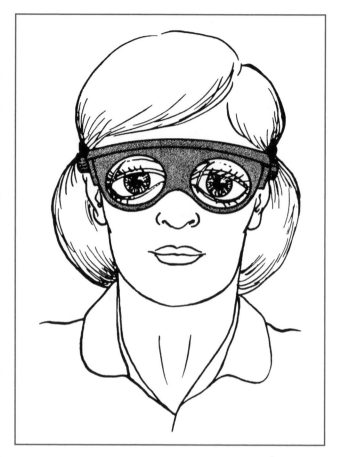

FIGURE 3–12. Illustration of a patient wearing Frenzel lenses. (Illustration by Mary Dersch from Pender, 1992, with permission of Daniel Pender)

Static Vestibular Imbalance

Spontaneous Nystagmus. The last step in the gross eye movement examination is to evaluate the eyes with vision denied (e.g., VNG goggles with the shield down) or distorted (e.g., Frenzel glasses) while the patient is mentally tasked. A patient with Frenzel lenses is shown in Figure 3–12. Spontaneous vestibular nystagmus is generated by a static imbalance of tonic neural activity at the level of the peripheral vestibular system (i.e., SCC-ocular reflexes).

Dynamic Vestibular Function

Head-Impulse Test. The head-impulse test (HIT) first described by Halmagyi and Curthoys (1988) for use to assess vestibular function is now a routine component in the bedside assessment of

vestibular function. It has become increasingly popular, due to the test's sensitivity to vestibular impairments, as well as the ease with which can be administered and interpreted. More recently, the development of video goggles has afforded the clinician a quantitative measurement of this bedside test (video head impulse testing or vHIT). The HIT evaluates an individual's ability to maintain visual fixation on a target during a high frequency head rotation. The test, which assesses the canal-ocular reflex (described in detail in Chapter 2), can provide insight into whether a patient has a significant unilateral or bilateral vestibular impairment.

In order to perform the test, the clinician should first instruct the patient to keep their eyes locked on the tester's nose while the head is rotated. The examiner should then gently grasp the patient's head and quickly move it to the left or right approximately 15 to 20 degrees. A normal functioning canal-ocular reflex should completely compensate for the head movement by rotating the eyes in the orbit 180 degrees the (ratio of eye velocity to head velocity is equal) out of phase thereby maintaining the fovea on the target. Accordingly, a negative HIT is when the patient's eyes continue to stay on the examiners nose throughout and after the head movement. A positive HIT is qualified by the presence of a catch-up saccade in the direction opposite the head is thrust (i.e., away from the impaired side) (Figure 3–13). Patients with significant bilateral peripheral vestibular impairments will demonstrate catch-up saccades opposite to the direction of head thrust in both directions.

Dynamic Visual Acuity. The clinician should be vigilant to patients that report symptoms of "blurred" vision or "bouncing" of the visual field when ambulating. These are descriptions that are often used by patients that have a significant unilateral or bilateral vestibular impairment. The clinical term that used for these symptoms provoked by dynamic actions is *oscillopsia* (i.e., "oscil-

lating vision") (Brickner, 1936). Oscillopsia is a consequence of an impaired canal-ocular reflex. The primary purpose of the canal-ocular reflex is to keep the fovea centered on a target of interest during head movement. As previously described in Chapter 2, the semicircular canals transduce head movement into equal and opposite eye movements in order to keep the retina fixed on a target. When the vestibular system is impaired, it only takes the canal-ocular reflex being off by a few degrees to degrade an individual's visual acuity (Westheimer & McKee, 1975). The natural response by a patient suffering from oscillopsia is to move their head very slowly so that the ocular motor system can be used to stabilize the retina on the object they are interested in viewing. In 1984, Hugh Barber described a test referred to as the "oscillopsia test" that could measure the above-described phenomenon in patients underlying vestibular impairments. The test consists of measuring a patient visual acuity with and without oscillation of the head. The test is based on the idea that if the canal-ocular reflex is impaired, a patient's visual acuity should be poorer when the head is moving versus when the head is stable. The current iteration of the oscillopsia test is now

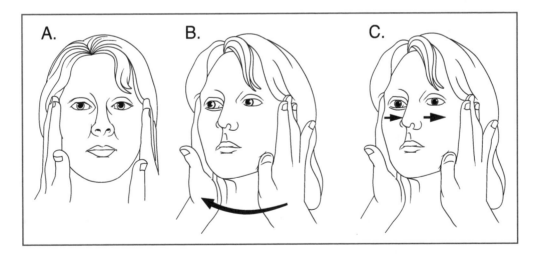

FIGURE 3–13. A. The patient is instructed to fixate on a target directly in front of him or her. **B.** When the patient's head is rotated abruptly 15 to 20 degrees to one side the eyes should deviate 180 degrees out of phase with the head thrust and remain fixed on the target. However, when the eyes cannot maintain fixation on the target due to an impaired vestibular system, the eyes travel with the head and come off the target. **C.** In order to reacquire the target, a saccadic eye movement is generated to bring the eye back to the point of visual fixation.

referred to in the literature as the dynamic visual acuity (DVA) test.

The test is performed by first determining a patient's best-corrected vision using a Snellen eye chart with the head still. When measuring visual acuity in this condition, it is recommended that the patient wear their glasses or contacts. The patient's visual acuity threshold is defined as the lowest line read on the chart with three or fewer errors. To perform the test, the clinician should first explain the test and then hold the patients head at the malar eminences. The patient's head is then oscillated back and forth at about 20 degrees of arc displacement in the yaw (i.e., horizontal) plane and at a frequency of about 5 Hz. The clinician should alter the direction that the patient reads the lines on the chart in order to avoid memorization. Interpretation of the test is as follows. A negative head-shaking test is typically considered a drop of no more than one line in best-corrected vision. A positive result is considered a drop in best-corrected vision of two or more lines.

Skull Vibration-Induced Nystagmus Test (SVINT)—The Vestibular Weber Test.

Over the last 10 years, the skull vibration-induced nystagmus test (SVINT) has become a staple in the direct vestibular office examination for detecting the presence of unilateral vestibular loss. In fact, the SVIN is the equivalent of the Weber test for the auditory system. When a 100-Hz vibration is applied to the mastoid to an individual with no vestibular impairment there typically no nystagmus or if there is some it is of very small amplitude. However, when the 100-Hz vibration is introduced to the skull in a patient with a significant vestibular paresis, a nystagmus where the fast phases beat toward the intact end organ will emerge. This response will begin immediately once the stimulus is initiated, be abolished once the stimulus is stopped and continue as long as the stimulus is delivered to the head (Figure 3–14). The nystagmus will beat in the same direction regardless of which mastoid is stimulated and it has been shown to be highly reproducible. Vibration induced nystagmus is able to be recorded in patients with unilateral peripheral weaknesses because the neurons from the semicircular canals are sensitive and can be activated by the bone-conducted vibration. In patients with equal SCC function, the response from the fibers will cancel out resulting in no observable nystagmus. Those individuals with an asymmetry will have a response that is unopposed to some degree due to incomplete cancellation. This asymmetrical stimulation of the labyrinths by the bone-conducted stimulus creates a neural pattern that is similar to a head turn toward the intact side. This in turn generates a nystagmus with the fast phases directed toward the healthy side. The attractiveness of this test is that it is very simple to perform, is non-invasive, and is sensitive in patients that are fully compensated. SVIN has been shown to be correlated with the degree of caloric hypofunction (Figure 3–15). In fact, it is able to be measured in nearly 90% of patients with a unilateral weakness of 50% of greater (Soper et al., 2018).

SVINT Test Technique:

1. Place either VNG or Frenzel goggles on the patient in order to inhibit fixation of the response.
2. Collect a baseline measure of spontaneous nystagmus with vision denied.
3. Apply the 100-Hz vibrator perpendicularly and firmly to the mastoid process posteriorly

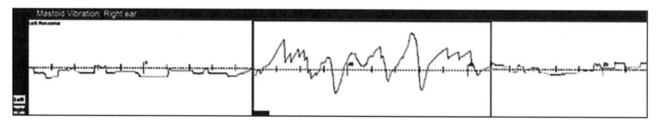

FIGURE 3–14. Example of left-beating vibration nystagmus applied to the left ear (i.e., right peripheral vestibular system weakness). *First panel:* no vibration; *second panel:* vibration administered; *third panel:* vibration stopped.

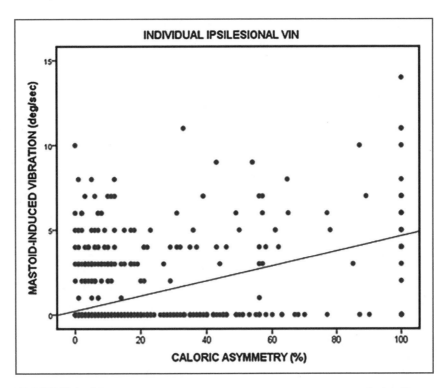

FIGURE 3–15. Vibration nystagmus and caloric asymmetry. A significant positive correlation was demonstrated for ipsilesional vestibular induced nystagmus ($r = 0.42$, $p < 0.000$) (Soper, 2018).

to the auricle and at the level of the external acoustic meatus with a pressure of approximately 1 kg.

4. Use the hand not holding the vibrator to brace the patient's head. (Figure 3–16)
5. Collect three 20-second stimulation trials from each mastoid.
6. If nystagmus is observed, calculate the intensity of the nystagmus and document the direction.

Provocative Maneuvers

Valsalva. A person's ability to purposefully change intracranial and middle ear pressure is referred to as the Val Salva maneuver (VM). In certain disorders, the VM can provoke eye movements that are specific to the pathology. The VM references Antonio Mario Valsalva (1666–1723) who was one of the tests early proponents. In the beginning of the 20th century, this concept of changes of pressure and eye movements was further described by Hennebert. Hennebert is cred-

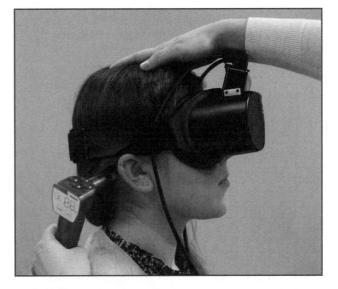

FIGURE 3–16. Mastoid vibration being administered with vision denied.

ited with providing detailed descriptions of the characteristic eye movements that can be induced by changes in middle ear pressure, which are today known as "Hennebert's sign." When positive pressure is introduced into a sealed external auditory meatus, a positive sign is when the eyes move slowly away from the ear with the impairment. Conversely, negative pressure will generate a movement of the eyes toward the impaired ear. This finding would be a positive Hennebert's sign. Disorders that will commonly manifest a positive Hennebert's sign are patients with superior canal dehiscence, Arnold-Chiari malformation, and perilymphatic fistula.

In most instances, the clinician will ask the patient to perform the VM. There are two generally accepted methods to performing the VM. One will act to increase the pressure in the middle ear and sinuses, whereas the other will increase the venous pressure in the head. In order to ensure that the eye movements are observed and to have a record, it is recommended that the clinician use VNG/Frenzel goggles. In addition to the objective eye movement recordings, it is also valuable to instruct the patient to report any symptoms (e.g., dizziness or changes in vision). When performing the test, is recommended that the clinician observe the eye movements prior to the maneuver in order to obtain a baseline as well as during and after the pressurization. The patient should first be given clear instructions about keeping their eyes open during the test. Then they should be instructed to breathe deeply, pinch the nose, close the mouth and then blow like they would when trying to "clear their ears" on a plane. If possible, the patient should maintain the increase in pressure for approximately 10 seconds. If there is a response, the patient should then be instructed to strain against their lips and a closed glottis. A negative test is considered no symptoms of dizziness and no observable eye movements. A positive test (i.e., positive Hennebert's sign) will be observable nystagmus "beats" (i.e., fast phase direction) toward the affected ear. The direction of the fast phase of nystagmus as well as the torsion will provide information regarding the location of the impairment. Torsional and down-beating nystagmus would be indicative of an affected anterior canal, whereas vertical up-beating nystagmus with torsion would indicate the posterior canal. A linear horizontal nystagmus that beats toward the affected ear would suggest impairment of the lateral semicircular canal.

Headshaking. The headshaking test was originally described by Robert Bárány in 1907 and refers to nystagmus (i.e., head-shaking nystagmus) that can be observed when the head is shaken vigorously in a patient with peripheral and central vestibular system impairments. Kamei and Kornhuber (1964) reported one of the first descriptions of how to utilize HSN clinically. The authors recommended having the patient wear Frenzel lenses while shaking the head back and forth 30 times in several different conditions (e.g., variations in direction and plane of the head movement). The emergence of nystagmus following the head being shaken was considered a positive test. Once the Frenzel lenses/VNG goggles have been fit to the patient, he or she is instructed to oscillate the head from side to side approximately 30 to 45 degrees from center for 25 cycles at a frequency of 2 Hz. This is considered the active procedure. If the clinician chooses to hold the patient's head, it is referred to as a passive procedure and the same procedures as the active evaluation. A headshake test is considered positive when a significant nystagmus emerges. The nystagmus can take a number of forms, including being monophasic or biphasic (i.e., it changes direction as it decays), beating toward or away from the impaired side and having a vertical component (referred to as crosscoupled nystagmus). In patients with peripheral impairments, the fast phase of the nystagmus is typically directed toward the contralesional ear. A negative result is no identifiable post-head-shake nystagmus following the head-shaking procedure.

OTOSCOPIC EXAMINATION

Following an examination of the patient's eye movements, the clinician should inspect the external auditory canal and tympanic membrane in order to determine if any accommodations need to be made before the caloric examination. The ear canal should first be examined for any obstructing cerumen (Figure 3–17). In most ears, there is some amount of wax. In cases where there is a cerumen impaction or enough wax that the clinician cannot see the tympanic membrane, the wax should be removed. A significant amount of wax can significantly impede the caloric stimulus and produce an erroneously reduced response. In cases where there is a significant amount of wax present, the examiner should prepare to remove the obstruction so that caloric testing can be performed. The clinician should also examine the ear canal for any anatomical anomalies that may affect caloric transmission. In cases of a surgical ear, caloric testing may be contraindicated. An otoscopic exam also provides the examiner with information about normal anatomical characteristics. For example, if the ear canals are tortuous, the clinician may need to retract the auricle and straighten out the ear canal in order to deliver an adequate caloric stim-

ulus. After a careful inspection of the ear canal, the tympanic membrane should be examined. The clinician should be concerned with ensuring that the tympanic membranes are intact. If a perforation exists, then the use of water for generating the caloric response is contraindicated. In cases of tympanic membrane perforations, air can be employed as the stimulus; however, this can produce a caloric response that beats in a paradoxical direction and can be confusing to the clinician. A detailed account of what to look for during the otoscopic exam prior to the caloric exam is presented in Chapter 6.

THE VNG ENVIRONMENT

The VNG examination room should be large enough to accommodate the examiner, patient, and a person accompanying the patient. This environment should also be large enough to allow the clinician to move around freely. An ideal room for VNG testing is at least 10 feet wide and 14 feet long. These dimensions provide for enough room to have a sink, casework for the equipment to sit on, an examination table, and a stool for the examiner. Figure 3–18 shows the layout of a typical VNG examination room. Besides the dimensions, there are some key features that should be in the room. First, the room should have appropriate ventilation and a thermostat so that the room can be heated and cooled as needed. For example, in a hospital setting, an inpatient may arrive at the appointment wearing only a gown, or in cases of patients with severe motion intolerance, a cool room helps mitigate the effects of nausea. Another key feature is the ability to have nearly complete darkness. Although most of the testing is done with dim light, there may be occurrences where it is desirable to have nearly complete absence of light (e.g., during the caloric testing or when there is a need to increase pupil size to help the VNG system track the eye). Table 3–15 shows equipment and Table 3–16 shows supplies that are required for the conventional ENG/VNG laboratory.

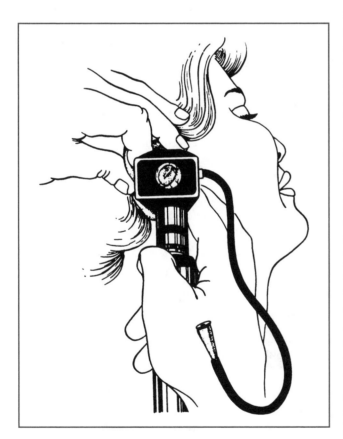

FIGURE 3–17. Illustration of a patient receiving an otoscopic examination. (Illustration by Mary Dersch from Pender, 1992, with permission of Daniel Pender)

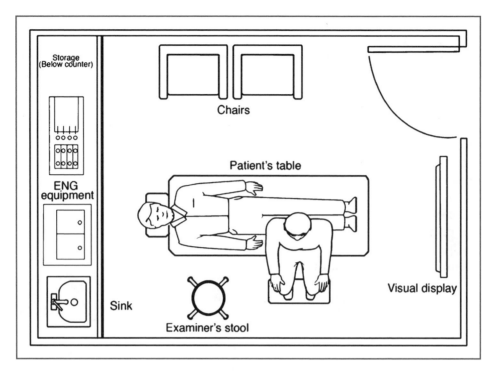

FIGURE 3–18. Illustration of a layout of a typical VNG laboratory.

Table 3–15. Equipment Used in a Conventional ENG/VNG Laboratory

Equipment	Use
Examination table	Should be either a hydraulic or mechanical table that allows for positioning the patient anywhere from sitting to supine. An additional feature is the ability to remove the headrest for tests such as the Dix-Hallpike maneuver.
Caloric irrigator	Deliver caloric stimulus; can be air or water.
Recording system	Should be capable of measuring and recording eye movements using VNG or ENG.
Cabinet for supplies	Storage of supplies and patient-counseling materials.
Examination stool	For examiner to sit with patient and take case history and deliver caloric stimulus.
Visual stimulation system	Should be capable of producing appropriate stimuli for oculomotor testing (e.g., light bar or projector).

Recommended Pre-Evaluation for VNG Examination:

1. Administer the Dizziness Handicap Inventory (DHI) and Dizziness Symptom Profile (DSP) while patient is in the waiting room.
2. Observe gait.
3. Directed Case History
4. Gross Eye Movement Examination
5. Head Impulse Testing
6. Cover/uncover—Cover/cross-cover
7. Headshake
8. Mastoid Vibration

Table 3–16. Supplies Used in a Conventional ENG/VNG Laboratory

Supply	Use
Disposable electrodes	Recording EOG (when VNG is not indicated or cannot be performed).
Dental napkins	When using water caloric irrigations, these act to catch any water that may come out of the ear canal.
Paper pillowcases or disposable pillows	Provide comfort for those patients with neck or back impairments.
Alcohol, abrasive gel, gauze, cotton swabs	Preparing patient's skin for the recording of EOG.
Wax-removal tools	To remove cerumen in cases where the ear canal is blocked.
Irrigator specula or water-delivery tubes	Each patient should have their caloric irrigation delivered through a clean system.
Bleach	If using water, the baths should be bleached regularly.
Laboratory thermometer, graduated cylinder, and stopwatch	To calibrate water bath.
Emesis basins	Catch water when performing caloric or for use if patient becomes sick.

EOG = electro-oculography.

4

Eye Movement Examination

In order to evaluate the integrity of the peripheral vestibular system, clinicians must be able to do sophisticated recording for each of the different functional classes of eye movements. Although it is difficult to obtain direct recordings from the peripheral vestibular system, the eye movement system affords the clinician a way to access the organs and nerves of balance via central nervous system connections located in the cerebellum and brainstem. Abnormalities identified during the eye movement examination can both provide the clinician with insight into the causes of a patient's reported dizziness, as well as avoid misinterpretation of recordings obtained during the caloric test. A comprehensive clinical evaluation of the oculomotor system also provides valuable information for the referring physician to use during his or her differential diagnosis. Although a multitude of techniques exist for studying eye movements, this chapter describes only ENG and VNG.

INSTRUMENTATION

Eye Movement Recording Systems

The quantitative assessment of the oculomotor system and vestibulo-ocular reflex (VOR) is accomplished using either electro-oculographic (EOG) or video eye-tracking systems. Over the past decade there have been rapid advances in the quality and sensitivity of video eye-tracking systems. The majority of new systems sold in the United States now incorporate some form video eye-tracking technology.

Video Eye-Tracking Systems

Video eye-tracking systems employ specialized infrared cameras that can exploit the reflective properties of the corneal surface in order to calculate pupil position and angle of gaze. These cameras are typically mounted to either the top

87

or side of a goggle system that is affixed to the head (Figure 4–1). An infrared illumination source that has the same orientation as the cameras is directed toward a mirror(s) composed of dichroic glass. Dichroic mirrors are simply glass that are coated with multiple layers of metal oxides that allow certain wavelengths of light to pass through (e.g., room light) or be reflected (e.g., infrared). Dichroic glass placed in front of the eyes at an angle enables the patient to look through the mirrors unobstructed while the infrared image of the eye is reflected to the cameras (Figure 4–2). The reflection of the eye that is received by the cameras is subjected to an analysis known as the "bright-pupil technique." This process causes the pupil to appear bright compared with the surrounding iris. The contrast between the iris and the pupil allows the video system to track the eye (Figure 4–3). This is accomplished by applying an algorithm that identifies either an elliptical portion of the pupil or the center of the pupil. In most systems, the clinician is afforded the ability to focus and adjust the pupil/iris "brightness" for maximum contrast. This ensures that the crosshairs of the tracking system stay locked on the pupils as the eyes move.

EOG/ENG: CORNEORETINAL POTENTIAL

EOG/ENG is the eye movement technique that involves converting the bioelectrical signal of the corneoretinal potential (CRP) into an electrical form that can be collected and analyzed using a recording system. The eye has an electrical charge that is similar to a battery. In other words, the front of the eye (cornea) is positively charged, while the back of the eye (retina) is negatively charged (Figure 4–4).

This dipolar electrical potential that exists between the retina and cornea of the CRP is maintained by metabolic activity in the retinal pigment epithelium (RPE). The RPE consists of a layer of hexagonal cells in the retina whose primary purpose is to protect the retina from excess incoming light (Carl, 1997; Marmor & Zrenner, 1993). The RPE cells are densely packed together, enabling the eye to maintain its dipolar orientation or its CRP. The CRP is a dynamic potential and has been shown to vary across levels of illumination. When light enters the eye and falls on the RPE cells, the metabolic activity level in these cells increases. In

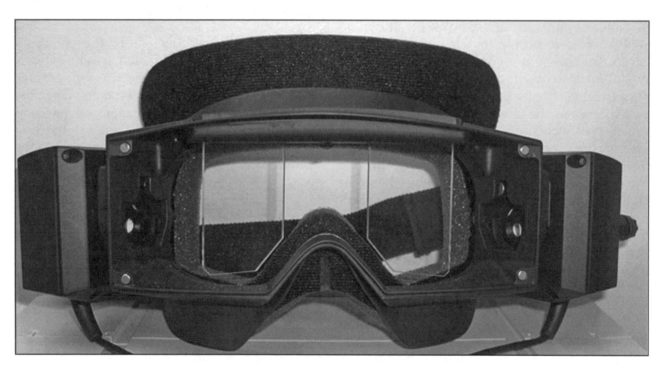

FIGURE 4–1. A binocular video eye movement recording system. (Interacoustics, Assens, Denmark)

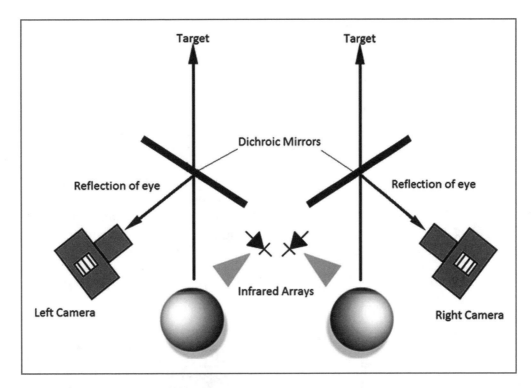

FIGURE 4–2. A basic illustration of the components and process of how a standard videonystagmography system operates.

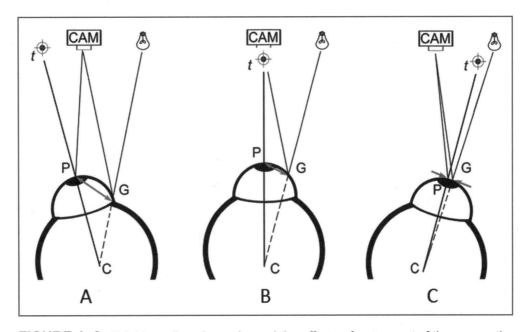

FIGURE 4–3. Bright-pupil oculography and the effects of movement of the eye on the magnitude of vector PG between the center of the pupil (*P*) and the center of the first Purkinje image (*G*). **A.** Movement away from the light source; **B.** eyes in the primary position; **C.** eye movement toward the light source. (From Jacobson, Shepard, Dundas, McCaslin, & Piker, 2008, p. 529)

this regard, if a patient is kept in a room with little or no light (dark adapted), the CRP potential will be smaller than if they were kept in a well-lighted room (light adapted).

Another factor has been reported to have a direct effect on the magnitude of the CRP. Some ENG systems allow the examiner to acquire an amplitude measurement of the CRP from the cali-

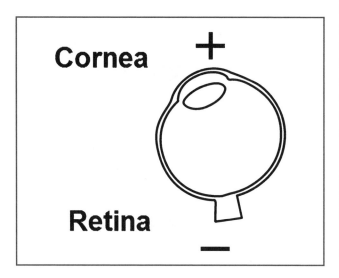

FIGURE 4–4. The electrical potential between the cornea and retina is shown.

bration data. According to Jacobson and McCaslin (2004), there is a population of patients that generate "noisy" eye movement recordings when they are being tested using ENG (Figure 4–5). When the authors measured strength of the CRP in this subset of patients, it was found to be exceedingly low. In fact, the "noise" that was being recorded in the tracings was the noise floor of the amplifier. Jacobson and McCaslin (2004) went on to report that this group of patients with low CRP magnitudes also had retinal disease when they were evaluated by an ophthalmologist. In this regard, the strength of amplification of the CRP during calibration after the patient has been dark adapted could be a marker for retinal disease. Table 4–1 outlines the percentile values of the CRP for both men and women.

USING THE CRP TO RECORD EYE MOVEMENTS

Concept

The CRP can be used to track a patient's eye movements by placing electrodes on the outer

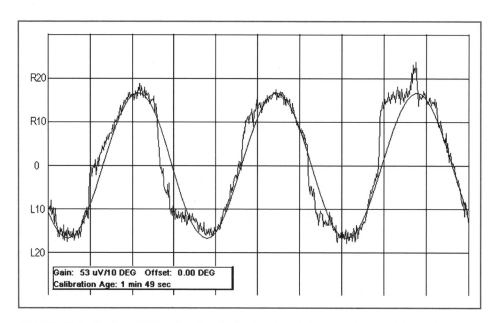

FIGURE 4–5. An ENG calibration in the horizontal plane obtained in an 80-year-old woman with advanced glaucoma and hypertensive retinopathy. (From Jacobson & McCaslin, 2004)

Table 4–1. Percentile Values Associated with Corneoretinal Potential Values Corresponding to 1° Eye Deviations from Midline

Sex	1st	5th	10th	15th	20th	50th	80th	85th	90th	95th	99th
M	7.1	8.2	9.2	9.5	10.4	13.8	17.3	19.1	19.9	21.8	25.8
F	9.0	10.8	11.4	13.0	13.2	17.2	21.7	22.2	24.5	27.3	28.2

Source: From Jacobson & McCaslin (2004).

canthi of the eyes. The process entails using differential amplification techniques to resolve the movement of the eyes. For example, in the case of a one-channel recording, if the non-inverting electrode is placed on the right side of the eye and the inverting electrode is placed on the left side of the eye, there is no voltage change while the eyes are in the primary position (Figure 4–6A); however, if the eye is moved to the right, the recording system will register an increase in voltage because the cornea (positive pole of the dipole) is being brought closer to the noninverting electrode (Figure 4–6B). If the eye is deviated to the left, the cornea will be brought closer to the inverting electrode. In this case, the increase in voltage will register as a decrease in voltage because the inverting electrode inverts the responses it records (positive becomes negative) (Figure 4–6C). This method is also employed to record vertical eye movements by placing a noninverting electrode above the eye and an inverting electrode below the eye. When recorded in this fashion the magnitude of the CRP can range from 0 to 7 uV per degree of horizontal eye deviation (Jacobson & McCaslin, 2004). Table 4–2 provides a comparison between VNG and ENG recording techniques.

Clinical Application

When Eye Movements Are Conjugate

The determination of how many recording channels to use depends on whether the patient had full, conjugate range of motion of the eyes during the gross eye movement examination. In the majority of cases it is adequate to record the EOG using a "bitemporal" array. In this electrode montage a pair of electrodes (channel 1) is placed at

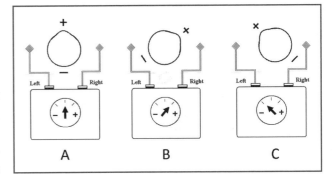

FIGURE 4–6. A–C. The corneoretinal potential and change in voltage registered at the electrodes with left and right eye movements. (From Jacobson et al., 2008, p. 28)

the outer canthus of each eye. These electrodes are used to record lateral (right and left) eye movement and should be positioned so that if an imaginary line were drawn between them, it would pass through the center of the pupils. In order to record vertical eye movements a second pair of electrodes (channel 2) should be placed above and *VOG* video-oculography; *EOG* electro-oculography a Bell's phenomenon is an upward and outward reflexive movement of the eyes that occurs during eye closure. This reflex can cause induced nystagmus (e.g., produced during caloric or positional testing) to become dysrhythmic. This distortion can make interpretation of the response difficult when ENG is being used to record eye movements below one of the eyes (Figure 4–7). The ground electrode should be placed on the forehead or nasion. A movement of the eyes to the right results in an upward deflection of the recording in the horizontal channel, whereas a movement of the eyes to the left creates a downward deflection in the same channel

Table 4–2. Comparison of VNG and ENG Recording Techniques

Variable	VOG/VNG	EOG/ENG
Spatial resolution	<0.5°	<1°
Vertical recording	Good (has capability to record and archive eye movements)	Occasionally interrupted by eye-blink artifact
Setup	Accomplished quickly	Takes longer than VOG due to electrode-preparation techniques
Cost	High cost	Low cost
Recording of torsional eye movements	Good	Poor
Effect of Bell's phenomenon[a]	None	Affected

VOG video-oculography; *EOG* electro-oculography.

[a]Bell's phenomenon is an upward and outward reflexive movement of the eyes that occurs during eye closure. This reflex can cause induced nystagmus (e.g., produced during caloric or positional testing) to become dysrhythmic. This distortion can make interpretation of the response difficult when ENG is being used to record eye movements.

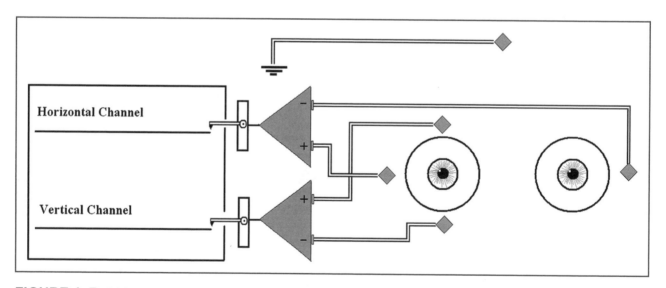

FIGURE 4–7. A bitemporal electrode montage and the connections to a two-channel differential amplifier electrode montage. (From Jacobson et al., 2008, p. 28)

(Figure 4–8). For vertical eye movements, an upward movement of the eyes generates an upward deflection in the recording and a down-ward eye movement drives the recording in a negative direction (Figure 4–9). Oblique eye movements change the voltage in both the ver-

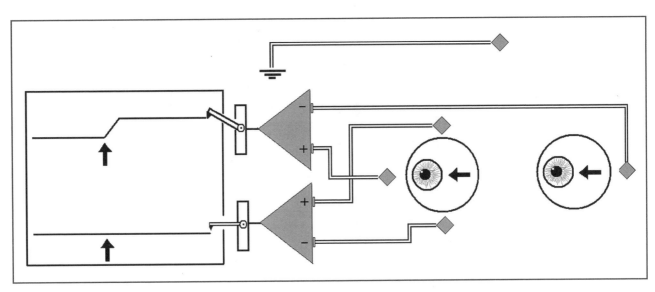

FIGURE 4–8. The horizontal and vertical amplifier outputs (*vertical arrows*) to a recording system for a rightward eye deviation (*horizontal arrows*). (From Jacobson et al., 2008, p. 28)

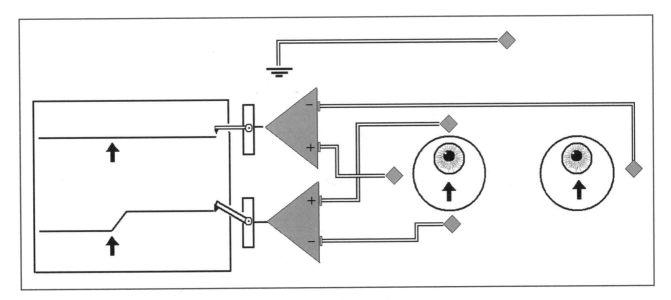

FIGURE 4–9. The horizontal and vertical amplifier outputs (*left arrows*) to a recording system for an upward eye deviation (*right arrows*). (From Jacobson et al., 2008, p. 28)

tical and horizontal channels at the same time (e.g., leftward and downward) (Figure 4–10). One of the limitations of recording with ENG is that the system is insensitive to purely torsional eye movements (e.g., counterclockwise or clockwise) (Figure 4–11).

When Eye Movements Are Not Conjugate

When a patient presents with disconjugate eye movements, the "bitemporal" recording method is not appropriate. This is because the CRP from each eye is averaged together when this electrode

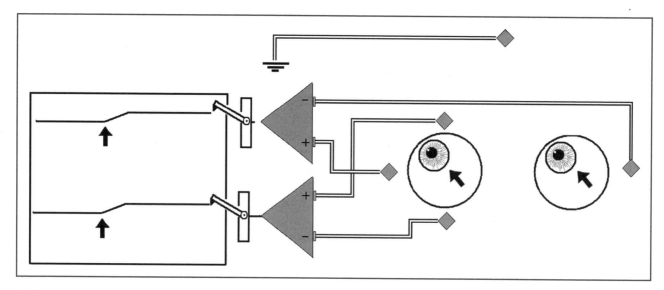

FIGURE 4–10. The horizontal and vertical amplifier outputs to a recording system for an oblique eye movement (*arrows*). (From Jacobson et al., 2008, p. 28)

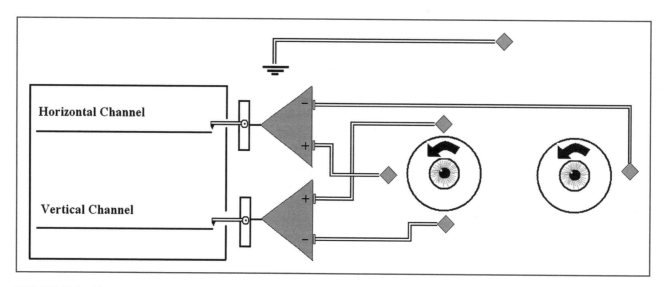

FIGURE 4–11. The horizontal and vertical amplifier outputs to a recording system for a completely torsional eye movement (*arrows*). (From Jacobson et al., 2008, p. 28)

array is used. In cases where a patient presents with disconjugate eye movements, a monocular electrode montage should be used. A monocular recording affords the clinician the ability to record the eye position of each eye separately. Figure 4–12 illustrates a four-channel recording that is capable of recording each eye independently. Each eye has a horizontal and vertical channel and the ground is placed on the forehead.

Calibration

The process of calibration involves converting eye movement into a digital representation that can be analyzed by the ENG/VNG computer. Early ENG systems recorded eye movement with red (vertical) and blue (horizontal) pens that would transcribe the eye movement in the horizontal or vertical plane on a paper-strip chart (i.e., pen

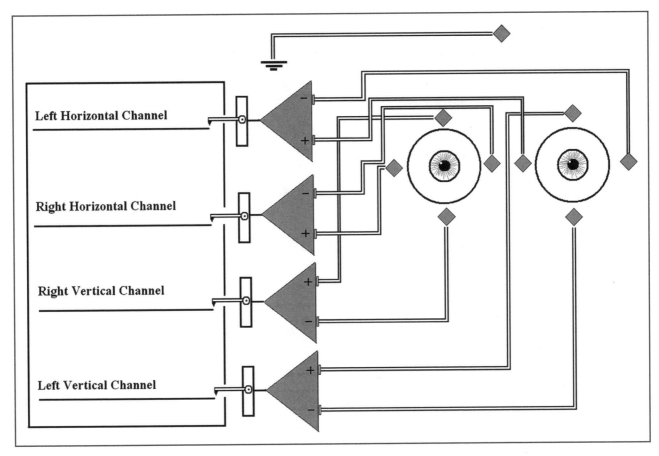

FIGURE 4–12. The horizontal and vertical amplifier outputs to a recording system for a four-channel monocular montage. (From Jacobson et al., 2008, p. 28)

deflection). Most contemporary computerized ENG/VNG systems continue to display data in a similar way but in an electronic form. The calibration of an ENG/VNG system is based on the fact that the patient will be at a known distance from the visual stimulator. A common distance that manufactures use for the distance between the targets and the patient is 4 feet. Visual targets (e.g., lights) are placed in both the horizontal and vertical planes in such a way that an eye excursion of a person 4 feet away will be 10° from primary gaze (center gaze). To ensure that the patient is an appropriate distance from the target, some systems employ active range finders that let the examiner know whether the patient is too close or too far. Once the calibration procedure is initiated and the patient acquires the target, the amplifier gain is adjusted so that the movement of the recording (horizontal and vertical) is equal in degrees to the eye movement (e.g., 10°). It is extremely important that the patient be the correct distance from the targets during the calibration process. If a patient is too close (less than 4 feet) or too far (greater than 4 feet), when the system is calibrated the conversion factor will be incorrect. For example, if a patient is 5 feet from the targets rather than 4 feet, the eye will move fewer than 10° (e.g., 6°) to acquire the target. The recording system will increase the gain to match the 6° eye movement to the target that is 10° from primary gaze. In this way the system overestimates the eye movement (e.g., a 6° eye movement is represented as a 10° eye movement). Alternatively, if the patient is only 3 feet from the target, the eye will need to move more than 20° to acquire the target (e.g., a 15° eye movement is represented as a 10° eye movement by the recording system). Data collected from an improperly calibrated system can lead to a misinterpretation (e.g., bilateral caloric weakness or hyperactive response) because of the over or underestimation of the eye movements.

Whether the examiner uses ENG or VNG, the procedure for calibrating the system remains the same. What is different is the number of times that the ENG system must be recalibrated during the examination compared with the VNG system. Given that VNG goggles rely on tracking the pupil, as long as the goggles are not moved there is no need to recalibrate; however, as described in the previous section, ENG relies on the recording of the CRP, which is a dynamic electrical potential. The amplitude of the CRP varies depending on the amount of light in the environment. This is because the level of metabolic activity in the RPE changes depending on the level of illumination. On average, there is nearly a twofold increase in the amplitude of the CRP when an individual that has been dark-adapted is moved to an illuminated environment and then light adapted (McCaslin & Jacobson, 2004. Lightfoot (2004) reported that approximately 6 to 9 minutes are required to fully light adapt an individual and 7 to 12 minutes to completely dark adapt. Accordingly, the recording system should be recalibrated approximately every 10 minutes until the CRP is stabilized, at which point the examiner should make every effort to ensure that the level of illumination is kept fairly constant for the duration of the test. A convenient time to calibrate is before the initial oculomotor subtest, again before positioning testing, and immediately before the first irrigation. Although the American National Standards Institute (ANSI,1999) and the British Society of Audiology (BSA) (1999) have recommended that the recording system be recalibrated prior to each caloric irrigation, it is the present author's opinion that this is unnecessary unless the level of illumination in the environment has changed, the electrodes have been moved, or there is an unexplained disagreement in the caloric responses.

VOLUNTARY SACCADE TEST

Saccade testing assesses specific structures composed of different populations of neurons in the brainstem to the cerebral cortex (see Chapter 1 for a detailed review). There are a several different types of saccadic behaviors that can be observed. For example, there are the saccades that are generated during vestibular or optokinetic nystagmus. Saccades are also generated in response to a novel stimulus that is presented unexpectedly (i.e., reflexive saccade) or they can be just randomly generated without any particular task being accomplished. There are memory-guided saccades that can be invoked to direct gaze to a point where a target was previously and there are predicative saccades, which are generated when an individual is anticipating a target to appear at a specific location. Antisaccades are voluntary fast eye movements that can be purposely generated in the opposite direction of a visual target that appears in the environment. The type of saccade that is most commonly evaluated during the ocular motor subtest of the ENG/VNG examination is what has been termed voluntary saccades. Voluntary saccades are extremely fast eye movements that an individual purposely generates in order to acquire a visual target (e.g., a target on a light bar).

Before the advent of computerized ocular motor testing, the assessment of voluntary saccades was accomplished with the examiner asking the patient to look at small dots fixed to the wall or ceiling. Today's computerized systems utilize projection systems and light bars and can present targets in a multitude of ways. Targets can now be presented at fixed and randomized times and locations. During the randomized paradigm, visual stimuli are presented in unpredictable locations in both the horizontal and vertical plane, and the patient's ability to acquire the targets is measured. When assessing saccadic function, the randomization of stimuli has been suggested to increase the sensitivity of the test to disorders compared with a fixed protocol (Isotalo, Pyykkö, Juhola, & Aalto, 1995). Currently, the randomized paradigm is the most common presentation for evaluating the saccade subsystem during ENG/VNG testing and is the focus of this section. Figure 4–13 illustrates eye recordings taken in a patient during the presentation of stimuli using a random saccade paradigm.

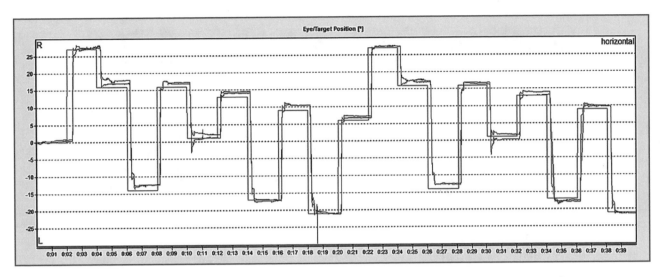

FIGURE 4–13. A recording of eye movements in response to a pseudorandom saccade paradigm.

Assessment of Voluntary Saccades

The procedure for the saccade test is as follows:

1. Perform a gross eye movement examination to determine whether the eye movements are disconjugate or conjugate.
2. Calibrate the patient using either individual eye recordings (if disconjugate eye movements were observed) or both eyes averaged together (if conjugate eye movements were observed).
3. Instruct the patient carefully (e.g., "Do not move your head and try not to anticipate where the target is going to show up next.").
4. Record the patient's saccades using a pseudorandom presentation where the targets are presented between 5° and 40° from midline with a fixed interstimulus interval.
5. Record and observe the eye movements for a duration that is sufficient to collect several patient responses for each saccade deviation (e.g., 30 s).
6. Analyze and inspect the data.
7. If abnormalities are noted, record for additional amount of time until it is confirmed that the abnormalities observed are repeatable and consistent (e.g., 30% to 50% of the responses are consistently abnormal).

Interpretation and Analysis

The three primary parameters that are used for the clinical analysis of visually guided saccades are how close the eye comes to acquiring the target (accuracy), the speed at which the eye moves to acquire the target (velocity), and the time it takes for the eye to move following a movement of the target (latency). The sections below provide definitions of the analysis parameters and summaries of the causes of abnormality.

Accuracy

Accuracy describes how far over or under the target the eye was following its excursion to the target. This is referred to as saccadic dysmetria. If the eye falls significantly short of the target, it is referred to as a hypometric response, and if the eye travels significantly past the target, it is hypermetric. There is often a small amount of saccadic dysmetria observed in normal individuals. Specifically, with very small excursions during small amplitude saccades there is typically some hypermetria observed and during large amplitude saccades there is often some degree of hypometia. Normative data in most VNG systems account for these variances. A normal saccadic tracing with accuracy within normal limits is presented in Figure 4–14.

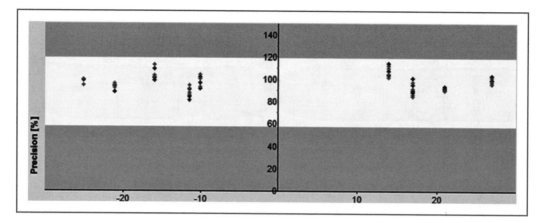

FIGURE 4–14. Saccade test accuracy data obtained in a normal individual. Shaded areas indicate abnormal accuracy.

Velocity

Velocity refers to how fast the eye moves toward the target once the saccade has been initiated. Most systems calculate the peak eye velocity, which is the maximum velocity reached during the eye movement. It is noteworthy that the farther the target is away from the midline (e.g., 0.5° versus 35°), the higher the velocity must be for a response to be normal. Accordingly, the peak velocity of a saccade will vary between 30° to 700° per second. This is because the eye movement system must overcome the viscoelastic forces that would normally keep the eyes in a neutral position. Once these forces have been overcome (i.e., as the eye moves further away from its starting point), the eye velocity increases. The relationship between saccade velocity (speed of the eye movement) and amplitude (degrees of eye movement) is termed the main sequence. The main sequence is a ratio that can be used to describe saccadic abnormalities. A normal saccadic velocity tracing is presented in Figure 4–15.

Latency

Latency reflects the difference in time (in milliseconds) between the presentation of a target and the initiation of the eye movement intended to acquire that target. The onset of the saccade will typically occur between 150 to 200 msec. A normal saccadic latency tracing is presented in Figure 4–16.

Saccade Abnormalities

As described in Chapter 1, a patient with impairment in the saccade eye movement system is unable to rapidly and accurately acquire a visual target or hold the eye on the target. This almost always involves abnormality of the pulse or step response (see Chapter 1 for a review).

The sections below provide descriptions of some common saccade disorders, cases illustrating these disorders, and a summary of each disorder's basic characteristics.

Velocity

Slow Saccades. Disorders of saccadic velocity involve a disorder in the pulse. The height of the pulse can be too big or too small, and the duration (width) can be too long or too short. The velocity of the saccade can also be asymmetric (each eye moves at a different speed). Abnormalities in the height and/or duration of the saccadic pulse affects the velocity of the eye when measured at the target. Although the velocity of saccades is in large part controlled by burst neurons located in the paramedian pontine reticular formation (PPRF) or medial longitudinal fasciculus (MLF), the superior colliculus and cortex have also been shown to contribute (Leigh & Zee, 2006). Disorders that can result in a patient having slow saccades are basal ganglia syndromes, cerebellar syndromes, peripheral oculomotor nerve or

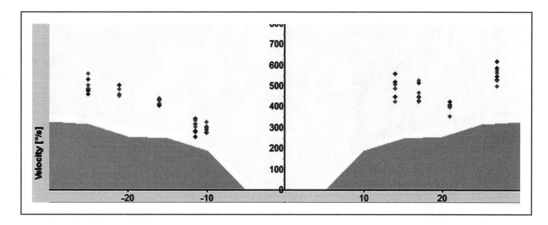

FIGURE 4–15. Saccade test velocity data obtained in a normal individual. Shaded areas indicate abnormally low velocity for a given target.

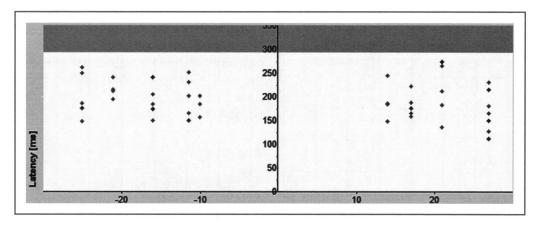

FIGURE 4–16. Saccade test latency data obtained in a normal individual. Shaded areas indicate abnormally long latency for a given target.

muscle weakness, and white matter diseases. One classic example of a disorder that can cause saccadic slowing is internuclear ophthalmoplegia (INO). There are varying levels of severity of INO ranging from simply slow movements of the adducting eye (the eye moving toward the nose) to total paralysis (Figure 4–17). INO can be either unilateral or bilateral and implicates impairment in the MLF (Leigh & Zee, 2006). Patients with a bilateral INO typically present with abducting nystagmus accompanied by weakness in the adducting eye. This disorder is typically observed in patients suffering from brainstem stroke. An INO should be able to be identified prior to testing during the gross eye movement examination and case history. Although the major-

ity of patients with an INO do not complain of dizziness, some may report double vision or even oscillopsia (Leigh & Zee, 2006). When abnormally low-velocity saccades are observed in a patient, the examiner must first rule out the contribution of medication and/or lack of alertness (Figure 4–18).

Fast Saccades. Patients can also present with abnormally high-velocity saccades. The causes of fast saccades can be a result of a mass or trauma to the eye, cerebellar impairments, and brainstem impairments. Calibration error should always be an initial consideration in patients who generate saccades that are too fast. If a patient continues to generate abnormally fast saccades

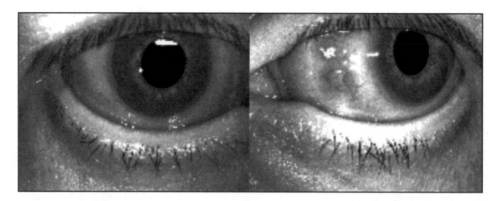

FIGURE 4–17. A patient with a right internuclear ophthalmoplegia demonstrates impaired adduction of the right eye. The target is located 30° to the left from primary gaze.

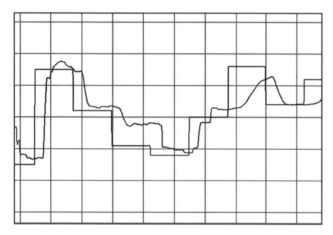

FIGURE 4–18. A recording of saccades in a patient who was heavily medicated and extremely drowsy at the time of testing.

following recalibration, the clinician should check whether the saccades are of normal amplitude and whether the patient has full range of motion for both eyes. The velocity of the eye during a saccade is proportional to the distance the eye must travel. In other words, the eye generates higher-velocity movements for targets farther away and slower velocity movements for targets that are closer. In cases where the eye has a restricted range of movement, the eye may be stopped before it reaches the target. According to Leigh and Zee (2006), the central nervous system calculates the size of the pulse based on the eye's position relative to the target. If the eye is stopped prematurely during the saccade, an analysis of the waveform will suggest that the

velocity is abnormally high. This is because prior to the eye being halted, it was traveling at a velocity calculated to acquire a target further away (required a higher velocity); however, because the eyes are stopped short of the target, the amplitude of the saccade is lower than normal for the target.

Accuracy

Saccadic Pulse Dysmetria. Another type of saccade abnormality is called saccadic pulse dysmetria. The cerebellum is largely responsible for the accuracy of saccades. Specifically, dorsal vermis, fastigial nucleus, and uncinate fasiculus are three key structures that, when impaired, can result in saccadic pulse dysmetria. The dorsal vermis is composed of four primary parts. These include the declive, pyramis, tuber, and folium. It receives neural input from the inferior olivary complex, vestibular nuclei, and paramedian pontine reticular formation (PPRF) (Figure 4–19). Activation of the dorsal vermis will generate smooth pursuit eye movements and contralateral saccades. The fastigial nucleus receive inputs from the inferior olivary nucleus, nucleus reticularis tegmenti pontis (NRTP), and dorsal vermis. When ipsilateral and contralateral saccades are being generated, neurons in the fastigial nucleus are active. The uncinate fasiculus (UC) is also a contributor to the accuracy of ipsilateral and contralateral saccades. When impaired, the UC will generate a characteristic set of findings (i.e. hypometric ipsilesional saccades and hypermetric contralesional saccades)

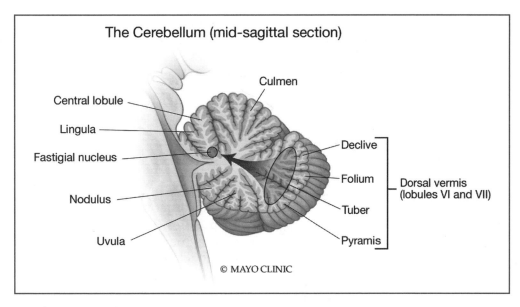

FIGURE 4–19. Illustration of a mid-sagital section showing the key features of the dorsal vermis. (Used with permission of Mayo Foundation for Medical Education and Research. All rights reserved.)

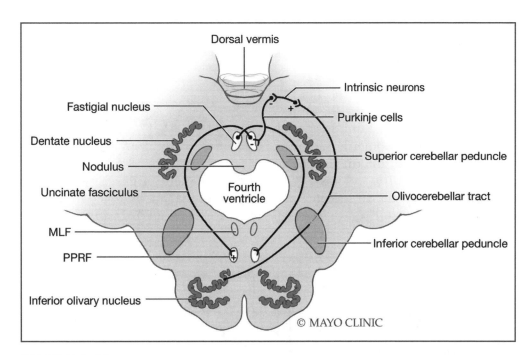

FIGURE 4–20. Illustration of the cerebellum showing the neural relationships between the dorsal vermis, the fastigial nucleus, and the uncinate fasiculus. (Used with permission of Mayo Foundation for Medical Education and Research. All rights reserved.)

(Figure 4–20).When these anatomical structures are impaired, , the cerebellum cannot correctly calculate the amplitude of the saccade that is needed to acquire the target. The pulse (velocity signal) of the saccadic pulse-step step system is defective, causing the patient to overshoot (hypermetric) or undershoot (hypometric) the visual stimulus. When the saccade is too large or too small, a corrective saccade is generated to bring the eye onto the target.

In the case of a hypermetric saccade, the eye has overshot the target and must be moved in the direction opposite the target. The main characteristic of hypermetric saccades is that the eyes overshoot the target, remain at a fixed point a few degrees beyond the target for approximately 150 to 200 ms, and then return to fixate on the target. The mechanism is incorrect calculation of what the pulse-step should be by the neural integrator. These findings are suggestive of an impairment in the cerebellar dorsal vermis. Whenever hypermetric saccades are observed, caution should be exercised to rule out a visual impairment (e.g., macular degeneration), blinking, and improper calibration. (Note that over or undershoots must be repeatable and consistent. If the patient generates normal saccades with only occasional over or undershoots, the test is interpreted as normal.) Figure 4–21 illustrates the recordings from a patient with bilaterally hypermetric (overshoots) saccades. The recordings show that the eyes consistently pass by the target (overshoot) but then quickly return to fixate on the target.

The main characteristic of hypometric saccades is that the eyes undershoot the target, remain at a fixed point a few degrees short of the target, and then move again to acquire the target. Hypometric saccades can be either unidirectional or bidirectional. Causes of hypometric saccades include cerebellar impairments, internuclear ophthalmoplegia, supranuclear palsy, and basal ganglia disorders. Whenever hypometric saccades are recorded, caution should be exercised to rule out

a visual impairment (e.g., macular degeneration), fatigue, medication, lack of alertness, and blinking. Figure 4–22 presents the eye recordings of a patient with consistent hypometric saccades.

Latency

Late Initiation of Saccades

Saccades can be initiated abnormally late (i.e., when the target moves to a new location, the eye has a prolonged latency before it starts to move); however, due to a vast number of pitfalls, latency is a relatively insensitive measure of saccade dysfunction when employed during the ENG/VNG battery. Factors affecting latency include age, lack of alertness, and inattention. Visual impairment has also been reported as a contributor to abnormally prolonged saccadic latency (Ciuffreda, Kenyon, & Stark, 1978). It is noteworthy that the abnormally prolonged initiation of saccades has been observed in patients with degenerative disorders (Fletcher & Sharpe, 1986; Leigh & Zee, 2006).

GAZE TEST

The assessment of gaze involves evaluating the structures that are involved in fixation (see Chapter 1 for a review). In other words, the test is

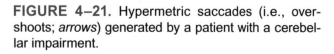

FIGURE 4–21. Hypermetric saccades (i.e., overshoots; *arrows*) generated by a patient with a cerebellar impairment.

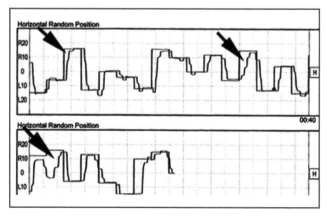

FIGURE 4–22. Hypometric saccades (i.e., undershoots; *arrows*) generated by a patient with a brainstem impairment.

designed to determine if there is any aberrant nystagmus with the head oriented in the midline and the eyes at center position and looking horizontally and vertically. The gaze test is one of the most informative oculomotor tests but can also be one of the most difficult to interpret. This is because impairments in gaze stabilization can stem from peripheral abnormalities, central abnormalities, or both simultaneously. The primary feature that the examiner should be looking for when conducting the gaze-stabilization test is impaired fixation. If visual fixation is impaired this indicates patient cannot keep their eyes on the target. When impaired visual fixation observed, the clinician must be able determine what type of eye movement occurred that *involuntarily* drew the eye off the target (i.e., fast or slow).

Key Questions to Determine When Evaluating the Gaze Test:

1. Did the eye slowly drift off the target and was then followed by a fast reacquisition of the target (e.g., gaze-evoked nystagmus)?
2. Was there an intrusive saccade that took the eye off the target (e.g., ocular flutter)?

Being able to answer these questions will provide critical information for the clinician to first describe the eye movement accurately in the report as well as provide localizing information regarding the impairment. Accordingly, a description of the characteristics, terminology and convention for reporting forms of nystagmus will be addressed in the following section.

Characteristics Associated with Measuring and Understanding Nystagmus

In order to differentiate nystagmus of central origin from peripheral, the clinician should be informed as to the different parameters that are measured and evaluated when nystagmus is observed. Nystagmus is a normal response when the head is moved (generated by the VOR) or when the optokinetic system is engaged. When abnormal nystagmus is present during the ocular

motor examination, the most common origin is from the above two systems but also can be connected to a lesion in the gaze-holding mechanism. When aberrant nystagmus is observed, there are several characteristics that should be described and these are summarize in Table 4–3.

The waveform of the nystagmus can be either pendular or jerk. Nystagmus that has a clearly defined fast and slow component is termed jerk nystagmus (see Chapter 2). It is convention to describe the direction of jerk nystagmus using the direction of the fast phase and the amplitude of the nystagmus using the slow phase. The slow component eye movement of jerk nystagmus can take on three different forms. These include constant velocity eye movements, a decreasing velocity eye movement, and an increasing velocity eye movement. Pendular nystagmus describes an eye movement where both phases are slow (Figure 4–23).

It is also important to identify, when nystagmus is observed, whether the eyes are moving in the same direction and whether both eyes have the same amplitude and frequency. Accordingly, the three primary questions that should be included in any report are as follows. First, in what direction does the nystagmus beat? Second, how does the intensity of the nystagmus change with visual fixation? Third, in what positions does the nystagmus occur? Answering these three questions correctly is critical for interpreting the ocular motor function and allows the examiner determine if the origin of the nystagmus is caused by a peripheral vestibular system impairment, a central eye movement system impairment, or both (Table 4–4). The following two sections provide the recommended assessment techniques for gaze stabilization and how to interpret and differentiate central from peripheral involvement.

Assessment of Spontaneous Peripheral Vestibular Nystagmus

Spontaneous peripheral nystagmus is most commonly a result of impairment to one of the vestibular end organs of nerves. It is noteworthy that a symmetrical bilateral reduction in vestibular function will not result in the generation of spontaneous peripheral nystagmus.

Table 4–3. Key Characteristics Used for Describing Nystagmus

Is the nystagmus jerk or pendular (e.g., the waveform)?	Pendular nystagmus typically is characterized by slow-phase sinusoidal oscillations Jerk nystagmus consists of a slow phase followed by a fast phase.
What plane/s and direction does the nystagmus beat (e.g., horizontal, vertical, or torsional,)?	Nystagmus is described by the plane perpendicular to the axis of rotation (e.g., horizontal plane rotation). Torsional direction is typically described by the ear toward which the top or upper pole of the eye rotates.
Are the eye movements conjugate during the eye movement?	Eye movements during nystagmus that move both eyes together in the same direction by the same amount are referred to as conjugate. When the eyes do not rotate in the same plane and direction the nystagmus is said to be disconjugate.
What is the amplitude of the nystagmus (e.g., this is commonly described using the slow component eye velocity)?	Jerk nystagmus amplitude refers to the magnitude (degrees) of eye movement from the base of the slow component eye movement to its peak
What is the frequency of the nystagmus?	This is typically not of diagnostic value for vestibular nystagmus. However, this parameter can be of value when observing disorders with nystagmus associated with certain frequencies, such as oculopalatal tremor.

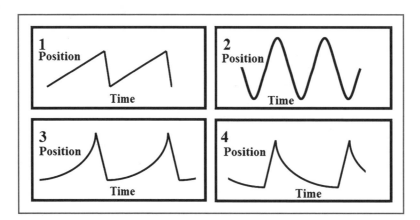

FIGURE 4–23. Examples of the different nystagmus waveforms (1) Constant velocity waveform. (2) Pendular nystagmus. (3) Increasing velocity waveform. (4) Decreasing velocity waveform.

The search for spontaneous vestibular nystagmus should be performed in the following manner:

1. Instruct the patient to keep the head midline and fixate on the target (remember to rein-struct the patient to not move their head). The patient should be in the sitting position.
2. Record the eye movements for at least 30 s while tasking the patient.
3. Occlude vision and continue recording for at least another 30 s.

Table 4–4. Differentiation Between Central- and Peripheral-Gaze Nystagmus

What Is the Direction of Nystagmus?	
Peripheral	*Central*
Direction-fixed horizontal nystagmus	Direction changing in one or more gaze positions
Primarily horizontal with a slight torsional component	Direction fixed but purely vertical (up-beating or down-beating)
	Demonstrates rebound nystagmus (i.e., the direction of the nystagmus is always in the last direction that the eye moved)

What Is the Effect of Visual Fixation?	
Peripheral	*Central*
Enhanced intensity with vision occluded (i.e., vision denied)	Is present or enhanced with fixation
Diminished intensity with fixation invoked	Intensity does not change significantly with *removal* of fixation

In What Positions Does the Nystagmus Occur?		
	Primary Position	*Eccentric Gaze*
Peripheral	Horizontal nystagmus with a slight torsional component	Follows Alexander's law (i.e., horizontal nystagmus amplitude increases when the patient gazes in the direction of the fast phase; amplitude decreases when the patient gazes in the direction of the slow phase)
Central	Horizontal nystagmus (rarely observed in primary position)	Horizontal nystagmus observed (typically bidirectional (right-beating on right gaze and left-beating on left gaze)
	Vertical nystagmus (can be present in primary position)	Vertical nystagmus observed (typically enhances with vision)

4. If nystagmus is observed, restore vision (or turn on a fixation light) and have the patient fixate on a target.

5. Record any changes in the nystagmus (reduction or increase in amplitude)

Peripheral Vestibular Nystagmus: Interpretation and Analysis

Nystagmus of peripheral origin (vestibular labyrinth or vestibular nerve) that changes intensity with gaze is most commonly generated by an uncompensated asymmetry in neural input from the two labyrinths. When interpreting the spontaneous nystagmus test it is important that the clinician have laboratory-specific normative data to compare with the patient findings. This prevents over interpretation and unnecessary referrals for additional studies. Peripherally generated nystagmus is characterized by a nystagmus with the fast phase directed away from the ipsilesional ear. The characteristic waveform of peripheral vestibular nystagmus (PVN) caused by unilateral disease is a combination of horizontal and torsional due to the fact that there is incomplete cancellation of the response generated by the vertical canals (i.e., anterior and posterior). For example, when the eye movements generated by stimulation of the right horizontal SCC, the right anterior canal, and the right posterior canal are summed, they produce a corresponding movement with the following characteristics (Figure 4–24).

PVN as a result of a unilateral vestibulopathy is direction fixed and has a constant velocity waveform. The intensity of the nystagmus increases when the eyes are deviated in the direction of the fast phase (Alexander's law). Alexander's law refers to peripherally generated nystagmus that is observed with the eyes open. It is qualified by degrees of severity (Figure 4–25). With the first degree, nystagmus is observed only during lateral gaze in the direction of the quick phase (Figure 4–26). With the second degree, nystagmus is present in the primary position with the lateral gaze in the direction of the quick phases (Figure 4–27). With the third degree, nystagmus is present in the primary gaze with the lateral gaze in both directions (Figure 4–28). A classic sign that the observed nystagmus is peripheral in origin is that it reduces in intensity with visual fixation and increases in intensity when vision is denied. When a patient exhibiting PVN fixates their gaze on a target the amplitude of the nystagmus will diminish and enhance with vision denied. If the compensation mechanisms are intact, this form of nystagmus will be extinguished in a few days.

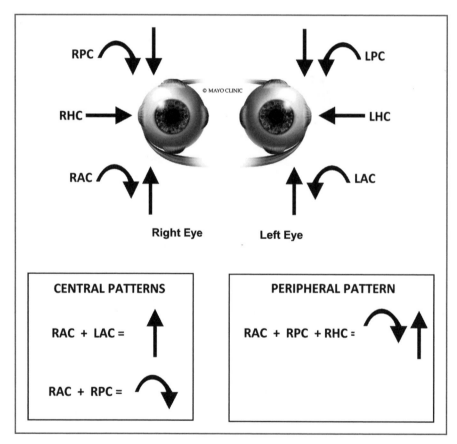

FIGURE 4–24. Activation of a single semicircular canal will generate a slow-phase eye movement in the same plane as the canal. A purely vertical or torsional nystagmus is considered central because in order to generate this form of eye movement, the same canal on both sides would be to be stimulated equally. Activation of all three canals on a single side generates a mixed horizontal-torsional nystagmus. R = right; L = left; PC = posterior canal; AC = anterior canal; and HC = horizontal canal. (Used with permission of Mayo Foundation for Medical Education and Research. All rights reserved.)

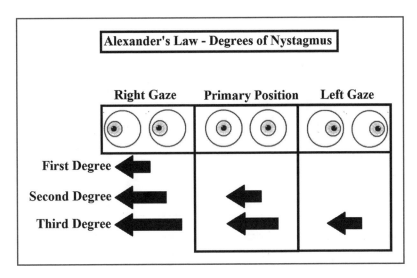

FIGURE 4–25. Degrees of nystagmus associated with Alexander's law. Arrows represent the direction of the fast phase of the nystagmus, and the length of the arrow represents the intensity.

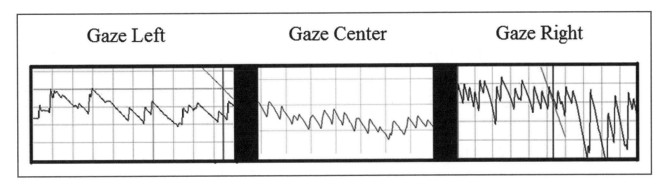

FIGURE 4–26. First-degree direction-fixed spontaneous vestibular nystagmus in the gaze positions. Note that the nystagmus is present only during right gaze (i.e., the direction of the fast phase). This case illustrates a 47-year-old man with a history of a left temporal bone fracture incurred 3 days before the recordings were taken. The patient reports both continuous disequilibrium and positional vertigo.

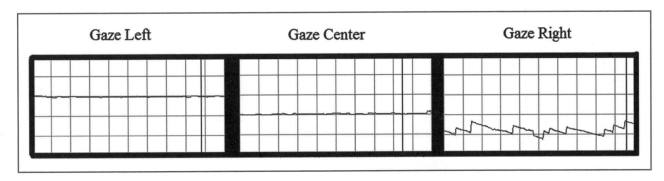

FIGURE 4–27. Second-degree left-beating direction-fixed spontaneous vestibular nystagmus. Note that the nystagmus is present in center and left gaze, but not when gaze is directed to the right. This case illustrates a 51-year-old man with a history of vertiginous episodes that occur approximately three times per week and last 30 to 40 min. The vertigo is accompanied by aural fullness and tinnitus in the right ear. The patient carries a provisional diagnosis of Ménière's disease.

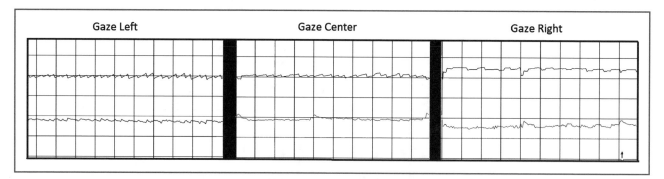

FIGURE 4–28. Third-degree right-beating direction-fixed spontaneous vestibular nystagmus. Note that the nystagmus is present in center, left, and right gaze. This case illustrates a 49-year-old man with a history of vertigo that has been ongoing for the past 5 years. The attacks of vertigo are followed by periods where the patient is asymptomatic. The patient's last attack was 1 day before the recordings were obtained.

(See Chapter 2 for a complete review.) K. Barin (personal communication) has reported that, spontaneous horizontal nystagmus with vision denied must be greater than 6° per second for ENG and 4° per second for VNG to be considered abnormal. Additionally, vertical nystagmus must exceed 7° per second with vision denied when using VNG. In cases where patients are seen acutely following an attack of peripheral vertigo, this form of nystagmus can be observed during the gaze test. In patients suffering from peripheral impairments, spontaneous nystagmus that is present with fixation is typically observed only acutely. Other symptoms that accompany peripheral vestibular nystagmus include diaphoresis, nausea, and vomiting.

Central Vestibular Nystagmus

Central vestibular nystagmus (CVN) is typically the result of impairment of the cerebellum (i.e., vestibulocerebellum) or the brainstem. One of the most common types of central nystagmus is one that increases in intensity as the eyes are brought from primary gaze position to eccentric gaze. CVN has nystagmus profiles that consist of purely vertical eye movements, reverse direction during gaze, are not suppressed by vision, and may be accompanied by other cerebellar signs (e.g., ataxia).

Central vestibular nystagmus should be assessed in the following manner:

1. Continue to have the patient keep the head midline and fixate on the target (remember to reinstruct the patient not to move their head). The patient should be in the sitting position.
2. Record at least 30 s of eye movement using targets placed at 30° from primary position (with vision present) for each of the subsequent gaze positions.
3. If nystagmus is found to be present, perform the test again to confirm that it is consistent. Additionally, the examiner should search for rebound nystagmus. Test sequence:
   a. Center gaze with eyes on target
   b. Center gaze with vision denied
   c. Right gaze with eyes on target (30°)
   d. Left gaze with eyes on target (30°)
   e. Up gaze with eyes on target (30°)
   f. Down gaze with eyes on target (30°)
4. If nystagmus is noted in any condition, repeat the examination until it is determined that the findings are consistent.

Centrally Mediated Nystagmus

Central nystagmus (CN) generated by impairments in structures such as the brainstem and vestibulocerebellum can take many forms (e.g., vertical, oblique, horizontal). The nystagmus will often be purely vertical, torsional, horizontal or some combination and can vary in intensity and direction. The velocity waveform of they nystagmus will vary (e.g., can be increasing, decreasing or linear). CN is most commonly jerk and one of the key features of this form of eye movement is that it is no suppressed by vision. CN may reverse direction with gaze which is referred to bidirectional nystagmus (i.e., right-beating on right gaze and left-beating on left gaze). Typically but not always, patients with CN will manifest other cerebellar signs (e.g., ataxia).

Nystagmus Generated by Eccentric Gaze

Gaze-Evoked Nystagmus. Significant GEN has been suggested to be nystagmus that is persistent during eccentric gaze of 30° or less (Hain, 1992). The main characteristic of bilateral GEN is small-amplitude nystagmus that is equal in intensity in all directions and observable when the eye is gazing eccentrically. The quick phase of the nystagmus beats away from the primary gaze position and is not suppressed by visual fixation. The causes of bilateral GEN are congenital nystagmus, and lesions in the cerebellum and/or brainstem. Bilateral GEN can also be caused by medications (anticonvulsants or sedatives) and/or alcohol.

The presence of GEN is often associated with a defect in the pulse-step relationship (described in Chapter 1). In other words, the burst neurons in the brainstem must generate an appropriate pulse to overcome the elastic restoring forces of the eye and bring the fovea to rest on the target. Once the eye reaches the target, neurons in the cerebellum and brainstem (i.e., neural integrator) generate a neural command to continually contract the extraocular eye muscles and hold the eye on the target (Leigh & Zee, 2006). This tonic response that keeps the eye from returning to its midline position is referred to as the step response (Leigh & Zee, 2006). Impairment in the neural integrator sets up a situation where the step response is inadequate and the eye slowly drifts off the target in the direction of primary gaze. Leigh and Zee (2006) have referred to this a "leaky" neural integrator (Figure 4–29). Once the oculomotor system detects that the fovea is no longer on the target, a saccade is generated in the direction of the gaze to reacquire the target. This pattern of the slow centripetal drift of the eye off the target followed by a saccade is the pattern of eye movement that is referred to as GEN (Figure 4–30). The clinician should be vigilant to the fact that GEN manifests during other tests of oculomotor function requiring eccentric gaze (e.g. saccade test) (Figure 4–31).

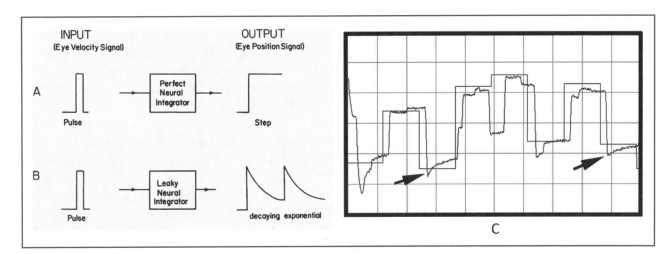

FIGURE 4–29. A simplified illustration of the neural integrator. **A.** A normal eye velocity signal (burst) and normal eye position signal (step response). **B.** A leaky neural integrator causes the eye position signal to decay. **C.** Recordings from a patient with a cerebellar impairment. The arrows designate where the eye begins to drift off the target due to an inadequate step response. (A and B adapted from Leigh & Zee, 2006)

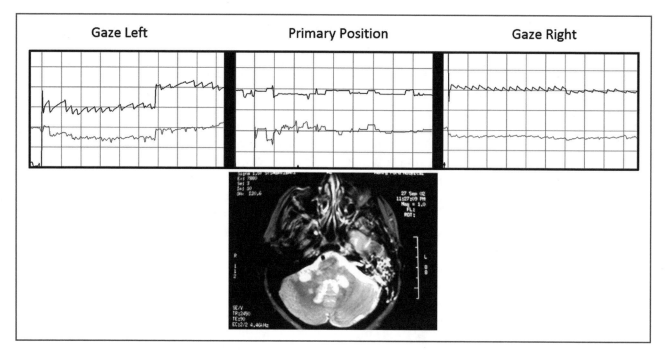

FIGURE 4–30. Bidirectional gaze-evoked nystagmus in three gaze conditions. The patient has an impairment affecting the cerebellum (i.e., multiple sclerosis).

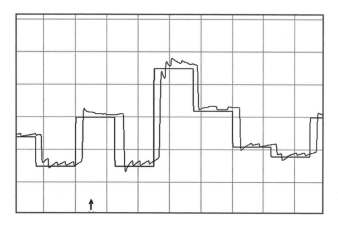

FIGURE 4–31. An example of how gaze-evoked nystagmus can be observed during other tests of ocular motility. In this case, bidirectional gaze-evoked nystagmus was observed during the saccade test.

Rebound Nystagmus. Patients with bidirectional GEN often generate rebound nystagmus. Rebound nystagmus is an aberrant form of nystagmus that is observed in patients with brainstem and cerebellar diseases (Hain & Rudisill, 2008; Lin & Young, 1999). When the patient's eyes are brought back to midline from eccentric gaze, a brief (5 s) burst of nystagmus beating in the opposite direction of that in which the eye was gazing may be observed. For example, if the nystagmus is beating in the direction of eccentric gaze (e.g., right-beating on gaze right), when the eyes are brought back to midline, the nystagmus will beat to the left. If the nystagmus is left-beating on leftward gaze, when the eyes are brought back to midline the nystagmus will be right-beating (Figure 4–32). Rebound nystagmus is typically observed in patients with cerebellar impairments.

Physiological End-Point Nystagmus. It is also important that the clinician distinguish between pathological GEN and a normal phenomenon known and "physiological end-point" nystagmus. This type of nystagmus is occasionally observed in neurologically intact patients during extreme lateral gaze (e.g., >40°) and will not often not be sustained (the examiner may only see a few beats of nystagmus) (Figure 4–33). If the physiological end-point nystagmus is sustained it will often be low frequency and low amplitude. This form

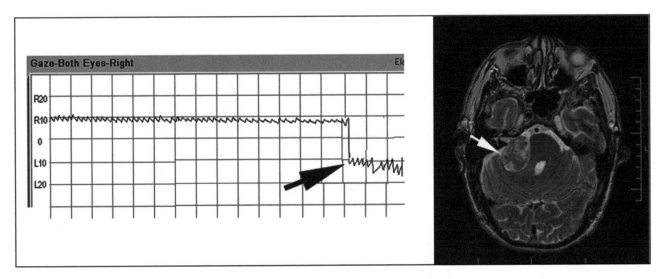

FIGURE 4–32. Rebound nystagmus in a patient with an impairment affecting the cerebellum. The arrow indicates the point where right-beating nystagmus shifts to left-beating nystagmus when the eyes move from right gaze to center gaze.

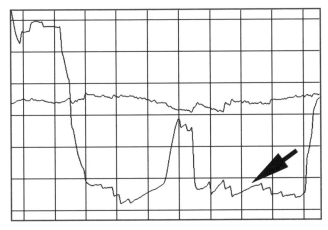

FIGURE 4–33. End-point nystagmus is shown (*arrow*).

nomas or acoustic neuromas) that are large enough to compress both the ipsilateral eighth cranial nerve and the cerebellar flocculus. When the patient directs gaze to the ipsilesional side, a large amplitude low frequency horizontal spontaneous nystagmus emerges. Conversely, when the patient looks eccentrically toward the contralesional side a small amplitude, high frequency nystagmus can be observed (Figure 4–34). The presence of Bruns' nystagmus typically indicates that the patient has a large tumor (>3.5 cm) (Baloh, Konrad, Dirks, & Honrubia, 1976; Lloyd, Baguley, Butler, Donnelly, & Moffat, 2009; Nedzelski, 1983; Okada, Takahashi, Saito, & Kanzaki, 1991). See Table 4–5.

of nystagmus accompanies an otherwise normal oculomotor examination and nystagmus typically occurs immediately after moving the eyes to the eccentric position. (Leigh & Zee, 2006).

Bruns' Nystagmus. Bruns' nystagmus is a variant of nystagmus that is characterized by a combination of both central and peripheral vestibular nystagmus (Bruns, 1908; Croxson, Moffat, & Baguley, 1988). Bruns' nystagmus is typically observed in patients suffering from large cerebellopontine-angle tumors (e.g., commonly vestibular schwan-

Down-Beating Nystagmus. Down-beating nystagmus (DBN) is commonly able to be observed in primary position and is typically conjugate. The direction of the plane of the nystagmus is vertical and the eyes are conjugate (Figure 4–35). It is characterized by the fast phase of the nystagmus beating downward. Visual fixation does not suppress it significantly and the slow phases may increase or decrease in intensity. Patients with down-beating nystagmus often complain of oscillopsia or severe unsteadiness (retinal slip caused by the slow phase) (Leigh & Zee, 2006. The involvement of the cerebellum also leads the patient to

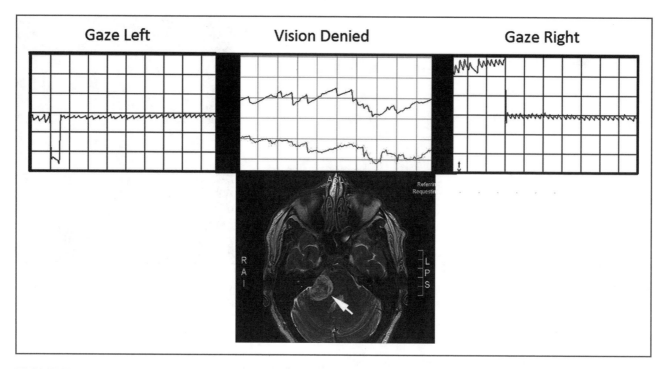

FIGURE 4–34. Bruns' nystagmus. The patient presented with a 3-cm mass in right cerebellopontine angle that extended into the internal auditory canal. Note the spontaneous peripheral vestibular nystagmus with vision denied. With lateral gaze, characteristics of the nystagmus change (i.e., low-amplitude high-frequency bidirectional nystagmus).

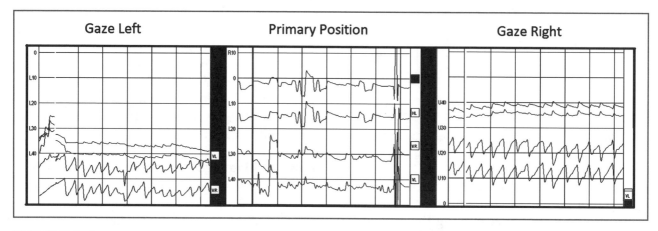

FIGURE 4–35. Down-beating nystagmus in different positions of gaze recorded in a 50-year-old patient diagnosed with midline cerebellar dysfunction (paraneoplastic).

complain of postural instability and generalized imbalance. The presence of down-beating nystagmus implicates the vestibulocerebellum and medullary region of the brain and their connections to the semicircular canals (Leigh & Zee, 2006). Specifically, the cerebellum (i.e., flocculus and ventral paraflocculus) inhibits responses from the anterior semicircular canal (produces slow upward eye movements) but not responses from the posterior semicircular canal (produces slow downward

Table 4–5. Summary Table for Central Vestibular Nystagmus

	Congenital Nystagmus	*Up-Beating Nystagmus*	*Down-Beating Nystagmus*	*Acquired Pendular Nystagmus*	*Periodic Alternating Nystagmus*
Nystagmus	Horizontal May have small vertical or elliptical movements	Upward Increases in amplitude with supramedial gaze	Downward with increases in amplitude on lateral and downward gaze	Horizontal May have small vertical or elliptical movements	Horizontal
Site of Lesion	Typically associated with visual impairments	Bilateral midline lesions in the ponto-mesencephalic or medullary junction Superior cerebellar peduncle	Cerebellum—Flocculus Pontomedullary junction	Pontomedullary	Cerebellum—nodulus/uvula
Waveform	Increasing velocity of the slow phase	Jerk—increasing or decreasing velocity of the slow phase	Jerk—increasing or decreasing velocity of the slow phase	Pendular—sinusoidal slow-phase	Jerk—constant velocity
Etiology	Visual system impairment; genetic	Cerebellar degeneration Cerebellar and brainstem strokes Multiple sclerosis	Arnold-Chiari malformation Cerebellar degeneration Multiple sclerosis Drugs	Visual loss Central myelin disorders (e.g., multiple sclerosis Oculopalatal tremor Acute brainstem stroke	Congenital Cerebellar degenerations multiple sCKEclerosis Arnold-Chiari Malformation
Management (not a comprehensive list)	Cycloplegic refraction Prisms	Baclofen	Baclofen Suboccipital craniotomy for Arnold-Chiari Malformation	Memantine Clonazepam Gabapentin	Baclofen

eye movements) (Baloh & Spooner, 1981; Ito et al., 1977). Because the vertical canals are paired (RALP and LARP), a loss of the inhibitory input to the anterior canals due to a cerebellar impairment causes the eye to slowly drift upward. The oculomotor system generates a downward saccade to reset the eye resulting in the pattern that is down-beating nystagmus. Down-beating nystagmus has been reported to be enhanced when patients are subjected to a "head-hanging" position (e.g., the Dix-Hallpike maneuver) (Marti, Palla, & Straumann, 2002). In this regard, care should be taken during the examination to not confuse down-beating nystagmus of central origin with benign paroxysmal positional vertigo (peripheral origin). The common disorders associated with of down-beating nystagmus are Arnold-Chiari malformation, head trauma, cerebellar degeneration, vertebrobasilar infarction, toxic-metabolic insults, and multiple sclerosis. Down-beating nystagmus can also be caused by drug intoxication (e.g., lithium, phenytoin, and carbamazepine).

Up-Beating Nystagmus. Up-beating nystagmus that is central in origin is characterized by a conjugate nystagmus with a fast phase beating upward when the patient's eyes are in the primary position (Figure 4–36) (Bojrab & McFeely, 2001). Impairments that cause this form of nystagmus are not as localized as those that cause down-beating nystagmus; however, it has been reported primarily in patients with impairments in the superior cerebellar peduncle, dorsal paramedian caudal medulla, and pontine and midbrain lesions (Leigh & Zee, 2006). The underlying mechanism is thought to be an impairment in the neural connections between the brainstem and the anterior semicircular canal. One important clinical note is that the examiner should differentiate a centrally generated up-beating nystagmus from posterior canal BPPV (benign paroxysmal positional vertigo, transient up-beating nystagmus with changes in head position). Up-beating nystagmus that is present in primary position often follows Alexander's law (largest intensity during upward gaze). Up-beating nys-

tagmus does not typically increase with lateral gaze as does down-beating nystagmus, although when the patient tilts their head upward, the nystagmus may reverse (Leigh & Zee, 2006). As with down-beating nystagmus, up-beating nystagmus of central origin is not fully suppressed by visual fixation and patients often complain of impaired gait, unsteadiness, and oscillopsia (Leigh & Zee, 2006). Up-beating nystagmus is commonly associated with lesions of the medulla, midbrain, and cerebellar degenerations (Leigh & Zee, 2006). Other causes of up-beating nystagmus are stroke, multiple sclerosis, congenital factors, and tumors. It can also be caused by tobacco abuse and middle ear disease, and it must be differentiated from posterior semicircular canal BPPV.

Torsional Nystagmus. A purely conjugate torsional nystagmus is characterized by the upper pole of the eye beating away from the lesioned side. This form of nystagmus can be observed in patients with impairments in the cerebellum or midbrain, but are more often associated with lesions in the pontomedullary junction. The most common causes are stroke, multiple sclerosis, Arnold-Chiari malformation, and venous angioma.

Periodic Alternating Nystagmus (PAN)

Periodic alternating nystagmus is an eye movement that is primarily horizontal and will oscillate in direction, amplitude, and frequency. For example, the nystagmus may be right-beating for approximately 2 to 4 minutes and then wane (referred to as the null period) for up to 20 seconds, during which there may be some downbeat nystagmus or no eye movement at all. The response then reverses direction and becomes left-beating for another 2 to 4 minutes (Figure 4–37). PAN follows Alexander's law (i.e., nystagmus increases in amplitude when gaze is directed in the direction of the fast phase). The disorders most commonly associated with PAN are Arnold-Chiari malformation, cerebellar degeneration, multiple sclerosis, and bilateral impairment in vision. Lesions in patients with PAN are located in the midline cerebellum (i.e., nodulus and uvula). These structures are responsible for modulating the rotational velocity storage mechanism and impairment leads

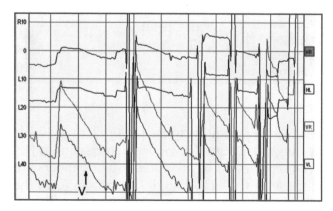

FIGURE 4–36. Up-beating nystagmus at center gaze is shown.

to increase gain in this system. PAN can be successfully treated using Baclofen (Lioresal).

Infantile/Congenital Nystagmus

Congenital nystagmus (CN) is a primarily horizontal nystagmus that is commonly conjugate and horizontal in all positions of gaze (including upward) (Figure 4–38). The waveform is typically a jerk nystagmus with a slow component eye movement that increases in velocity. The plane of the nystagmus will stay the same in all positions of gaze (i.e., uniplanar). Interestingly, patients do not complain of oscillopsia. This is important to note because it differentiates CN from nystagmus that is generated by brainstem or cerebellar impairments. The examiner, in some instances, may observe a small torsional or vertical component. When a patient with CN has his or her eyes near a certain orbital position, he or she has an eccentric neutral zone, or "null zone," where the nystagmus slows or is abolished and the patient's visual

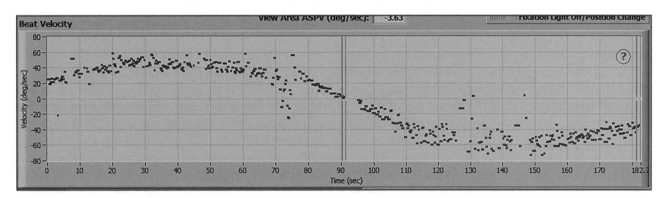

FIGURE 4–37. The velocity (deg/sec) of periodic alternating nystagmus at center gaze is displayed on the ordinate. Time in seconds is displayed on the abscissa. The center line indicates where the nystagmus changes direction. (Courtesy of Doug Garrison, Duke University)

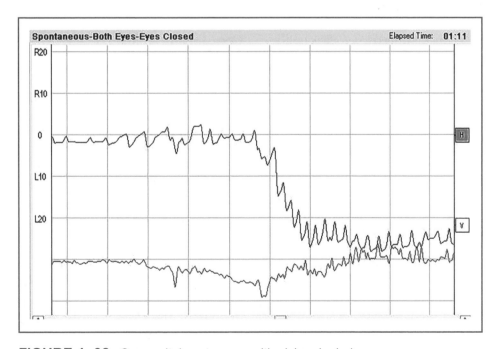

FIGURE 4–38. Congenital nystagmus with vision denied.

acuity is the best. The patient may turn his or her head in order to keep the eyes in this zone. During converging eye movements CN nystagmus typically decreases. The decrease in CN intensity during convergence can be evaluated by having the patient fixate on a target 6 feet away and then bringing the target to 2 feet away. The intensity of the nystagmus should decrease or even stop. CN is more intense with arousal or visual attention, and CN may change direction with vision denied (e.g., during VNG). Finally, when the examiner is performing the gross eye movement examination, it is a good practice to simply ask the patient "How long have your eyes moved that way?" The answer is typically "all my life." Typically treatment consists of prisms to reduce nystagmus amplitude or a surgery known as the Kestenbaum procedure to orient the eyes so that primary position and the null zone are the same.

Acquired Pendular Nystagmus

Acquired pendular nystagmus (APN) is one of the more common forms of nystagmus that is characterized by quasi-sinusoidal oscillations of the eyes, which subsequently impairs gaze holding and visual acuity. Patients with APN often complain of oscillopsia. The plane of the nystagmus in patients with APN can consist of vertical, torsional, and horizontal components. It is not uncommon to see patients where the nystagmus trajectory is oblique, which occurs when the vertical and horizontal components are in phase and elliptical when the two components are out of phase (180°). The nystagmus may be conjugate, disconjugate or disassociated but frequency is, in most instances the same in both eyes. The most common causes of acquired pendular nystagmus include demyelinating disorders such as multiple sclerosis, Pelizaeus-Merzbacher, and oculopalatal tremor. Additional etiologies include acute brainstem stroke and spinocerebellar degeneration. The pathophysiology underlying this form of eye movement has been suggested to be from an impairment in the neural integrator that regulates the feedback circuits between the cerebellum, orbital proprioception, and vision (Kang & Shaikh, 2017). An abnormality in this process can result in the involuntary eye movements associated with this disorder.

Saccadic Intrusions

These types of eye movements refer to involuntary saccades that occur when the patient is performing the gaze test. Although covering every type of saccadic dyskinesia is beyond the scope of this book, the most common forms will be briefly reviewed.

Square Wave Jerks

Square wave jerks are small intrusive saccades (0.5°–3°) that occur when a patient is asked to fixate on a target during the gaze test. The name is taken from the waveform of these eye movements because the tracings appear as little squares (Figure 4–39). During a square wave jerk, the eyes are involuntarily taken off the target and then quickly returned. The time between the initial eye movement and the return saccade is approximately 150 to 200 msec. This time period is referred to as the intersaccadic interval. It is important to note that SWJs are generated by neurologically intact people at a rate of approximately 4 to 6 per minute, especially with vision denied. When square wave jerks exceed a rate of >15 to 20 per minute an abnormality should be suspected. The most common causes of an abnormal number of SWJs are basal ganglion (progressive supranuclear palsy), cerebellar (cerebellar degeneration), and cerebral cortex (frontal eye filed impairment) disease. Occasionally a patient will be noted to have what look like SWJs but they are much larger amplitude. These have been termed macrosquare wave jerks. These involuntary saccades are similar to SWJs only they consist of much larger saccades and occur in bursts (eye excursions of up to 50°). Treatment for both SWJs and macrosquare wave jerks consists of medication including but not limited to diazepam and phenobarbital.

Macrosaccadic Oscillations

Macrosaccadic oscillations are involuntary large saccades that are generated in both directions around the target of interest. This is a form of saccade hypermetria where the eyes repeatedly overshoot the target while attempting acquisition. That saccade interval is approximately 150 to 200 msec while the patient is gazing eccentrically.

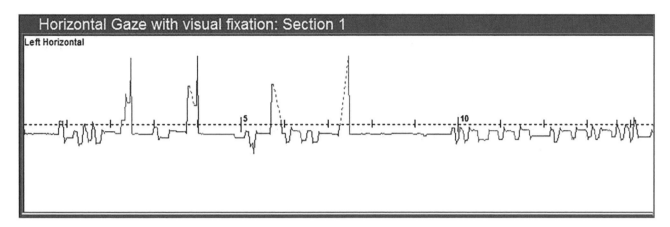

FIGURE 4–39. Example of an eye movement tracing illustrating square wave jerks.

This form or eye movement is also triggered when the patient performs saccades. Once notable characteristic of macrosaccadic oscillations is that they will be extinguished with vision denied. Patients presenting with macrosaccadic oscillations will often have deep midline cerebellar impairments (i.e., vermis). Diseases such as multiple sclerosis and paraneoplastic syndromes are commonly associated with these aberrant eye movements.

Ocular Flutter and Opsoclonus

Oscillating eye movements that occur repetitively with no intersaccadic interval are key characteristics of ocular flutter and opsoclonus (i.e., "dancing eyes"). These very fast intrusions are typically large amplitude conjugate eye movements that can have a high degree of variability. They are typically high frequency (10 to 25 Hz) and are able to be observed during visual fixation. One of the key distinctions between ocular flutter and opsoclonus is the plane in which they occur. Ocular flutter is most commonly constrained to one plane and horizontal (Figure 4–40). Opsoclonus is multidirectional (horizontal, vertical, and torsional) and is observed during the pursuit test and can even be seen while the patient has their eyes closed. Opsoclonus and myoclonus (involuntary quick movements of the limbs) are often observed together. One theory regarding the pathophysiological mechanism of opsoclonus and ocular flutter is centered around cerebellar dysfunction. Specifically, saccadic intrusions have been sug-

gested to be due to a disinhibition of the fastigial nucleus that is a consequence of impairment in the Purkinje cells in the dorsal vermis. The dorsal vermis exerts an inhibitory influence on the fastigial oculomotor which in turn controls the omnipause neurons located in the pons. A loss of neural drive to the omnipause neurons frees the saccadic burst neurons to oscillate resulting in opsoclonus or flutter. The most common etiologies of opsoclonus and ocular flutter are parainfectious encephalitis, paraneoplastic effects, meningitis, hydrocephalus, and intracranial tumors (Leigh and Zee, 2006).

SMOOTH PURSUIT TRACKING TEST

The testing of the functional eye class smooth pursuit is accomplished by recording the patient's eye movements while they track a target moving in a sinusoidal trajectory in the horizontal plane. Although today's targets are typically displayed on a light bar or projected onto a wall in front of the patient, smooth pursuit can be evaluated by have the patient track a small hand held target (e.g., tip of a pen).

Assessment of Smooth Pursuit

In order to perform smooth pursuit testing, the patient should be instructed to maintain the head

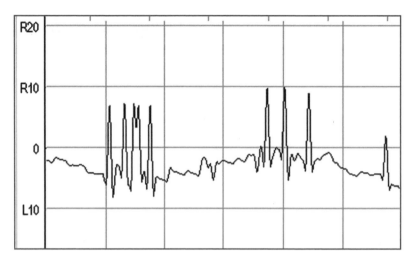

FIGURE 4–40. Example of an eye movement tracing illustrating horizontal ocular flutter.

in the midline position and follow the target with their eyes. It is important to communicate to the patient that they should keep their attention directed toward the stimulus for the duration of the test. The visual stimulus should make an excursion of 30° to the right and 30° to the left at a range of frequencies (0.2 to 0.8 Hz). Smooth pursuit performance degrades with age; thus, when testing, age-corrected normative data should be employed. When an abnormality (e.g., saccadic pursuit) is observed, the test should be repeated.

Interpretation and Analysis

The three primary parameters that are used for the clinical analysis of pursuit are how close the eye movement is to the movement of the target, the difference in percent between the left eye and right eye, and whether the eye is leading or lagging the target. When interpreting the smooth pursuit test, the recordings should be examined for the presence of any GEN, spontaneous vestibular nystagmus, or saccadic intrusions. The sections below provide the primary parameters that are used for the analysis of smooth pursuit.

Velocity Gain

Velocity gain is the relationship between the velocity of the eye and the velocity of the target at a given time. Specifically, velocity gain describes how closely the output signal (eye) matches the input signal (target) at a certain point in time. If the eye velocity (in degrees per second) is equal to the target velocity (in degrees per second) at the time of measurement, the gain is 1. If the eye falls behind the target, when the measurement is made the target (input) velocity will be greater than the eye (output) velocity and the value will be less than 1. As is seen in Figure 4–41, abnormal gain is in the lower region (<1). This is typically considered to be a sign of central impairment. The abnormal region represented by the shaded area and displays two standard deviations from mean age-corrected normative data.

The following equation defines velocity gain:

$$\text{Velocity gain} = \frac{\text{Peak eye velocity (degrees/second)}}{\text{Peak target velocity (degrees/second)}}$$

Asymmetry

Asymmetry reflects the difference in velocity gain (described above) between rightward eye movements and leftward eye movements. This can often be abnormal in cases where a patient is generating spontaneous nystagmus. For example, if the patient has right-beating spontaneous nystagmus, the patient typically manifests abnormally reduced velocity gain on the right.

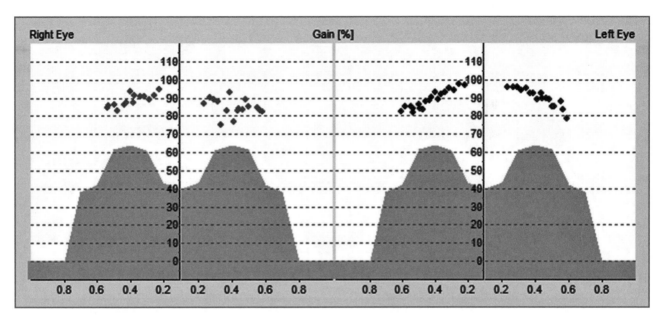

FIGURE 4–41. An image of how pursuit velocity gain is plotted. (Interacoustics, Assens, Denmark)

Phase Angle

Phase angle refers to the measurement of how much the eye is leading or lagging the visual target. The value is calculated in degrees and provides a measure of how in phase the eyes are with the target (e.g., an eye movement that is 180° out of phase with the target suggests that the eye is moving in the opposite direction (Figure 4–42). When the patient's eyes are continually ahead of the target, they should be reinstructed.

Pursuit Abnormalities

Patients with impairments affecting the pursuit system most commonly replace the smooth pursuit of the target with a series of saccadic eye movements. Saccadic pursuit occurs when the patient's eyes lag behind the target and the oculomotor system must generate a saccadic eye movement to reacquire it. This series of events results in a stepped response rather than the smooth sinusoidal response that is observed in normal patients. Saccadic pursuit is typically analyzed as reduced gain (eye velocity divided by target velocity) and is often referred to in the literature as "cogwheeling." Saccadic pursuit is also occa-

sionally observed in normal patients. Specifically, if the clinician notices that the patient's eyes are being taken off the target and jumping ahead, it may indicate a lack of concentration or alertness and reinstruction regarding the task should be administered. The pursuit pathway sends projections to numerous regions of the brain and brainstem and thus has limited clinical utility for localizing the site of lesion. For example, abnormal pursuit is observed in patients with impairments affecting the vestibular nuclei, cerebellum, dorsolateral pontine nuclei, striate cortex, middle temporal areas of the cortex, and the frontal eye fields (Kandel, Schwartz, & Jessell, 2000); however, abnormal pursuit can also be the result of medications, inattention, and cooperation. When a pursuit impairment is confirmed, Leigh and Zee (2006) report that it is typically more severe when the lower-level generators are involved (i.e., brainstem).

Bilaterally Saccadic Pursuit

Overall, bilaterally reduced smooth pursuit is of little or no diagnostic utility. Bilaterally low-gain pursuit responses are found in patients with disorders affecting the visual system as well as the central and peripheral vestibular systems. For

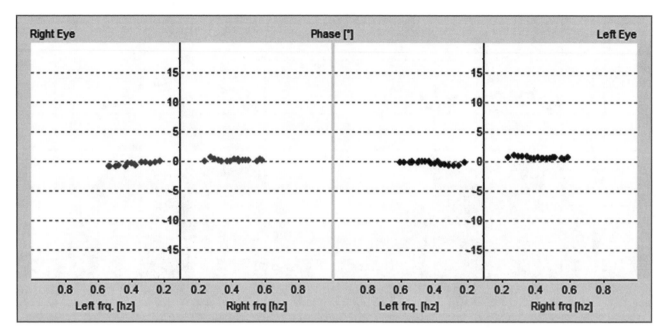

FIGURE 4–42. An image of how pursuit asymmetry is plotted. (Interacoustics, Assens, Denmark)

this reason, the examiner should exercise caution when attempting to diagnose impairments based on findings from pursuit testing alone. Hain (1992) has suggested categorizing bilaterally reduced pursuit responses into three types. First, pursuit is considered normal if the gain parameter is greater than 0.8 Hz. Second, pursuit gains of greater than 0.2, but less than 0.8, are considered to be in a "gray zone." In these cases interpretation should include findings from other tests before making a decision regarding whether the examination is normal or abnormal. Finally, patients with a gain of less than 0.2 are considered to have significant pursuit abnormalities (Hain, 1992). Impairments can range from the level of the cortex to the cerebellum and brainstem (a very diffuse circuit making localization of the impairment difficult). Bilaterally saccadic pursuit can be caused by brainstem disease, cerebellar impairments, and cerebral hemisphere impairments. When bilaterally saccadic pursuit tracing are encountered, caution should be exercised to rule out medication, inattention, fatigue, inattentive head movement, and congenital nystagmus. Figure 4–43 shows a pursuit recording of a patient with multiple sclerosis in the brainstem and cerebellum. There is a significant degree of saccade pursuit bilaterally.

Unilaterally Saccadic Pursuit

When a patient generates pursuit that is asymmetric, the clinician must determine if the origin is central or peripheral. When spontaneous nystagmus originating from an acute peripheral vestibular disorder is present, the oculomotor system is generating a sawtooth waveform (slow and fast phase). In other words, the asymmetry in tonic neural activity between the two vestibular systems activates the VOR and the eyes are driven slowly toward the impaired ear until they reach a point in the orbit and are quickly reset in the direction of the intact ear. Patients with spontaneous vestibular nystagmus often produce unilaterally impaired tracking waveforms (asymmetric low gain) because the oculomotor system is unable to integrate the fast phase of the aberrant spontaneous nystagmus and the smooth pursuit movement generated by the tracking system. When the patient is instructed to follow the smooth pursuit target in the direction of the slow phase of the nystagmus, the gain (eye movement/target movement) is essentially equivalent; however, when the patient is requested to pursue targets in the direction of the spontaneous nystagmus fast phase, the resulting pursuit waveform will either be low in amplitude (i.e., low pursuit gain) or absent entirely (Figure 4–44). In

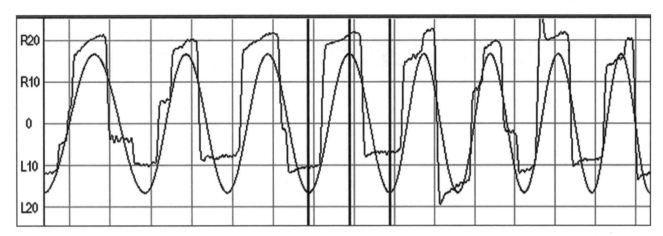

FIGURE 4–43. A recording of bilaterally saccadic pursuit is shown.

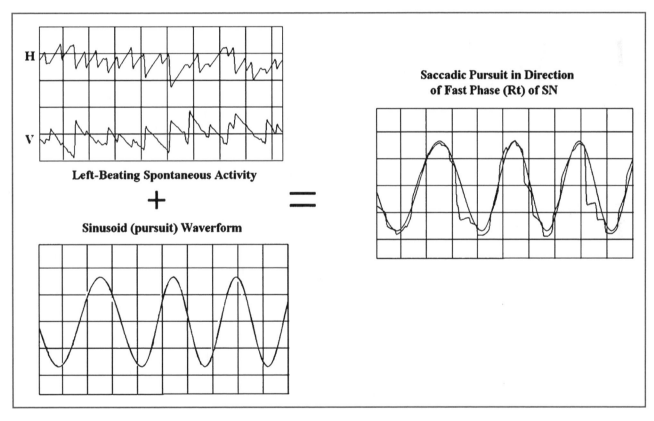

FIGURE 4–44. The effect that spontaneous vestibular nystagmus has on the pursuit test. Note that the eye movement system cannot integrate both a smooth and a fast eye movement. SN = Spontaneous nystagmus; H = horizontal; V = vertical. (From McCaslin & Jacobson, 2009)

central cases, the pursuit system cannot accurately compute the target velocity resulting in the use of saccades to track the target (Heide, Kurzidim, & Kömpf, 1996). Central causes of unilaterally saccadic pursuit include impairments in the cortex (parietal and frontal lobe), thalamus, midbrain, cerebellum, and dorsolateral pontine nuclei. Cortical impairments typically degrade smooth pursuit performance in the direction ipsilateral to the impairment (Heide et al., 1996) (Table 4–6).

Table 4–6. Summary of Pursuit Deficits

Sites of Lesion	Clinical Finding
Striate Cortex or Middle Temporal Area	Bilaterally abnormal horizontal pursuit
Medial Superior Temporal Visual Area	Impaired horizontal pursuit toward the side of the lesion
Dorsolateral Pontine Nuclei—Nucleus Prepositus Hypoglossi	Impairments in ipsiversive horizontal pursuit
Cerebellum—Vermis	Impairments ipsiversive horizontal pursuit
Cerebellum—Fastigial Nucleus	Impairments in contraversive pursuit
Cerebellum—Ventral Paraflocculus and Flocculus	Bilateral impairments in horizontal and vertical pursuit. Impaired VOR cancellation

OPTOKINETIC TEST

The optokinetic test (OKN) is accomplished by having a patient watch a series of stimuli moving horizontally across their visual field while recording their eye movements. The primary purpose of the OKN system is to stabilize objects of interest when the head is moving (originally referred to as "railway" nystagmus). In this regard, in order to generate a "true" OKN nystagmus the observer's visual field should be 90% or more filled with stimuli. Using a full-field visual stimulus will evoke circular-vection (i.e., the subjective perception of circular motion) (Leigh & Zee, 2006). Full-field stimulation of the visual field cannot, in most instances, be achieved using the light bars that come with many commercially available ENG/VNG systems. OKN responses generated using stimuli delivered via a light bar are volitional and are activating primarily the pursuit system. These responses are referred to as "look" OKN responses (Shepard & Schubert, 2008). In contrast, the true reflexive, brainstem-mediated OKN response generated using full-field visual stimulation is known as "stare" OKN. In order to generate "stare" OKN responses, most systems employ a projector system or present the stimuli inside a rotational chair enclosure. OKN stimuli consist of high contrast patterns that consist of stripes or circles. Recently, stimuli employing images (e.g., trains or playground scenes) have been employed for use with children and have been shown to produce OKN responses equivalent to conventional stimuli (D. L. McCaslin, C. Bahner, and B. Wengar, unpublished findings) (Figure 4–45). The instructions provided to the patient are important in obtaining robust OKN responses. Patients who choose to "look through" the OKN pattern can significantly reduce the gain. Patients should be instructed to keep their head very still and simply look at the pattern as it passes by. Because of the diffuse projections, OKN ("stare") testing, like pursuit, is of limited diagnostic utility; however, unlike the pursuit system, the response is reflexive and is not as heavily influenced by inattention or medication. The two primary paradigms for evaluating the OKN system are fixed and sinusoidal.

The section below outlines the technique for the fixed paradigm. (Readers are referred to Shepard and Schubert [2008] for a more comprehensive discussion regarding the assessment of OKN [e.g., sinusoidal and optokinetic after-nystagmus paradigms].)

Assessment of the Optokinetic System

In order to perform optokinetic testing, the patient should be instructed to maintain the head in the

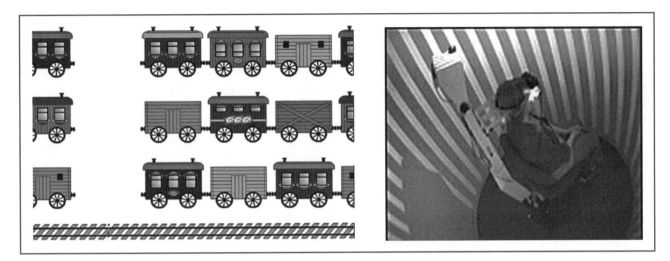

FIGURE 4–45. A. An example of the type of stimuli that can be employed using projectors for the generation of optokinetic stimuli. **B.** An example of a patient in the rotary chair being subjected to a full-field optokinetic stimulus.

midline position and look *straight ahead* at the pattern as it moves across the screen or wall. Furthermore, the patient should be asked to "look" and focus on the stimuli as they pass by, and not to ignore them. It is important to communicate to the patient that they should be careful not to select one stimulus and follow it as that will invoke the smooth pursuit system. The visual stimulus should consist of a full-field stimulus moving at a constant velocity at 20° per second and 35 to 40° per second in both directions. Recordings should be taken for a minimum of 30 s. When an abnormality (e.g., reduced gain) is observed the test should be repeated.

Interpretation and Analysis

As with pursuit testing, the primary parameter that is evaluated during the assessment of OKN is velocity gain. A gain measure is calculated for targets moving to the right and left and then compared using an asymmetry formula. There are two primary OKN abnormalities when the fixed paradigm is employed. First, gain can be bilaterally reduced. Secondly, gain can demonstrate a significant asymmetry (e.g., the response to the rightward-moving field is smaller than the response to the leftward-moving field. The calculated asymmetry should not exceed 25% (Shepard & Schubert, 2008). It is noteworthy that each clinician should have normative data, as the calculations and analysis methods used to calculate these values are often proprietary and vary between manufacturers.

Velocity Gain

Velocity gain is the relationship between the velocity of the eye and the velocity of the OKN stimulus. Specifically, velocity gain describes how closely the slow phase of the nystagmus (eye) matches the velocity of the optokinetic field.

The following equation defines OKN velocity gain:

$$\text{OKN velocity gain} = \frac{\text{Peak eye velocity (degrees/second)}}{\text{Peak target velocity (degrees/second)}}$$

Asymmetry

Asymmetry reflects the difference in velocity gain (described above) between rightward and leftward eye movements. This can often be abnormal in cases where a patient is generating spontaneous nystagmus. For example, if the patient has right-beating spontaneous nystagmus, the patient typically manifests abnormally reduced velocity gain on the right.

Optokinetic Abnormalities

An abnormality in the OKN system has been reported to occur when the gain for a 60° per second stimulus is less than 0.56 (Baloh & Furman, 1989). It is important to note that normal OKN gain is not the same for all target velocities. Specifically, OKN gain decreases as the speed of the targets is increased.

Bilaterally Reduced Optokinetic Responses

Symmetrically reduced optokinetic responses can occur for a number of reasons. First, the presence of a disorder in the pursuit system manifests bilaterally reduced gain. When performing the pursuit task, the fovea must be kept directly on the target; however, the OKN response is evoked by both central (foveal) and peripheral (extrafoveal) vision and is the reason that a full-field stimulus is used. In patients with impairments in central vision, the examiner commonly observes reduced OKN gain at the beginning of the test and increasing OKN as the test progresses (Baloh, Yee, & Honrubia, 1980). In patients with impairments in their peripheral vision, but have normal central vision, this increase in gain is not observed. Another abnormality that contributes to symmetrically reduced OKN gain is a saccade impairment. Patients with disease in the brainstem, where the pulse neurons for the generation of saccades are located, are unable to generate the fast phase that is required to reset the eye during the OKN response. This inability of the patient to quickly bring the eye back to center results in the gain of the OKN response being significantly reduced (Figure 4–46). This inability to generate saccades is often observed during caloric and rotational testing and can be mistaken for a weakness in the bilateral peripheral vestibular system. Other sources of bilaterally reduced optokinetic responses include impairments in the cortex to the cerebellum. Whenever bilaterally reduced OKN is observed caution should be exercised to rule out medication, visual impairments, inattention, and inattentive head movement.

Unilaterally Reduced Optokinetic Responses

The finding of a significant asymmetry during optokinetic testing can suggest either a central nervous system impairment or the presence of spontaneous vestibular nystagmus. As explained in the previous section detailing abnormalities in

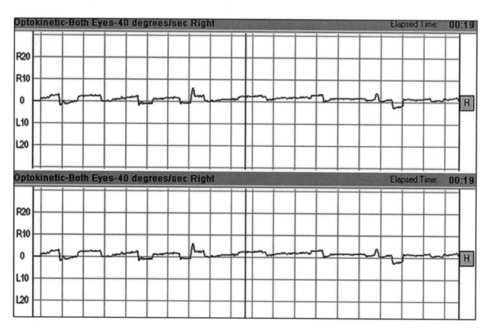

FIGURE 4–46. Bilaterally reduced optokinetic gain is shown.

the pursuit system, the oculomotor system has difficulty integrating the fast phase of the spontaneous nystagmus and the slow movement of the target (Figure 4–47). This can lead to asymmetrically reduced OKN gain when the direction of the OKN stimulus beats in the opposite direction of the fast phase of the spontaneous nystagmus; however, it is noteworthy that asymmetric pursuit can be observed in patients with impairments in the temporal lobes, unilateral parieto-occipital disorders, and the brainstem. If a central cause is suspected, other tests of oculomotor function (e.g., gaze and saccades) should be carefully inspected and the presence of any spontaneous nystagmus should be ruled out.

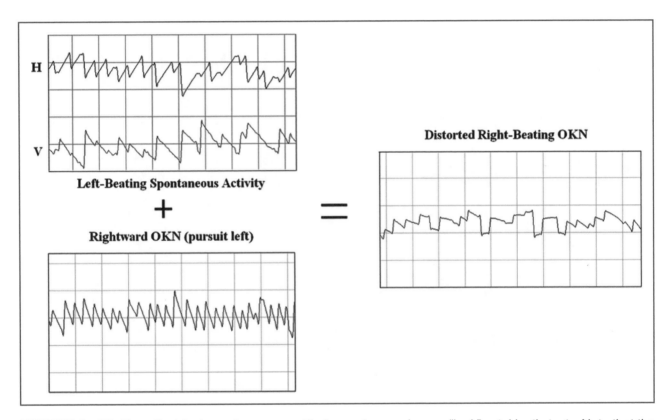

FIGURE 4–47. The effect that spontaneous vestibular nystagmus has on "look" optokinetic tests. Note that the eye movement system cannot integrate both a smooth and a fast eye movement. OKN = Optokinetic nystagmus; H = horizontal; V = vertical. (From McCaslin & Jacobson, 2009)

‖‖ 5 ‖‖

Positional and Positioning Testing

STATIC POSITIONAL TESTING

Introduction

The purpose of positional testing is twofold. First, the test is performed to document the patient's complaint of position-induced vertigo and/or dizziness. The second reason is to record the effect that gravity, and static body positions, has on the tonic afferent neural output originating from the peripheral vestibular system. Patients with both peripheral and central vestibular system impairments can generate position-induced nystagmus.

Background

Static positioning testing involves recording a patient's eye movements with the head placed in a sequence of different positions. Each position changes the orientation of the head with respect to the earth gravitational vector and can subsequently modulate the baseline "neural tone" in the vestibular system (Coats, 1993); thus, the purpose of this test is to document (through eye recordings) the presence or modulation of position-induced nystagmus, and, to the extent possible, determine whether the nystagmus is

originating from the peripheral vestibular system or the central vestibular system (Baloh & Honrubia, 2001; Brandt, 1990; Leigh & Zee, 2006). A comprehensive list of the causes of nystagmus associated with changes in head position is provided in Table 5–1. It is noteworthy that not all positional nystagmus is of clinical significance. There continues to be disagreement in the literature as to whether there is a high percentage of the normal population that presents with positional nystagmus (Barber & Wright, 1973; Coats, 1993; McAuley, Dickman, Mustain, & Anand, 1996). For example, in a landmark study examining positional nystagmus in normal subjects, Barber and Wright (1973) reported that 82% of their randomly selected sample of 112 participants had measureable positional nystagmus. This finding that positional nystagmus is observed in the majority of normal subjects has been supported by others (McAuley et al., 1996). In contrast to these findings, Van Der Stappen, Wuyts, and Van De Heyning (2000) and Hajioff, Barr-Hamilton, College, Lewis, and Wilson (2000) reported positional nystagmus in their control sample of 7.5% and 27%, respectively. In a recent report by Martens, Goplen, Nordfalk, Aasen, and Nordahl (2016), the investigators evaluated 75 adult participants without a history of a balance impairment or vertigo. Each subject was evaluated in six different standardized positions using a TRV

Table 5–1. Nystagmus and Vertigo Associated with Changes in Head Position

Vertigo and/or Nystagmus Associated with Head Motion or Changes in Head Position Relative to the Gravitational Vector
Central vestibular (pontomedullary brainstem of vestibulocerebellum)
Positional down-beating nystagmus
Down-beating nystagmus/vertigo
Up-beating nystagmus/vertigo
Central positional nystagmus without major vertigo
Central positional vertigo with nystagmus
Basilar insufficiency
Vestibular nerve
Neurovascular compression ("disabling positional vertigo")
Peripheral labyrinth
Benign paroxysmal positional vertigo
Cupula/endolymph gravity differential (buoyancy mechanism)
Positional alcohol vertigo/nystagmus
Positional "heavy water" nystagmus
Positional glycerol nystagmus
Positional nystagmus with macroglobulinemia
Perilymph fistula
Ménière disease
Vestibular atelectasia
Physiologic "head-extension vertigo" or "bending-over vertigo"
Vestibular head-motion intolerance (oscillopsia and unsteadiness of gait)
Bilateral vestibulopathy
Oculomotor disorders (defective vestibulo-ocular reflex)
Neurovascular cross-compression ("vestibular paroxysmia")
Vestibulocerebellar ataxia
Perilymphatic fistula
Post-traumatic otolith vertigo
Vestibulocerebellar intoxication (e.g., alcohol, phenytoin)

Source: From Brandt, 1993.

positioning chair (Figure 5–1). Interestingly, in this normal population of subjects, 88% were shown to have measurable positional nystagmus. Nystagmus, in this study, was classified as measurable when there were >5 beats of nystagmus within a 30-second time period using VNG goggles. The position with the most common occurrence of positional nystagmus was the Dix-Hallpike position (55% demonstrating positional nystagmus). Using VNG goggles, the investigators calculated the 95th percentile (i.e., a significant finding if exceeded) of the maximum slow-phase velocity to be 5.06 deg/sec in the horizontal plane and 6.48 deg/sec in the vertical plane. Although this rigor-

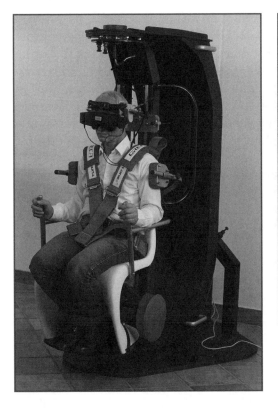

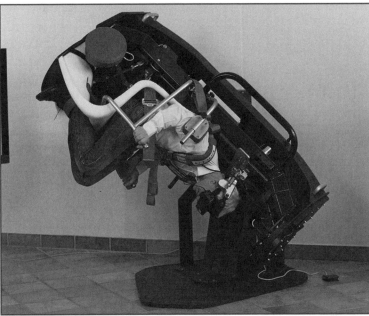

FIGURE 5–1. Patient situated with the TRV chair with restraints and goggles.

ous study demonstrates how common positional nystagmus is in the normal population, the failure to find consensus in previous studies is related to investigators using a multitude of different positions and analysis techniques. For these reasons the observation of nystagmus or vertigo induced by static position testing is, in most instances, of minor diagnostic utility.

The one factor that does discriminate between central and peripheral positional nystagmus is fixation ability. Positional nystagmus due to impairment in the peripheral vestibular system can almost always be significantly attenuated with visual fixation. For this reason, static positioning testing is initially performed without fixation (vision denied). If nystagmus is observed during a position with vision denied (no fixation), the test should be repeated with fixation. The patient should be given mental alerting tasks during the test.

Technique

The technique for static positional testing (Figure 5–2) is as follows:

1. Perform the search for spontaneous nystagmus (sitting) and positioning testing before assessing static positional testing.
2. Prepare to provide a mental-alerting task for the patient for each position. The patient should be wearing videonystagmography goggles or Frenzel glasses with eyes open.
3. Lay the patient in the recumbent position (supine) with vision denied for 30 s.
   a. If nystagmus is present following 30 s of recording, maintain the patient in this position for 2 min (allows differentiation between positional nystagmus and benign paroxysmal positional vertigo).
   b. If the nystagmus continues at a constant intensity, instruct the patient to fixate on a target.
   c. Record the effect of fixation on the nystagmus (i.e., determine if fixation significantly reduces the observed nystagmus).
4. Repeat the sequence in Step 3 for head right or body right (body right can be used if patient presents with cervical spondylosis, osteoarthritis, did not have any measurable nystagmus during spontaneous testing, or has a restricted cervical range of motion).

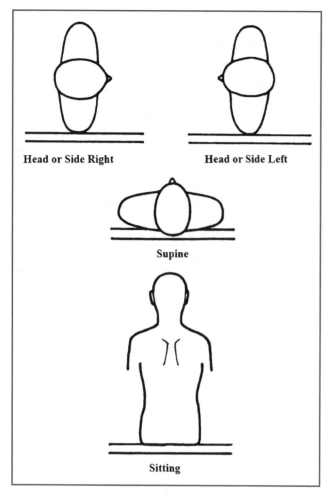

Head or Side Right **Head or Side Left**

Supine

Sitting

FIGURE 5–2. The primary positions used during the static position test. (Adapted from Brandt, 1993)

5. Repeat the sequence in Step 3 for head left or body left.
6. Repeat the sequence in Step 3 with the patient supine with neck flexion at 30°.

Interpretation

When interpreting positional nystagmus, it is important that the findings be correlated with the quantitative vestibular function test results as well as the case history. In order to appropriately determine if static positional nystagmus is pathologic (i.e., peripheral or central), the examiner should be able to answer four primary questions. First, what is the peak amplitude of the observed nystagmus (e.g., average of three beats)? When recording using VNG, if the slow-phase velocity of any observed horizontal nystagmus is greater than 4° per second (7° per second for vertical nystagmus) in any of the static positions, then further analysis should be undertaken (Barin, 2008b). Second, how long does the response last (intermittent or persistent)? This question serves to determine if the nystagmus observed is a form of benign paroxysmal positioning vertigo (BPPV) or if it is positional nystagmus generated by an asymmetry in the vestibulo-ocular reflex (VOR) pathway. Third, is the nystagmus direction fixed or direction changing in one or more head positions? The presence of a positional nystagmus that changes direction in a single head position is diagnostic for intracranial disease, usually affecting the cerebellar system (i.e., cerebellum and pons). When horizontal nystagmus is not observed during either the sitting or supine positions but is measurable during the head left or head right position, the examiner should consider the effect of neck rotation. The effect of neck rotation can be ruled out by retesting the patient in the body left and body right positions. If there is no measurable nystagmus during the body right or body left position, the observed nystagmus is most likely due to neck torsion (e.g., "cervicogenic dizziness/nystagmus"). Finally, what is the effect of fixation on the intensity of the positional nystagmus? A positional nystagmus that cannot be attenuated with visual fixation implicates abnormal function of the reciprocal connections between the midline cerebellar structures and pons. In many instances, a significant horizontal positional nystagmus that can be attenuated with visual fixation is found in the presence of a unilateral peripheral vestibular system impairment. Tables 5–2 and 5–3 present a summary of potential findings for each of the questions and their significance.

Two flow charts recently reported by Barin (2008b) have summarized the interpretation of both horizontal (Figure 5–3) and vertical nystagmus (Figure 5–4) during the static positional test. These decision pathways can be used as a simple and effective way to guide the clinician through the process of interpreting whether observed positional nystagmus is of clinical significance.

Table 5–2. Duration of Observed Nystagmus

Finding	Significance/Comments
Intermittent nystagmus	Rule out BPPV and patient lack of alertness
Persistent nystagmus	Significant if peak SPV is >6° per second for ENG (no fixation)
	Significant if peak SPV is >4° per second for VNG (no fixation) (Barin, 2008b)
	Significant if nystagmus of any intensity does not diminish with fixation

BPPV = benign paroxysmal positioning vertigo; SPV = slow-phase velocity.

Table 5–3. Characteristics of the Nystagmus and the Effect of Fixation

Finding	Fixation	No Fixation	Significance/Comments
Direction-fixed horizontal nystagmus	Decreases significantly (50%) or is abolished	Enhances	Peripheral (vestibular nystagmus)
Direction-fixed horizontal nystagmus	Decreases significantly (50%) or is abolished	Present	Normal
Vertical nystagmus	No decrease	Present	Central abnormality (up-beating or down-beating) (Baloh & Honrubia, 1990; Pierrot-Deseilligny & Milea, 2005).
Vertical nystagmus <7° per second (VNG)	Decreases significantly (50%) or is abolished	Present	Normal (Barin, 2008b)
Direction-changing horizontal nystagmus (apogeotropic)	Decreases significantly (50%)	Present	Right oblique positional alcohol nystagmus and HSC BPPV
Direction-changing horizontal nystagmus (geotropic)	Decreases significantly (50%)	Present	Right oblique positional alcohol nystagmus and HSC BPPV
Direction-fixed horizontal nystagmus	No decrease in intensity	No increase in intensity	Suggests central impairment
Direction-changing horizontal nystagmus in a single head position	Present	Present	Rule out periodic alternating nystagmus; central finding
Direction-changing horizontal nystagmus in a single head position	Abolished	Present	Central finding

HSC = horizontal semicircular canal; *BPPV* benign paroxysmal positioning vertigo.

Positional Alcohol Nystagmus

As discussed in the previous section, nystagmus resulting from impairment in the peripheral ves-tibular system is typically direction fixed; however, one type of nystagmus that is peripheral in origin and changes direction with different head positions is positional alcohol nystagmus (PAN).

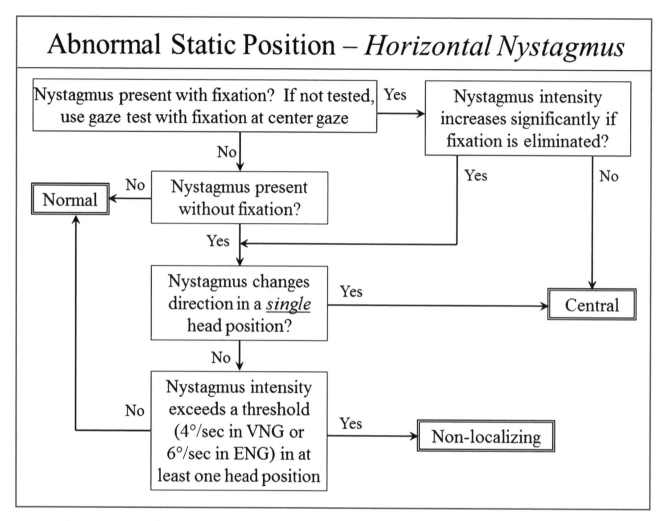

FIGURE 5–3. Algorithm for the interpretation of horizontal nystagmus observed during the static position test. (Courtesy of Kamran Barin)

Caution should be exercised when using the acronym PAN so that positional alcohol nystagmus is not confused with periodic alternating nystagmus. Alcohol consumed by a patient initially enters the bloodstream and then the cupula and endolymph. The mechanism behind PAN involves the ingested alcohol reaching the cupula before it reaches the endolymph. Because the density of alcohol is lighter than surrounding endolymph, the cupula becomes lighter and will float (like a bobber). This action will produce nystagmus during positional testing and has been termed PAN I. The main characteristic of PAN I (i.e., resorption phase of PAN) is direction-changing geotropic nystagmus with head right or left (Figure 5–5A). Alternatively, alcohol is absorbed by the body earlier in the cupula than in the endolymph causing the cupula to sink (like a sinker) and has been referred to as PAN II. PAN II (i.e., reduction phase of PAN) generates an apogeotropic nystagmus during positional testing (Figure 5–5B). Approximately 2 to 5 hours following the ingestion of a significant amount of alcohol, there will be a "window" between PAN I and PAN II where there is no observable positional nystagmus. This "intermediate period" exists when alcohol has diffused into both the cupula and the endolymph and the specific gravity becomes equal again.

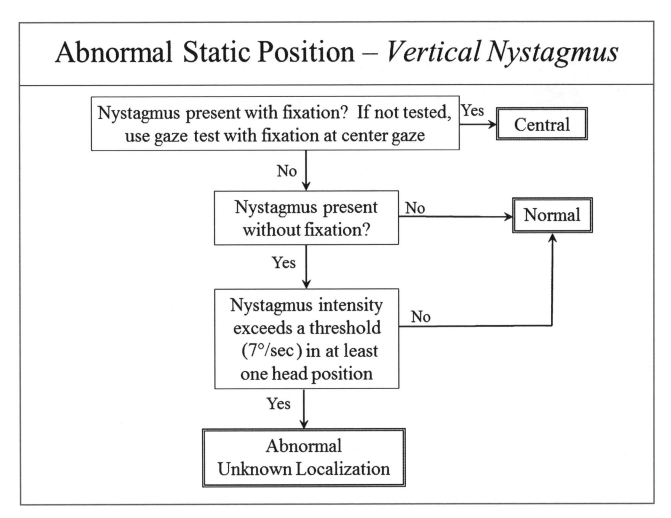

FIGURE 5–4. Algorithm for the interpretation of vertical nystagmus observed during the static position test. (Courtesy of Kamran Barin)

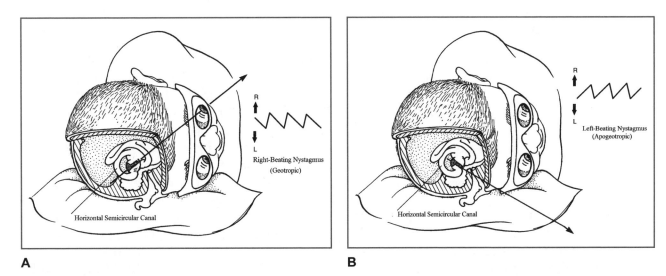

A   B

FIGURE 5–5. Eye movements and physiologic mechanism of positional alcohol nystagmus (PAN). **A.** PAN I generates geotropic nystagmus. **B.** PAN II generates apogeotropic nystagmus. (Courtesy of Daniel Pender, adapted from Pender, 1992)

Background

Benign paroxysmal positioning vertigo (BPPV) is one of the most common forms of vertigo (Bhattacharyya et al., 2008; Drachman 1998; Furman & Cass, 1999; Hotson & Baloh, 1998). Barany (1907) provided the initial description of this type of dizziness that is characterized by intense, but brief, vertigo and nystagmus provoked by changes in the position of the head. BPPV is the term most commonly used to describe the disorder with this specific set of symptoms. "Benign" refers to the fact that the disorder is peripheral and can often be successfully treated. The word "paroxysmal" means a brief, violent outburst. "Positioning" refers to the fact that in order to provoke the symptoms, the head, (and consequently the semicircular canals) must be moved into certain positions. Finally, "vertigo" implies that the patient perceives his or her surroundings to be moving when he or she is not moving. During the case history, patients with BPPV often report that the dizziness occurs when they roll over in bed, look up, or bend over. In this vein, Whitney, Marchetti, and Morris (2005) reported that five items on the Dizziness Handicap Inventory (DHI) can help the clinician in the identification of patients with BPPV. The five items include the following:

1. Does looking up increase your problem?
2. Because of your problem, do you have difficulty getting into or out of bed?
3. Do quick movements of your head increase your problem?
4. Does turning over in bed increase your problem?
5. Does bending over increase your problem?

Patients with BPPV had significantly higher mean scores than those who did not have BPPV. Specifically, the authors reported that scores on the five-item abbreviated BPPV DHI were predictive of patients with BPPV (Whitney et al., 2005).

The confirmation of BPPV is based on a set of maneuvers designed to induce the nystagmus and vertigo in each of the canals. The first maneuver described to specifically provoke BPPV was reported by Margaret Dix and Charles Hallpike in 1952 using their sample of 100 patients at Queen Square Hospital (Dix & Hallpike, 1952). In this maneuver, the patient sits on the exam table with the head turned 45° toward the side being tested and then is brought to the supine position with the head extended off the edge of the table. The authors reported a torsional vertical nystagmus beating toward the dependent ear that was brief in duration and reversed direction upon having the patient sit up. This maneuver, known as the Dix-Hallpike maneuver, continues to be part of the assessment of the dizziness patient.

Epidemiology

Several groups of investigators have reported on the incidence (the risk of developing a condition within a specified period of time) and prevalence (the total number of cases of the condition in the population at a given time) of BPPV in the general population. Approximately 6 million people per year enter the United States health care system with complaints of dizziness. According to Bhattacharyya et al. (2008), 17% to 42% of these patients are diagnosed with BPPV. Accordingly, the prevalence of BPPV ranges from 10.7 to 64 per 100,000 in the general population with a lifetime prevalence of 2.5% (Bhattacharyya et al., 2008). Findings are similar in other countries as well. For instance, Mizukoshi, Watanabe, Shojaku, Okubo, and Watanabe (1988) described the incidence of BPPV in Japan to be 10.7 to 17.3 per 100,000. von Brevern et al. (2007) conducted a cross-sectional study of the general population in Europe and reported a lifetime prevalence of 2.4%. Age is also a significant factor to be considered when reporting on the incidence and prevalence of BPPV. Froehling et al. (1991) presented data from a retrospective review of medical records in health care systems in the United States of patients presenting with BPPV. The authors reported that the patients seeking medical attention for BPPV increased by 38% with each decade of life (mean age 51 years). There are other studies supporting the fact that BPPV is more prevalent in the elderly (Baloh,

Honrubia, & Jacobson, 1987; von Brevern et al., 2007). Hilton and Pinder (2004) reported that the peak incidence of BPPV occurs between 50 and 70 years. In elderly patients, BPPV can have serious consequences. In a cross-sectional investigation by Oghalai, Manolidis, Barth, Stewart, and Jenkins (2000), elderly patients presenting with BPPV were shown to limit their activity level and have a greater incidence of falls. Furthermore, 9% of the participants in their study had unrecognized BPPV (Oghalai et al., 2000). Originally, the term "benign" in BPPV was included because this type of vertigo is peripheral and can be managed in most instances; however, those who experience it would agree that, when triggered, the sensation of BPPV is anything but "benign." Also, because elderly persons with BPPV are at a greater risk of falling, the term "benign" is a misnomer. BPPV does occasionally occur in younger patients who have suffered a head trauma, present with migraine, or have had a procedure that keeps them bedridden for an extended period of time.

The majority of patients with positioning vertigo present with BPPV that affects either the posterior (PSC-BPPV) or the horizontal semicircular canal (HSC-BPPV). PSC-BPPV has been reported to make up 85% to 90% of all BPPV cases (Parnes, Agrawal, & Atlas, 2003). HSC-BPPV accounts for 5% to 15% of cases of BPPV (Cakir et al., 2006; Parnes et al., 2003). The incidence of BPPV among

the three semicircular canals (SCCs), according to Roberts and Gans (2008), is given in Table 5–4. BPPV affecting the anterior semicircular canal (ASC-BPPV) and multiple canals is much less common accounting for no more than 5% of cases (De la Meilleur et al., 1996; Moon et al., 2006;).

As described above, the prevalence and clinical presentation of BPPV is well known, yet the condition often goes undiagnosed or is treated inappropriately. Also, because BPPV represents a "mechanical" impairment in the vestibular end organ, the condition may disappear spontaneously and go through long periods of remission. It is important that clinicians in the balance clinic work closely with the referring professional in order to identify and treat patients with BPPV in a timely and appropriate manner.

Pathophysiology

Our understanding of the pathophysiologic mechanism of BPPV has evolved significantly over the past 40 years. The initial pathophysiologic mechanism for BPPV was provided by Harold Schuknecht (1962). Using photomicrographs, he uncovered basophilic particles that had attached to the cupula. He proposed that these densities were displaced otoconia from the utricular maculae and the primary source of BPPV (Schuknecht,

Table 5–4. Incidence of Benign Paroxysmal Positional Vertigo Among Semicircular Canals

Study	Number	PC	HC	AC
Herdman, Tusa, & Clendaniel (1994)	59	63.6	1.3	11.7
Fife (1998)	424	91	6	3
Wolf, Boyev, Manokey, & Mattox (1999)	107	95.3	1.9	2.8
Honrubia, Baloh, Harris, & Jacobson (1999)	292	93.5	5.1	1.4
Ruckenstein (2001)	86	96.5	2.3	1.2
Korres & Balatsouras (2004)	122	90.2	8.2	1.6
Cakir et al. (2006)	169	85.2	11.8	1.2
Jackson, Morgan, Fletcher, & Krueger (2007)	260	66.9	11.9	21.2

PC = posterior canal; HC = horizontal canal; AC = anterior canal.
Source: From Roberts & Gans (2008, p. 181).

1969; Schuknecht & Ruby, 1973). The cupula is a gelatinous mass housed in the ampullated end of each SCC. The role of the cupula is to transduce angular head accelerations into increases or decreases in neural firing rate. The cupula is normally a neutrally buoyant structure due to the fact that it has the same specific gravity as the surrounding endolymph. When the head is subjected to acceleration, the hydrodynamic pressure from the endolymph distorts the cupula and triggers a response from the hair cells embedded in the base. This displacement of the cupula and shearing of the hair cells generates a neural code associated with movement. If the acceleration continues, the viscoelastic nature of the cupula returns it to its original position; however, when otoconial debris is displaced from the utricle, it can adhere to the cupula and change its density. This creates a situation where a sustained movement in the plane of the impaired canal causes the cupula to remain in a position where the debris exerts a force that keeps it deflected toward the earth. The description of this series of events led Schuknecht to coin the term "cupulolithiasis." This theory persisted until the early 1990s and was the model used to develop the early Cawthorne and Brandt-Daroff treatments (Cawthorne, 1944; Brandt & Daroff, 1980). At the time of this writing, it continues to be one of the two prevailing pathophysiologic mechanisms of BPPV.

Approximately 30 years later, John Epley (1992) postulated the "canalithiasis" theory of BPPV based on models of the labyrinth he developed. He set forth that the characteristic symptoms of BPPV (i.e., the fatigability and latency of the response) were more consistent with loose particles floating in the canals rather than attached to the cupula as Schuknecht had earlier proposed. This theory also supported the observed findings described by Dix and Hallpike (1952). In the very same year, Parnes and McClure (1992), located at the University of London in Ontario, observed free-floating particles in the endolymphatic space of a patient undergoing a posterior semicircular canal (PSC) fenestration procedure. The particulate matter found in the PSC was hypothesized to be otoliths (which normally rest on the otolith membrane of the utricle and saccule) that

had migrated from the utricular maculae and entered the PSC by way of the ductus reuniens. Otoliths (or canaliths if they have become free floating in the canal) are "heavier" than the surrounding endolymph. This means that, when at rest, the otoliths "sink" to the lowest level of the gravitational vector. When the head changes position, the otolith debris also changes position en masse, and in so doing displaces the endolymph. The endolymph displacement deflects the cupula (which is attached to the cristae) that normally occurs when the head is moving and, in so doing, sends a set of signals to the brain that normally would occur if the person were rotating. Parnes and McClure suggested that once enough of these otoliths accumulate in the PSC, they would form a large enough mass that would alter the physiologic characteristics of fluid motion in the SCCs. The authors added further support to this concept of free-floating particles by observing and documenting the symptoms of patients with BPPV.

These observations of the pathophysiology provided by Parnes and McClure, along with Epley's models of the vestibular system, provided the understanding that led to the development of the current canalith repositioning procedures (CRP) to treat patients with BPPV (Epley, 1992; Parnes & Price-Jones, 1993). The cupulolithiasis and canalithiasis pathophysiologic mechanisms as proposed by Schuknecht and Epley, respectively, continue to be the two primary theories explaining BPPV. Canalithiasis has been reported to be far more common than cupulolithiasis (Parnes et al., 2003).

Canalithiasis

Figures 5–6 and 5–7 illustrate how free-floating densities known as "canaliths" have been theorized to create aberrant endolymphatic flow with changes in the position of the head. In this set of figures, the patient is sitting supine and the canaliths have collected in the bottom of the PSC. When the head is turned and the patient is laid in the supine position (e.g., Dix-Hallpike maneuver), the right PSC and ASCs are placed in a position where the canaliths can fall. Because the canaliths

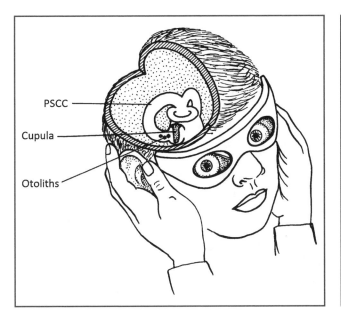

FIGURE 5–6. An illustration of canalithiasis. The particles are located in the posterior semicircular canal with the patient sitting. PSCC posterior semicircular canal. (Courtesy of Daniel Pender, adapted from Pender, 1992)

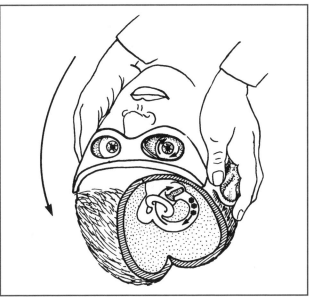

FIGURE 5–7. An illustration of canalithiasis. Following a provocative maneuver, the particles drop and trigger the vestibulo-ocular reflex. (Courtesy of Daniel Pender, adapted from Pender, 1992)

are denser than the surrounding endolymph, they are under the influence of gravity and will begin to drop. Endolymph is very thick and there is a short delay between the movement of the particles and when gravity begins to act on them. Once the canaliths begin to settle in the canal, the hydrodynamic drag caused by the movement induces endolymph flow and consequently deflects the cupula (Figure 5–8). In the vertical canals, the stereocilia in the cupula are oriented away from the utricle, and endolymph flow created by the falling densities when the patient is placed in the supine position creates an excitatory response from the vestibulo-ocular reflex (VOR). Because the VOR is being activated and the patient is not moving, the perception by the patient is of vertigo. Once the canaliths have gravitated to the lowest point in the canal, endolymph flow stops, the cupula returns to its neutral position, the neural drive to the VOR returns to its tonic resting rate, and the perception of vertigo by the patient ceases (Parnes & McClure, 1992). When the patient is brought back to the sitting position, the canaliths again begin to drop, and in this instance, the cupula is

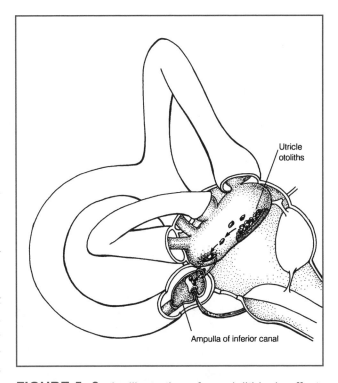

FIGURE 5–8. An illustration of cupulolithiasis affecting the posterior semicircular canal. (Courtesy of Daniel Pender, adapted from Pender, 1992)

deflected in the opposite direction, generating an inhibitory response (typically smaller) from the VOR and a reversal in the perceived movement by the patient (i.e., the nystagmus beats in the opposite direction).

Cupulolithiasis

In the cupulolithiasis variant of BPPV, the displaced otoliths are attached to the cupula, causing it to become heavier and, therefore, sensitive to gravity. This condition is less common than the canalithiasis type and is more resistant to treatment. The response patterns (direction of the nystagmus) are very similar to those of canalithiasis (described above), but the characteristics of the responses can be different. For example, because the otoliths are attached directly to the cupula, the response is often immediate (no latent period) (Figure 5–8). Additionally, in cases of cupulolithiasis, the nystagmus may continue for a longer time if the head is maintained in a provocative position.

Diagnosis

The correct diagnosis of BPPV and the identification of the canal(s) that are involved are dependent on the clinician being able to interpret the pattern of responses that occur following the movement of the patient into a position that provokes his or her vertigo. There are several maneuvers that have been designed to orient each SCC into a position where any displaced otoconia will be subject to the pull of gravity and stimulate the canal. How-

ever, it is not enough to just provoke the vertigo. The examiner must also have a thorough understanding of the semicircular canal ocular reflexes in order to correctly characterize the nystagmus and identify the location of the displaced particles. Each SCC is connected to a pair of eye muscles in such a way that when the canal is stimulated, the eyes move in the plane of that canal (see Figure 5–8). This is the premise of Ewald's first law, which states that the direction of the nystagmus should match the anatomic axis of the SCC that is stimulated (Ewald, 1892). These disynaptic connections between the SCCs and the eyes allow the clinician to accurately identify the location of the canaliths and form a correct treatment plan. Table 5–5 summarizes the excitatory actions of each of the canals and the associated nystagmus.

Posterior Semicircular Canal BPPV

The Dix-Hallpike maneuver is the gold standard for identifying PSC-BPPV (Dix & Hallpike, 1952). Before the maneuver is performed, the patients should be counseled regarding how they will be moved during the positioning and that they may experience some dizziness. It is important to reassure the patient that the dizziness will be transient (less than 60 s). The traditional Dix-Hallpike maneuver begins with the patient sitting on the exam table and the head turned 45° from midline toward the side that is being assessed. With the neck supported, the examiner guides the patient back into the supine position with the head hyperextended approximately 30° below the horizontal plane. The clinician should be in a position where

Table 5–5. Excitatory Actions of Each of the Canals and the Associated Nystagmus

Canal	Eye Muscles Activated	Associated Nystagmus (Fast Phase)
Posterior	Ipsilateral superior oblique Contralateral inferior rectus	Torsional/up-beating
Horizontal	Ipsilateral medial rectus Contralateral lateral rectus	Horizontal
Anterior	Ipsilateral superior rectus Contralateral inferior oblique	Torsional/down-beating

the patient's eyes can be clearly viewed. A positive response is indicated by vertigo and a torsional up-beating nystagmus in the supine position directed toward the dependent ear (Figure 5–9). The characteristics of PSC BPPV are described in Table 5–6 and an example of a VNG recording is

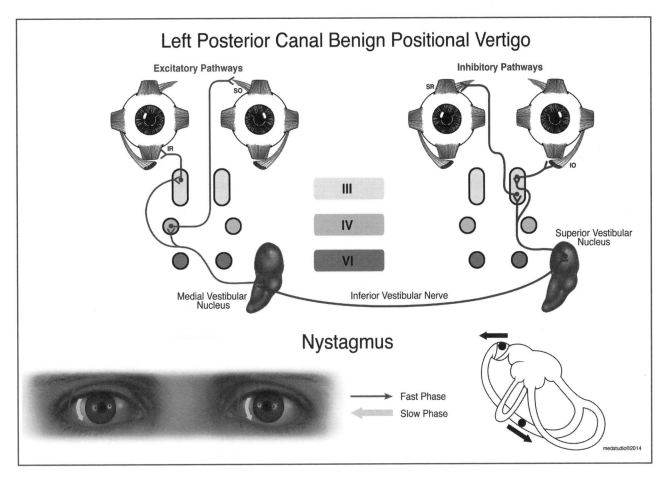

FIGURE 5–9. Figure illustrating left ear posterior canal BPPV and the excitatory and inhibitory receptor connections to the extraocular muscles and the direction of nystagmus. Nystagmus generated by posterior canal BPPV is typically described as a mixed torsional and vertical eye movement with the upper pole of the eye beating in the direction of the dependent ear. In this example, the response is an up-beating nystagmus with a torsional component to the left when the head is placed in the head-down left position. When a response is documented the patient should be asked if they perceive the perception of vertigo. When the patient is returned to the upright position, a reversal (typically smaller amplitude) of the response may be observable.

Table 5–6. Characteristics of Posterior Semicircular Canal Benign Paroxysmal Positioning Vertigo

Duration	Usually less than 40 s
Direction change	Down-beating when returning to the sitting position
Fatigability	Intensity reduces when the maneuver is repeated
Temporal course	Initial increase in intensity and then slowly declines
Direction of nystagmus	Torsional/up-beating when placed in the initial provocative position

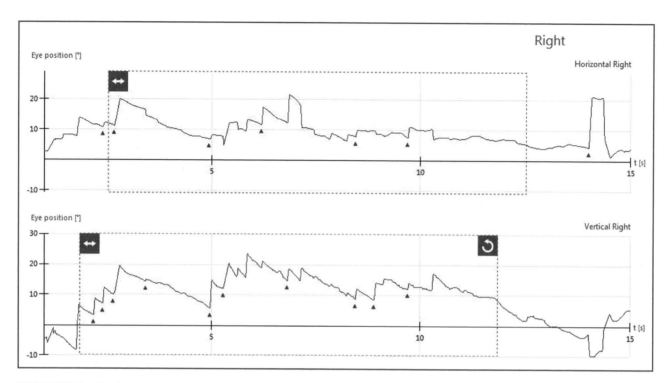

FIGURE 5–10. Up-beating torsional nystagmus during the Dix-Hallpike maneuver in a patient with canalithiasis affecting the right posterior semicircular canal. Up-beating torsional nystagmus during the Dix-Hallpike maneuver in a patient with canalithiasis affecting the right posterior semicircular canal. The panel on the top represents the horizontal eye movement tracing and the lower panel represents the vertical eye movements.

presented in Figure 5–10. Before performing the Dix-Hallpike maneuver, the examiner should have a thorough understanding of the patient's medical history. For instance, in order to avoid injuring the patient, caution should be exercised when assessing patients presenting with a history of vascular or orthopedic disorders (e.g., vertebrobasilar insufficiency, cervical spondylosis, Down syndrome, kyphoscoliosis, or cervical radiculopathy). In patients where hyperextension of the neck is contraindicated, a modified procedure known as the side-lying maneuver is an alternative technique to the Dix-Hallpike maneuver to assess the PSC (Herdman & Tusa, 1996). Humphriss, Baguley, Sparkes, Peerman, & Moffat (2003) compared the sensitivity of the Dix-Hallpike maneuver to the side-lying maneuver for the identification of PSC-BPPV. The investigators reported no significant difference between the two assessments.

Instruction Set Delivered to Patient Prior to the Maneuver

The instructions to be given to the patient are as follows:

In just a moment, we are going to make believe you are laying down in bed with your head turned to the right (or left). I would like you to cross your arms over your chest like this (demonstrate), turn your head to the right (or left), and then I will count to three. On three, I want you to let me guide you back so that you are lying on your back with your head just a bit over the edge of the table. We will stay there for about half a minute. It is critical that you keep your eyes open all of this time. You may or may not have a sensation of movement when you lie down. If you do, it is likely that your eyes will be moving a little bit and how they move tells us which maneuver we need to do to rid you of this positional vertigo. So no matter what sensation you experience, please keep your eyes wide open. Are you ready? I will count to 3 and on 3, we will lay back: 1—2—3.

Technique for the Dix-Hallpike Maneuver

The technique for the Dix-Hallpike maneuver is as follows:

1. The patient begins the maneuver seated in the upright position and the clinician stands on the side that is to be tested. It is important to ensure that the patient is oriented so that when they are put into the supine position the head will hang off the edge of the table.
2. The clinician should have the patient turn his head 45° toward the examiner and make sure that the hands are placed in a position where the neck is supported. Before the maneuver is initiated, patients should be instructed to make sure that they keep their eyes open.
3. The examiner lays the patient back maintaining the 45° head turn and extends the patient's head approximately 20° below the horizontal plane.
4. The examiner observes the patient's eyes for 30 s.
5. The nystagmus should be up-beating and torsional with the upper pole of the eye beating toward the dependent ear. After the nystagmus stops, the patient should be returned to the upright position. Once the patient is in the upright position, the patient will often experience dizziness again and the nystagmus should reverse direction.
6. If the Dix-Hallpike maneuver is positive it should then be repeated for the other side, and complete the same series of steps as outlined above (Figure 5–11).

Technique for the Side-Lying Test

The technique for the side-lying test is as follows:

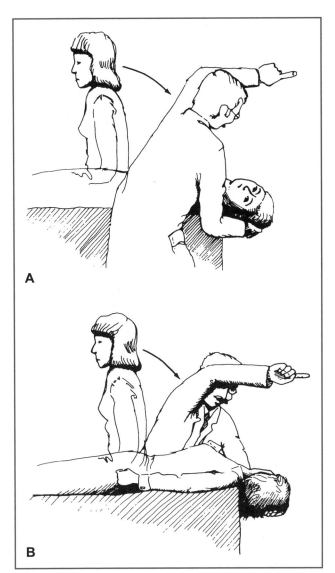

FIGURE 5–11. Illustration of the technique of the Dix-Hallpike maneuver to the right and left. **A.** The clinician stands on the left side, rotates the patient's head 45°, and supports the neck. The patient is then moved into a supine left-ear-down position with the head hyperextended and eyes open. **B.** The clinician stands on the right side, rotates the patient's head 45°, and supports the neck. The patient is then moved into a supine right-ear-down position with the head hyperextended and eyes open. (From Barber and Stockwell, 1980)

1. The patient is seated on the exam table facing the clinician.
2. The head is turned 45° away from the ear that is intended to be assessed.

3. While maintaining the head position, the patient is quickly moved to the side-lying position (avoid hyperextension) and the legs are brought up onto the exam table.

4. This position is held for approximately 30 s.

5. Patient is returned to the seated position (Figure 5–12).

Mechanism

The Dix-Hallpike and side-lying maneuvers place the posterior canal in the vertical plane (aligned with earth vertical), causing the canaliths to drop when the head is hung 30° over the end of the exam table. The orientation of the stereocilia in the posterior canals is such that when the otoliths gravitate, they create ampullopetal flow of the endolymph and deflect the cupula. This induces an excitatory response from the canal and activates the VOR. The VOR contracts the ipsilateral superior oblique and contralateral inferior rectus extraocular muscles, and a consequent nystagmus is generated. The slow phases of the nystagmus are directed in such a way as to drive the eyes downward with intorsion of the eye toward the lower ear and extorsion of the upper eye. The upper poles of the eyes beat up and toward the dependent ear during the fast corrective phase of the nystagmus (torsional up-beating). Upon

sitting, the canaliths again move, creating endolymph flow in the opposite direction and pressure on the cupula (ampullofugal), which generates a nystagmus that beats in the opposite direction (i.e., down-beating).

Horizontal Semicircular Canal BPPV

In contrast to PSC-BPPV, there are two forms of horizontal semicircular canal BPPV (HSC-BPPV). Each variant of HSC-BPPV produces different responses that are used to design the treatment. The classic sign of HSC-BPPV is nystagmus that is purely horizontal with no torsional component evoked with lateral head turns in the supine position. The most common type of HSC-BPPV generates a nystagmus, with the fast phase directed toward the ground (i.e., geotropic for the right side) (Figure 5–13). Figure 5–14 illustrates a VNG recording of a patient with HSC-BPPV that generates a geotropic response with lateral head turns. HSC-BPPV can also produce apogeotropic nystagmus (fast phase directed away from the ground). Figure 5–15 is a VNG recording of a patient with HSC-BPPV that produces apogeotropic nystagmus with lateral head turns. The direction of the nystagmus affords the clinician the ability to localize where the canaliths are in the horizontal canal.

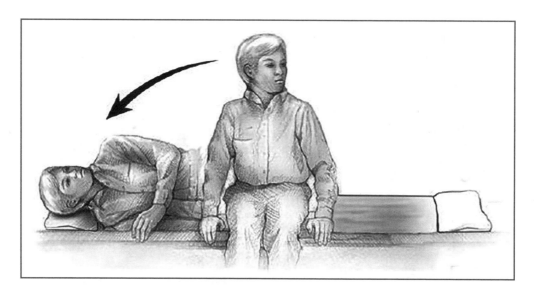

FIGURE 5–12. Illustration of the side-lying maneuver for the right side. (Used with permission of Mayo Foundation for Medical Education and Research. All rights reserved.)

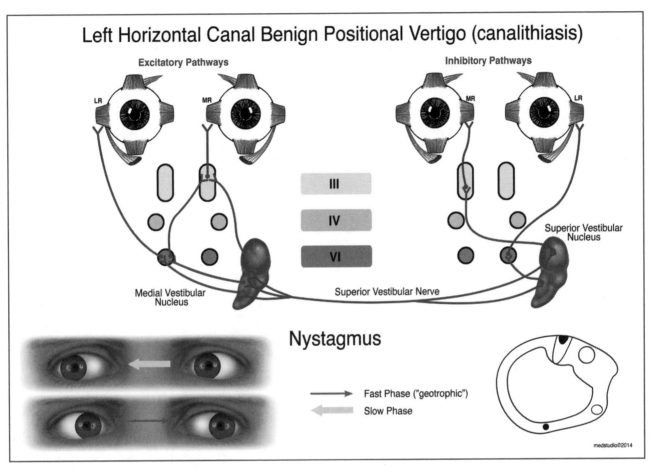

Left Horizontal Canal Benign Positional Vertigo (canalithiasis)

FIGURE 5–13. Figure illustrating left ear horizontal canalithiasis BPPV and the excitatory and inhibitory receptor connections to the extraocular muscles and the direction of nystagmus. In this case, a geotropic horizontal nystagmus is observed when the patient undergoes the supine head roll test (i.e., Pagini-Lempert Roll Test). The response (nystagmus amplitude) is largest when the head is turned to the left and the left ear is down. Note that the fast phase of the nystagmus is directed toward the left ear (geotropic). The most common form of horizontal canal BPPV is the geotropic variant.

In other words, geotropic nystagmus indicates that there are particles located in posterior arm of the HSC, whereas apogeotropic nystagmus is suggestive of otolithic debris in the anterior arm. The test for diagnosing HSC-BPPV is the supine head roll maneuver (i.e., Pagnini-McClure maneuver).

Technique for Supine Roll Test (Pagnini-Lempert or Pagini-McClure Roll Test)

This assessment consists of the examiner placing the patient in the supine position on an exam table with the head elevated approximately 30° (i.e., the same position used for caloric testing) and rotating it to the right and left. The supine head roll test provides two critical pieces of information that

the examiner later uses to treat the disorder. First, the maneuver enables the clinician to identify the affected side (i.e., right or left). Localization of the affected ear is based on a comparison of the intensity of the nystagmus between the left and right head turns. This is based on Ewald's second law, which sets forth that excitation (ampullopetal flow of endolymph) of the HSC (i.e., horizontal) produces a more robust (nystagmus) response than inhibition (ampullofugal flow of endolymph) of the HSC (Ewald, 1892); however, there occasionally are patients in whom the right and left head turns produce symmetric responses, making it difficult to identify the affected side. Reasons for this may include a different angle with which the supine head roll is done from left to right, or

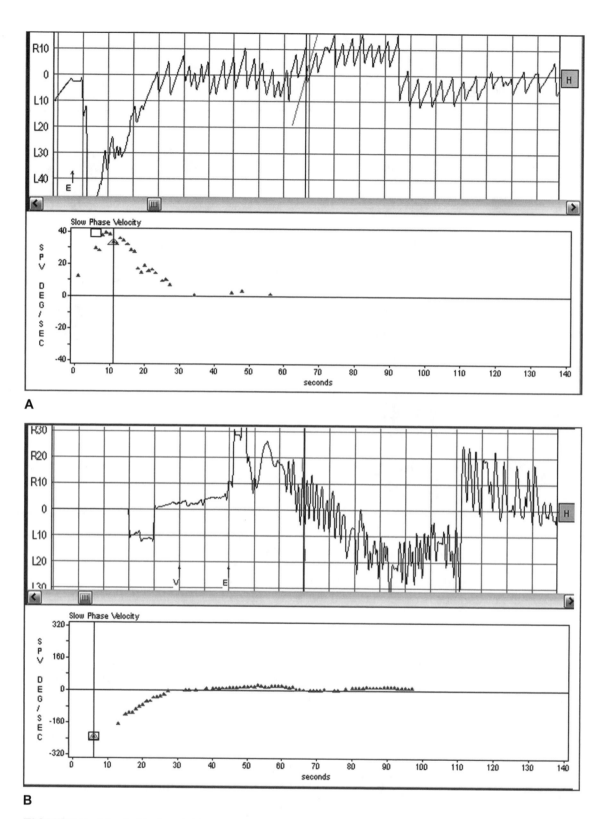

FIGURE 5–14. A. Horizontal nystagmus during the roll maneuver to the left in a patient with cana-lithiasis affecting the right lateral semicircular canal. The particles are located in the posterior arm. Note that the response is smaller than the response from the right (affected side). SPV slow-phase velocity. **B.** Horizontal nystagmus during the roll maneuver to the right in a patient with canalithiasis affecting the right lateral semicircular canal. The particles are located in the posterior arm. Note that the response is larger than the response from the left (unaffected side). SPV slow-phase velocity.

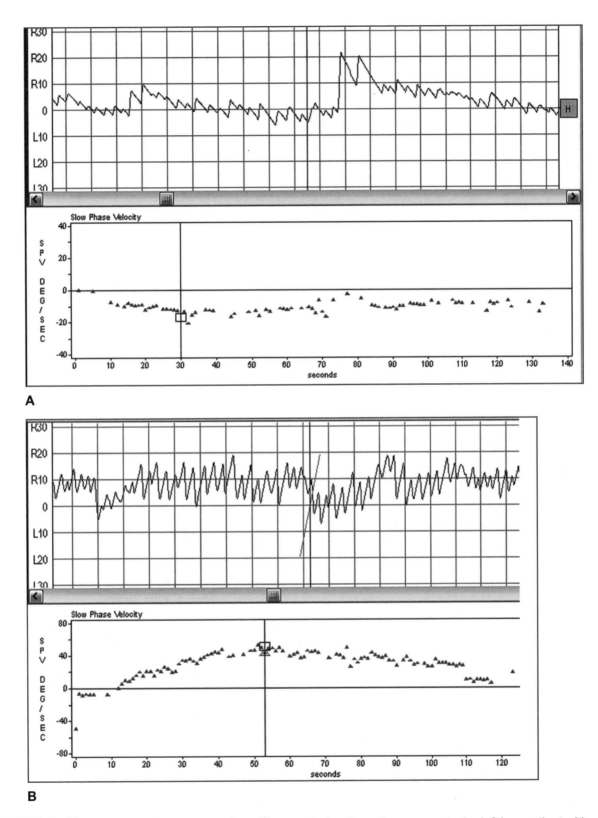

FIGURE 5–15. A. Horizontal apogeotropic nystagmus during the roll maneuver to the left in a patient with canalithiasis affecting the left lateral semicircular canal. The particles are located in the left anterior arm of the horizontal canal. Note that the response is smaller than the response from the right (unaffected side). SPV slow-phase velocity. **B.** Horizontal apogeotropic nystagmus during the roll maneuver to the right in a patient with canalithiasis affecting the left lateral semicircular canal. The particles are located in the left anterior arm of the horizontal canal. Note that the response is larger than the response from the left (affected side). SPV slow-phase velocity.

where the otolithic mass is positioned when the head is rolled (Strupp, Brandt, & Steddin, 1995). In these cases, there are alternative techniques that can be employed to determine which ear is impaired (e.g., the "bow and lean" test). Second, the direction of the nystagmus (i.e., geotropic or apogeotropic) that is provoked localizes where the otolithic debris resides in the HSC (i.e., anterior or posterior arm). A positive response is indicated by vertigo and nystagmus with lateral head turns, the characteristics of which are described in Table 5–7.

Instruction Set Delivered to Patient Prior to the Maneuver

The instructions given to the patient are as follows:

In just a moment, we are going to make believe you are turning your head side to side while lying in bed. I will count to three. On three, I want you to turn your head quickly all the way to the right and hold it there until I ask you to return it to the center. We will stay there for about half a minute. It is critical that you keep your eyes open all of this time. You may or may not have a sensation of movement after you turn your head. If you do, it is likely that your eyes will be moving a little bit and how they move tells us which maneuver we need to do to rid you of this positional vertigo. So no

matter what sensation you experience, please keep your eyes wide open. Are you ready? I will count to 3 and on 3, we will lay back: 1—2—3.

Technique for the Supine Head-Roll Test

The technique for the supine head-roll test is as follows:

1. The patient is moved into the supine position with the head elevated 30° and then asked to rotate his head 90° to one side.
2. Following the head movement, the examiner should observe the patient's eyes for any nystagmus for a period of 30 s. If nystagmus is observed, the direction and duration should be noted.
3. The head should be returned to the center (patient is facing up and forward) and held in this position until there is no longer any measurable nystagmus.
4. The head is rotated 90° to the opposite side and again the eyes should be observed for 30 s and the characteristics of any nystagmus noted (Figure 5–16).

Lateralizing the Impaired Ear Using the Supine Head Roll Test

With geotropic nystagmus, the affected ear is presumed to be the side with the larger amplitude and the particles located in the posterior arm of the HSC. With apogeotropic nystagmus, the affected ear is presumed to be the side with the smaller amplitude and the particles located in the anterior arm of the HSC.

Technique for the "Bow and Lean" Test

The technique for the "bow and lean" test is as follows:

1. The supine roll test is performed and the nystagmus direction is noted (geotropic or apogeotropic).

Table 5–7. Characteristics of Horizontal Semicircular Canal Benign Paroxysmal Positioning Vertigo

Duration	Usually less than 60 s
Direction change	Reverses direction on lateral head turns
Fatigability	Intensity reduces when the maneuver is repeated
Temporal course	Initial increase in intensity and then slowly declines
Direction of nystagmus	Linear–horizontal (can be geotropic or apogeotropic)

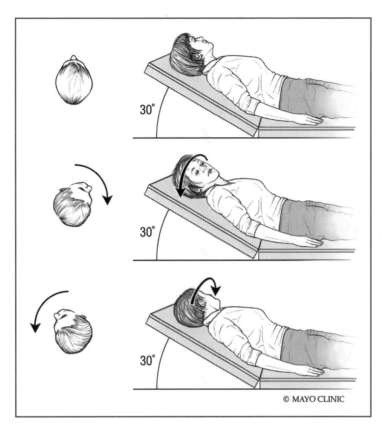

FIGURE 5–16. The supine head roll maneuver (Pagnini-McClure maneuver), to the right and then left, is shown. (Used with permission of Mayo Foundation for Medical Education and Research. All rights reserved.)

2. The patient then sits on the exam table facing the clinician.
3. The patient is asked to bow his head 90° forward, and the direction, amplitude, and duration of any nystagmus is recorded.
4. The patient tilts his head backward 45°, and again the characteristics of the nystagmus are documented.

Lateralizing the Impaired Ear Using the "Bow and Lean" Test. When the supine head-roll test generates geotropic nystagmus, the affected ear is the same as the direction of the fast phase of the bowing nystagmus and the opposite of the direction of the fast phase of the leaning nystagmus (Figure 5–17). When the supine head-roll test generates apogeotropic nystagmus, the affected ear is the opposite of the direction of the fast phase of bowing nystagmus and the same as the direction of the fast phase of the leaning nystagmus (Figure 5–18).

Mechanism

In order to treat HSC-BPPV, the canal where the particles are located must be determined. To accurately identify the affected canal requires that the examiner understand the biomechanics behind the various physiologic responses that occur when a patient has HSC-BPPV. When the head is moved, canaliths in the HSC cause the endolymph to move in a predictable way based on where they are located in the HSC. Ampullopetal flow of endolymph is excitatory and generates a larger response than ampullofugal flow, which is inhibitory (Ewald's second law). The clinician is

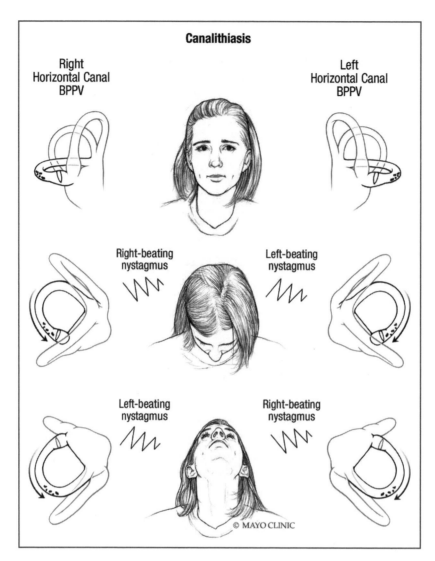

FIGURE 5–17. The "bow and lean" test for diagnosing the affected ear in cases of horizontal canal canalithiasis. In this example, the nystagmus will beat toward the affected ear when bowing. The nystagmus will beat away from the affected ear when leaning. (Used with permission of Mayo Foundation for Medical Education and Research. All rights reserved.)

able to identify the impaired canal by recording the direction and amplitude of the responses from the right and left and then comparing them. There are three patterns of HSC-BPPV: bilateral geotropic, bilateral apogeotropic that can be converted to bilateral geotropic and bilateral apogeotropic that cannot be converted to bilateral geotropic.

Geotropic HSC

Geotropic HSC, a variant of HSC-BPPV, is the most common form and produces a bilateral geotropic nystagmus during lateral head turns (Caruso & Nuti, 2005). The pathophysiologic mechanism of the geotropic variant of HSC-BPPV is the presence

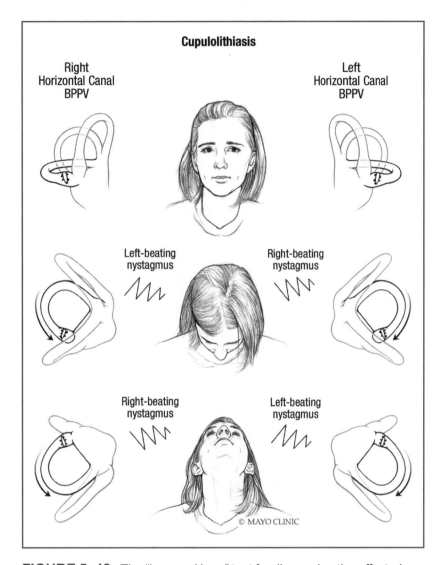

FIGURE 5–18. The "bow and lean" test for diagnosing the affected ear in cases of horizontal canal cupulolithiasis. In this instance, the nystagmus beats in the opposite direction as the bowing nystagmus and the same direction of the leaning nystagmus. (Used with permission of Mayo Foundation for Medical Education and Research. All rights reserved.)

of dislodged otoconia, most likely from the utricle, located in the posterior arm of the HSC (Figure 5–19A) (Nuti, Vannucchi, & Pagnini, 1992). The location of these particles is such that when the head is moved toward the affected ear, ampullopetal flow of the endolymph is induced and a corresponding vertigo and nystagmus occurs. When the head is turned toward the unaffected side, ampullofugal flow occurs in the affected canal, which again generates vertigo and a nystagmus that beats in the opposite direction. The reason for this is that when the is head turned toward the affected ear, the particles drop and move the endolymph in a way that produces an excitatory

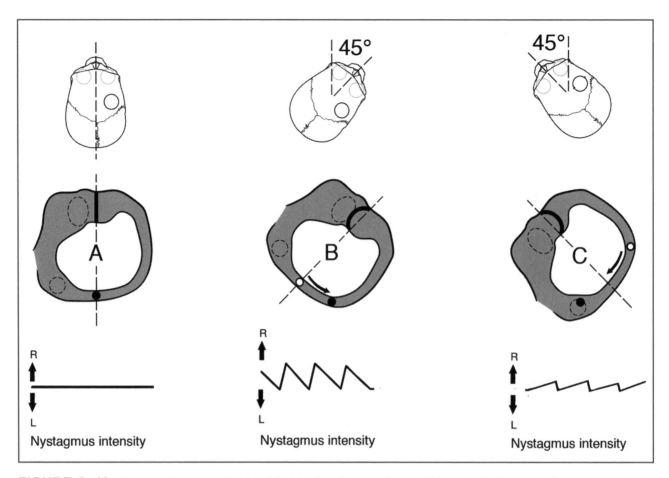

FIGURE 5–19. The mechanism of right-sided horizontal canal canalithiasis with the particles located in the posterior arm of the canal. **A.** Supine with no nystagmus. **B.** Head turn to the right generates a larger-amplitude right-beating nystagmus (geotropic). **C.** Head turn to the left generates a smaller left-beating nystagmus.

response resulting in a large-amplitude horizontal nystagmus, with the fast component beating toward the ground (lower ear) (Figure 5–19B). When the head is turned in the opposite direction toward the unaffected side, the nystagmus will again be geotropic but smaller in amplitude due to the inhibitory action of the endolymph flow (Figure 5–19C).

Apogeotropic HSC

Apogeotropic nystagmus has been theorized to be attributed to particles located in the superior arm of the HSC. Casani, Giovanni, Bruno, and Luigi (2002) have reported the characteristics of two different types of apogeotropic HSC-BPPV.

The first variant consists of otoliths attached to the cupula on the utricular side of the canal (Figure 5–20). The second type of apogeotropic HSC consists of debris on the canal side of the cupula (Figure 5–21). In cases of apogeotropic BPPV, when the head is turned in the direction of the unaffected ear, the canaliths either move (canalithiasis) and create endolymph flow, or the cupula is weighted (cupulolithiasis) in such a way that the movement produces an ampullopetal (excitatory) deflection of the cupula. This generates an intense apogeotropic nystagmus. Conversely, a head turn toward the impaired ear causes the particles to deflect the cupula in an ampullofugal (inhibitory) manner resulting in the generation of an apogeotropic horizontal nystagmus that is less

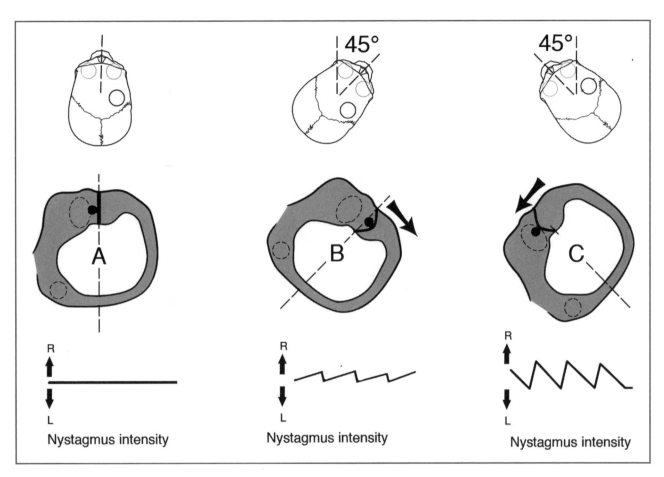

FIGURE 5–20. The mechanism of right-sided horizontal canal cupulolithiasis with the particles located on the utricular side of the cupula in the anterior arm of the canal. **A.** Supine with no nystagmus. **B.** Head turn to the right generates a smaller-amplitude left-beating nystagmus (apogeotropic). **C.** Head turn to the left generates a larger right-beating nystagmus.

intense than when the head is turned toward the healthy side (Asprella Libonati, 2005; Han, Oh, & Kim, 2006; Koo, Moon, Shim, Moon, & Kim, 2006).

Anterior Semicircular Canal BPPV

The assessment of the anterior semicircular canal (ASC) can be done using the traditional Dix-Hallpike maneuver described previously or a straight-back head-hanging maneuver. This has consistently been reported in the literature as one of the rarest forms of BPPV (Herdman & Tusa, 1996; Honrubia, Baloh, Harris, & Jacobson, 1999; Korres et al., 2002). Because of the vertical

orientation of the ASC, it has been suggested that canaliths entering this canal often "self-clear" and migrate into either the vestibule or the PSC (Crevits, 2004). The anterior canal is oriented superiorly with its posterior arm connecting at the bottom of the common crus. Although the Dix Hallpike is the maneuver of choice to evaluate a patient for PSC-BPPV, patients with ASC-BPPV will also commonly manifest nystagmus during this maneuver. The orientation of the ASC is such that when the head is rotated to the contralateral side 45° (as in the Dix-Hallpike maneuver), the ASC canal is oriented in the vertical plane. When the patient is placed in the head-hanging position, the ampulla is located anteriorly with the posterior

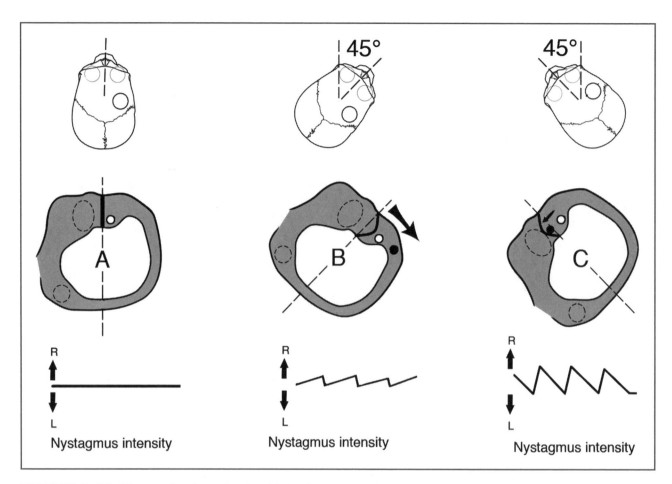

FIGURE 5–21. The mechanism of right-sided horizontal canal canalithiasis with the particles located on the canal side of the cupula in the anterior arm of the canal. **A.** Supine with no nystagmus. **B.** Head turn to the right generates a smaller amplitude left-beating nystagmus (apogeotropic). **C.** Head turn to the left generates a larger right-beating nystagmus.

arm located inferiorly. With this orientation of the ASC, the canaliths are subject to gravity and are able to drop posteriorly through the canal. A positive response is indicated by vertigo and a torsional/down-beating nystagmus in the supine position directed toward the dependent ear (Figure 5–22). The characteristics of ASC-BPPV are described in Table 5–8 and an example of a VNG recording is presented in Figure 5–23. However, identifying the involved side can be challenging in patients with ASC-BPPV for two reasons. First, the torsional component is typically very small or absent and, therefore, is not as helpful for use in identifying the affected side as is the case with PSC-BPPV (Bertholon, Bronstein, Davies, Rudge, & Thilo, 2002). Second, anatomic differences in

the ASC of patients can lead to the affected side producing larger responses in the ear oriented upward or the ear oriented downward (Crevits, 2004). For this reason, the straight-back head hanging (SBHH) maneuver is a useful alternative to use for the assessment of ASC-BPPV (Yacovino, Hain, & Gualtieri, 2009). During the SBHH, the patient is laid straight back with the head hanging at least 30° below the horizontal plane, thereby aligning the posterior arm of the anterior canal with earth vertical (see Figure 5–23, Position 1 and 2). Using this technique provokes a more robust response than the Dix-Hallpike maneuver in most patients because of the ability to achieve a lower head position (Crevits, 2004). When the head is turned laterally 45° during the Dix-Hallpike maneuver,

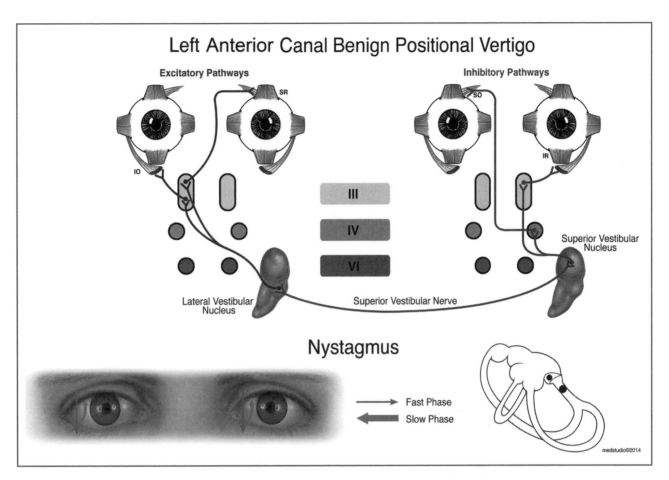

FIGURE 5–22. Figure illustrating left ear anterior/superior canal BPPV and the excitatory and inhibitory receptor connections to the extraocular muscles and the direction of nystagmus. Nystagmus generated by anterior/superior canal BPPV is typically described as a mixed down-beating torsional and vertical eye movement with the upper pole of the eye beating in the direction of the affected ear. In this example, the response is a down-beating nystagmus with a torsional component to the left when the head is placed in the head-down position. When a response is documented the patient should be asked if they perceive the perception of vertigo. When the patient is returned to the upright position, a reversal (typically smaller amplitude and up-beating) of the response may be observable.

Table 5–8. Characteristics of Anterior Semicircular Canal Benign Paroxysmal Positioning Vertigo

Duration	Usually less than 40 s
Direction change	Up-beating when returning to the sitting position
Fatigability	Intensity reduces when the maneuver is repeated
Temporal course	Initial increase in intensity and then slowly declines
Direction of nystagmus	Torsional/down-beating when placed in the provocative position (torsional component may be difficult to identify)

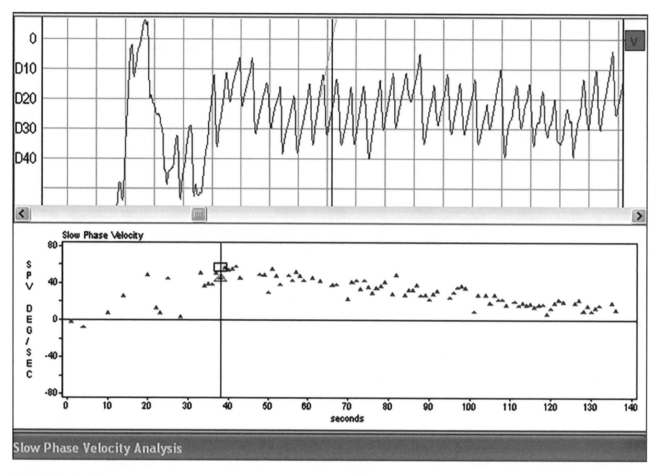

FIGURE 5–23. Down-beating nystagmus recorded during the Dix-Hallpike maneuver in a patient with canalithiasis affecting the right anterior semicircular canal. The top panel illustrates the vertical tracing. Note the abrupt onset and then decline of the response in the lower panel. SPV = slow-phase velocity.

the ability to hang the head vertically is limited. The SBHH maneuver provides appropriate information regarding the disorder in order to prepare the patient for the treatment phase. The examiner must be vigilant to the presence of down-beating nystagmus, as it is also a strong central sign. Down-beating nystagmus must be observed very carefully to differentiate between ASC-BPPV and the more serious form that involves the cerebellum and/or brainstem. Down-beating nystagmus of central origin typically does not have a latent period before the response emerges, and it will not habituate.

Set of Instructions to the Patient

The instructions given to the patient are as follows:

In just a moment, we are going to make believe you are lying down in bed with your head hanging over the edge. I would like you to cross your arms over your chest like this (demonstrate), and then I will count to three. On three, I want you to let me guide you back so that you are lying on your back with your head hanging over the edge of the table. We will stay there for about half a minute. It is critical that you keep your eyes open all of this time. You may or may not have a sensation of movement when you lay down. If you do, it is likely that your eyes will be moving a little bit and how they move tells us which maneuver we need to do to rid you of this positional vertigo. So no matter what sensation you experience please keep your eyes wide open. Are you ready? I will count to 3 and on 3, we will lay back: 1—2—3.

Technique for the Straight-Back Head-Hanging Maneuver

The technique for the SBHH maneuver is as follows:

1. The patient begins the maneuver seated in the upright position and the clinician sits or stands directly behind the patient. It is important to ensure that the patient is oriented so that when he or she is put into the supine position, the head will hang off the edge of the table at least 30°. A thorough questioning of the patient regarding any cervical spine disorders should be undertaken before performing the maneuver.

2. The clinician should have the patient's head oriented straight ahead and ensure that the hands are placed in a position where the neck and head are supported. Before the maneuver is initiated, the patient should be instructed to make sure that he or she keeps his or her eyes open.

3. The examiner lays the patient back and extends the patient's head approximately 30° below the horizontal plane.

4. The examiner observes the patient's eyes for 30 s.

5. The nystagmus should be a primarily down-beating vertical eye movement with a slight torsional component. The torsional component may not always be evident.

6. After the nystagmus stops, the patient should be returned to the upright position. Once the patient is in the upright position, the patient often experiences dizziness again and the eyes reverse direction (up-beating nystagmus).

7. In ASC-BPPV, it is important to document the latency, duration, and amplitude of the response. Locating the affected side for treatment is not as critical and is discussed in the treatment section of this chapter.

Mechanism

The ASC is positioned superiorly over the vestibule with the posterior arm oriented directly over the common crus and the utricle. In theory, any particles that migrate into the ASC should clear on their own when the patient lies supine; however, because of the geometry of the canal in some patients, it is thought that debris can accumulate in the anterior arm near the cupula. During the SBHH maneuver, the head is hung over the end of an exam table aligning the posterior arm with the gravity vector. This allows gravity to act on the particles that are heavier than the surrounding endolymph causing them to move from the anterior arm through the posterior arm toward the common crus. The movement of the particles generates an ampullofugal deflection of the cupula (excitatory response) that activates the vestibulo-ocular reflex (VOR). The ASC sends projections through the brainstem to the contralateral inferior oblique and the ipsilateral superior rectus extraocular muscles. This excitatory activation of the ASC and corresponding contraction of the extraocular muscles produces a down-beating nystagmus.

When BPPV Has Been Diagnosed

The following is an example of how a patient could be counseled in lay terms regarding the mechanism of BPPV:

The inner ear organs of balance function like electrical generators, and there are 5 organs on each side for a total of 10. When you are sitting still, each inner ear system, the left and right ones, produce 1 million electrical signals per second. When the brain receives 1 million signals per second from each side, that is an electrical code that tells the brain you are sitting still. When you turn your head to the right, the electricity from the right inner ear goes up and the electricity from the left inner ear goes down. "High right" and "low left" is an electrical code that tells the brain you are turning your head to the right. If you turn your head to the left, the opposite happens. The electricity from the left inner ear goes up and the right inner ear goes down. "High left" and "low right" is an electrical code that tells the brain you are turning your head to the left. Now if you are sitting still and instead of the brain receiving equal electricity from each side it actually receives low electricity from the left side because disease has damaged the left inner ear, well, that is the code the brain normally receives when the head is turning toward the right (high right, low left). The brain then makes you feel like you are turning. So when you feel like you are moving and are not, that usually means that, at least for a period of time, the electrical output from one of the inner ears has either temporarily or permanently been reduced and the sensation you get because of that change is called "vertigo."

Now let's look a little closer at the organs in the inner ear that produce the electricity. Three of the generators are located in half-circles filled with fluid. As they are half-circles, call these things semicircular canals. Inside each one, there is a device that is like gelatin and it "bends" when fluid pushes up against it. It is the bending of this device by the fluid that makes the electricity go up or down. The device moves when we turn our heads. The last two generators look a little different. They are made of calcium crystals that sit in a "net." Nerve fibers pass through the net up to the crystals. Just like gravel at the bottom of an aquarium would "shift" if we shook an aquarium back and forth or side to side, in the same way, the "gravel" in the inner ear shifts from side to side if we accelerate or decelerate in a car or go up and down in an elevator. It is the shifting of the calcium crystals (the "gravel") over the nerve endings that changes the electrical pattern coming from these devices that tells the brain what direction we are moving.

For various reasons, about which we are still not completely clear, these crystals can leave the "net" that normally holds them in place and drift to the semicircular canal system where they cause trouble. The crystals tend to clump together. If they are in the semicircular canal that reacts to forward and backward movement and you tip your head back at just the right angle, because the crystals are heavier than the inner ear fluid they will sink in the semicircular canal pushing the fluid ahead of them and bending the device in the semicircular canal that creates electricity. The result is that the sinking of the crystals in the semicircular canal produces the same electrical code that happens when we are turning, and that is the sensa-

tion we get. We call this positional vertigo because it occurs when we change position of the head or head and body together. It is the most common form of vertigo we see in the clinic, and almost all of the time it does not mean that the person has a serious disease. It is referred to as "benign," "paroxysmal" because the vertigo sensation is big, "positional vertigo" because it occurs when we change the position of the head, or head and body together. We abbreviate this condition as "BPPV."

So, how do we get rid of this problem? Well, we can get rid of the problem if we can find a way to move or "reposition" the crystals to a different part of the inner ear where they cannot cause trouble. There are many different types of "repositioning maneuvers" that have been invented to do just that, and they are referred to as "particle repositioning maneuvers" or "canalith repositioning maneuvers." The one that we choose for you will be customized for which semicircular canal we think the crystals are in.

TREATMENT OF BENIGN PAROXYSMAL POSITIONING VERTIGO

In many instances, BPPV self-remits with no intervention or treatment (Imai et al., 2005); however, some patients seek treatment before the BPPV resolves on its own. In these cases, the clinician can treat the BPPV in the office at the time of the VNG/ENG. The treatment of BPPV is accomplished by using simple and effective maneuvers or exercises designed to move otoconial debris out of the impaired canal(s) and into the utricle where they do not generate aberrant canal responses. The two primary types of treatment that are discussed in the following section are liberatory maneuvers (e.g., Semont, Freyss, & Vitte, 1988) and canalith repositioning procedures (CRP). The purpose of these techniques is to use a set of specific head positions that are based on the anatomy of the vestibular system to dislodge the displaced mass of otolithic debris and move it into a safe part of the end organ. When a treatment is successful, the symptoms of BPPV are resolved because the mass no longer creates abnormal endolymph flow and cupular displacement during head movements.

There are patients that will experience nausea during the treatments and vestibular suppressants can be helpful in these instances. Common medications that are classified as antivertiginous (e.g. Dramamine® or Transderm-Scop®) provide significant relief of symptoms during a canalith repositioning maneuvers (Brandt, Zwergal, & Strupp, 2009).

Posterior Semicircular Canal BPPV

The two most commonly reported CRP treatments for PSC canalithiasis are the modified Epley and Semont maneuvers (Epley, 1992; Semont, Freyss, & Vitte, 1988). Most CRP treatments of PSC-BPPV are based to some degree on Epley's original description of the treatment, with some modifications (Epley, 1992; Parnes & Price-Jones, 1993); however, there are occasions where the clinician encounters a patient who is unable to be treated using the conventional CRP (i.e., shoulder injury or in the morbidly obese). In such cases, the Semont maneuver is an excellent alternative because it has been shown to have a similar efficacy when it comes to treating PSC-BPPV (Cohen & Jerabeck, 1999; Cohen & Kimball, 2005; Herdman, Tusa, Zee, Proctor, & Mattox, 1993; Salvinelli et al., 2004).

Modified Epley Canalith Repositioning Maneuver for PSC-BPPV

The modified CRP for PSC-BPPV is as follows (Figures 5–24A and B):

1. The patient is placed in the upright position with the head turned 45° toward the affected ear (the ear that was positive on the Dix-Hallpike testing).
2. The patient is rapidly laid back to the supine head-hanging position, which is maintained for approximately 90 s, starting when the sensation of vertigo has stopped.
3. The head is turned 90° toward the other (unaffected) side and held for approximately 90 s, starting when the sensation of vertigo has stopped.
4. Following this rotation, the head is turned a further 90° (usually necessitating the patient's body to also move from the supine position to the lateral decubitus position) such that the patient's head is nearly in the face-down position (i.e., nose pointing toward the ground). This position is also held for 90 s, starting when the sensation of vertigo has stopped.
5. The chin is tucked down and the patient is then brought into the upright sitting position, completing the maneuver.

Semont Liberatory Maneuver for Treatment of PSC-BPPV

The procedure for the Semont maneuver for the treatment of BPPV (Figures 5–25A and B) is as follows:

1. The patient is seated on the examination table with legs hanging over the side.
2. The patient's head is rotated 45° toward the unaffected side.
3. While maintaining the head position the patient is quickly moved to the side-lying position.
4. This position is held for approximately 90 s, and then the patient is rapidly moved to the opposite side-lying position without pausing in the sitting position and without changing the head position relative to the shoulder.
5. This position is maintained for 90 s and then the patient gradually resumes the upright sitting position.

Home Treatment Procedure for PSC-BPPV

There are situations where it may be useful to have patients perform their own CRP (e.g., location or frequently recurring BPPV). BPPV has been reported to reoccur in patients at a rate of approximately 15% to 18% (Nunez, Cass, & Furman, 2000; Sakaida, Takeuchi, Ishinaga, Adachi, & Majima, 2003). In fact, there are several reports in the literature documenting that the addition of self-treated BPPV using CRP, in addition to seeing a professional, resulted in better outcomes than just CRP administered in the clinic by the provider (Radtke et al., 2004; Tanimoto, Doi, Katata, & Nibu, 2005).

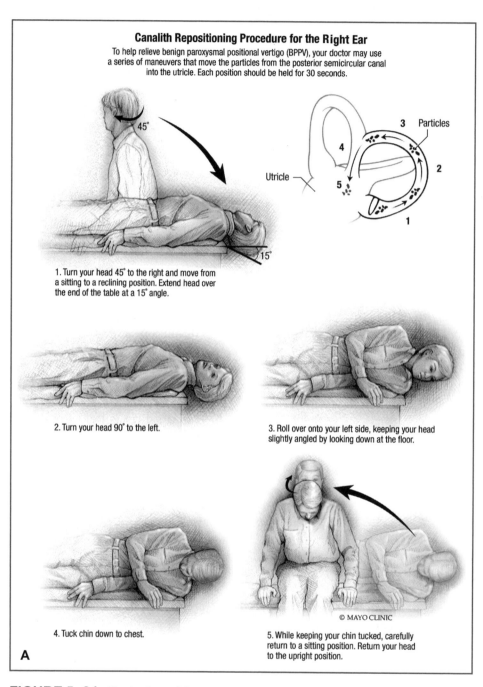

Canalith Repositioning Procedure for the Right Ear

To help relieve benign paroxysmal positional vertigo (BPPV), your doctor may use a series of maneuvers that move the particles from the posterior semicircular canal into the utricle. Each position should be held for 30 seconds.

45°

15°

3 Particles

4

Utricle

5

2

1

1. Turn your head 45° to the right and move from a sitting to a reclining position. Extend head over the end of the table at a 15° angle.

2. Turn your head 90° to the left.

3. Roll over onto your left side, keeping your head slightly angled by looking down at the floor.

© MAYO CLINIC

4. Tuck chin down to chest.

5. While keeping your chin tucked, carefully return to a sitting position. Return your head to the upright position.

A

FIGURE 5–24. Illustration of the canalith repositioning procedure (modified Epley maneuver) to treat right (**A**) and left (**B**) posterior semicircular canal benign paroxysmal positioning vertigo (BPPV). (Used with permission of Mayo Foundation for Medical Education and Research. All rights reserved.) *continues*

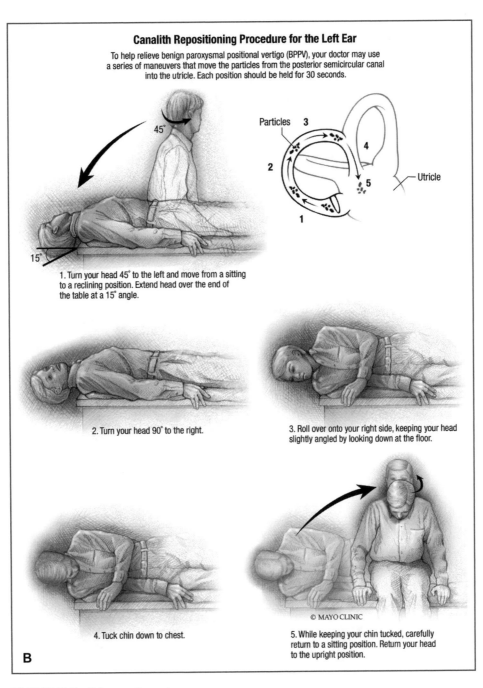

Canalith Repositioning Procedure for the Left Ear

To help relieve benign paroxysmal positional vertigo (BPPV), your doctor may use a series of maneuvers that move the particles from the posterior semicircular canal into the utricle. Each position should be held for 30 seconds.

45°

15°

Particles 3

2

4

1

5

Utricle

1. Turn your head 45° to the left and move from a sitting to a reclining position. Extend head over the end of the table at a 15° angle.

2. Turn your head 90° to the right.

3. Roll over onto your right side, keeping your head slightly angled by looking down at the floor.

4. Tuck chin down to chest.

5. While keeping your chin tucked, carefully return to a sitting position. Return your head to the upright position.

© MAYO CLINIC

B

FIGURE 5–24. *continued*

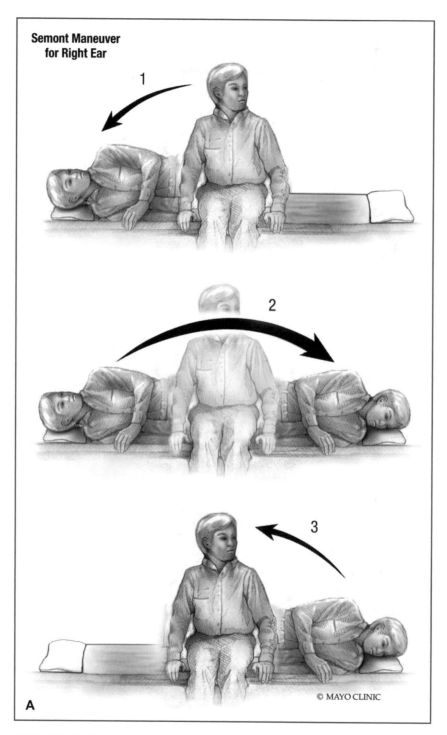

FIGURE 5–25. Illustration of the Semont maneuver used to treat right-sided (**A**) and left-sided (**B**) BPPV. (Used with permission of Mayo Foundation for Medical Education and Research. All rights reserved.) *continues*

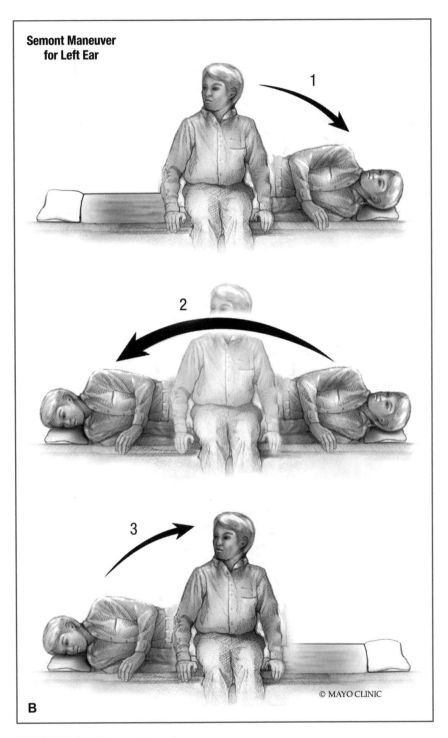

Semont Maneuver for Left Ear

© MAYO CLINIC

B

FIGURE 5–25. *continued*

A recent report by Kim and Kim (2017) described the characteristics of BPPV (i.e., canal and type) in patients with a recurrent form of the disorder. Specifically, they sought to determine if patients with recurrent BPPV have a tendency to develop BPPV that is similar to the initial type, or if it is a different. Their findings revealed that only 24% of the reoccurrences of the BPPV were the same as the previous type. That is, if patients had used a self-applied CRP to address the same form of BPPV as the initial episode they were diagnosed with, they would have been incorrect 76% of the time. This discordance between types of BPPV in patients with a recurrent form of the disorder suggests that providing the patient with a clear understanding of how to identify the canal and side of the BPPV is critical. Below is the method recommended CRP to self-identify and treat posterior canal BPPV. The self-applied modified CRP for left and right PSC-BPPV is as follows (Figure 5–26).

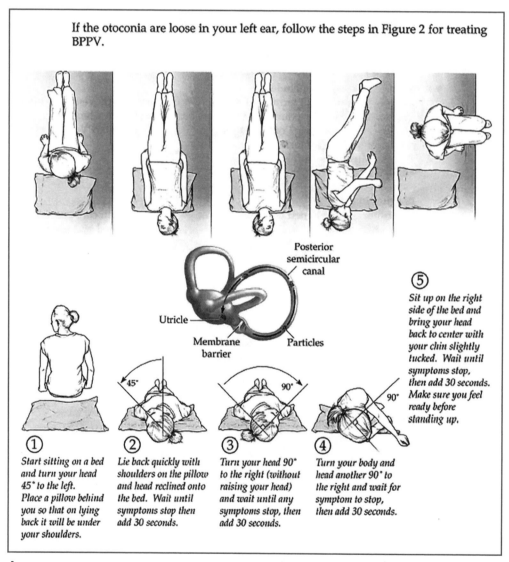

FIGURE 5–26. Illustration of self-treatment of posterior canal benign positional vertigo for the left (**A**) and right (**B**) ear. (Used with permission of Mayo Foundation for Medical Education and Research. All rights reserved.) *continues*

Treatment of Geotropic HSC-BPPV

The geotropic form of HSC-BPPV has been associated with the presence of canaliths in the posterior (nonampullar) arm. The treatment of this variant involves moving otolithic material from the posterior arm of the HSC into the vestibule. At the time of this writing, there is no consensus in the literature regarding the "best" treatment for HSC-BPPV; however, there are two primary canalith repositioning (CRP) methods that have been thoroughly reported. The first method involves positioning the patient in the supine position and then rotating the head and body 270° to 360° (Casani et al., 2002; Lempert, 1994). These types of treat-ments have been referred to as "roll maneuvers" ("log" or "barbeque") and use gravity to move the canaliths in an ampullofugal direction until they reach the vestibule. A second type of CRP has been proposed by Asprella Libonati (2005). This is a liberatory maneuver that has been reported to be successful in treating geotropic HSC-BPPV and has been praised in the literature for both its simplicity and success in treatment.

One reported way to increase the success rate of each of the above CRPs is to employ a technique known in the literature as "forced prolonged positioning" (FPP) (Casani et al., 2002; Nuti, Agus, Barbieri, & Passali, 1998). This method involves having the patient lie on the healthy side

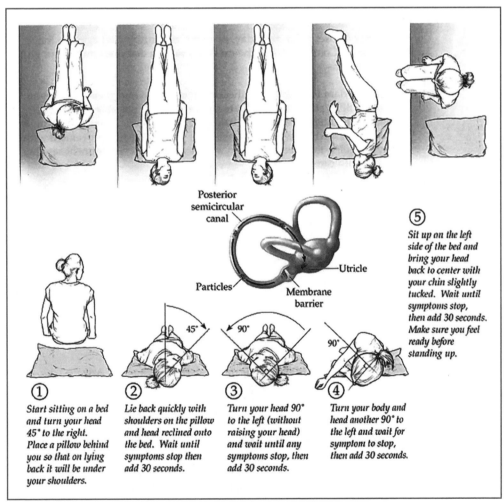

B

FIGURE 5–26. *continued*

for approximately 12 hours (Parnes et al., 2003; Vannucchi, Giannoni, & Pagnini, 1997). Lying on the healthy side aligns the HSC in a manner that subjects it to the pull of gravity (Figure 5–27). The patient maintains this position for approximately 12 hours the night following the CRP (Parnes et al., 2003). Several reports suggest the use of FPP in combination with canalith repositioning maneuvers in order to increase the success rate of treatment. It is also noteworthy that in patients who are unable to undergo a CRP (e.g., patients who experience severe nausea during the maneuvers), the FPP can be used in isolation with a high degree of success (Chiou, Lee, Tsai, Yu, & Lee, 2005).

Lempert 360° Roll Canalith Repositioning Maneuver

The procedure for the roll canalith repositioning maneuver (Figure 5–28) (Casani et al., 2002) is as follows:

1. The patient is placed in the supine position.
2. The patient is rotated 90° onto the side of the healthy ear. The patient is held in the position for 90 s starting when the feeling of vertigo has stopped.
3. A second rotation of 90° is made in the same direction placing the patient in the prone position. The patient is held in the position for

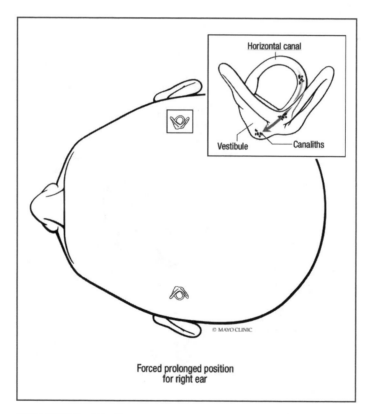

FIGURE 5–27. The "forced prolonged position" for a patient with right-sided horizontal canal BPPV. Note how the otolithic debris moves out of the horizontal canal and into the vestibule. (Adapted from Vannucchi et al., 1997; Used with permission of Mayo Foundation for Medical Education and Research. All rights reserved.)

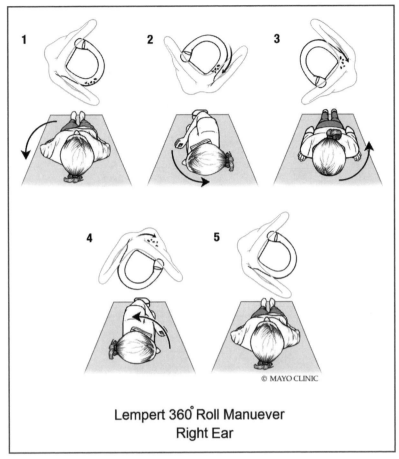

A

FIGURE 5–28. The Lempert 360° Roll (i.e., "barbecue") canalith repositioning procedure in a patient with right-sided (**A**) and left-sided (**B**) horizontal semicircular canal (HSC) BPPV. This maneuver is used in cases where the observed nystagmus is geotropic and the canaliths are located in the posterior arm of the horizontal canal. (From Casani et al., 2002; Used with permission of Mayo Foundation for Medical Education and Research. All rights reserved.) *continues*

90 s starting when the feeling of vertigo has stopped.

4. Another 90° rotation is made in the same direction placing the patient on the side of the impaired ear. The patient is held in the position for 90 s starting when the feeling of vertigo has stopped.

5. The patient finishes the maneuver by making a final 90° rotation when in the supine position. The patient is held in the position for 90 s starting when the feeling of vertigo has stopped.

6. The patient is instructed to sleep in the FPP the night of the CRP.

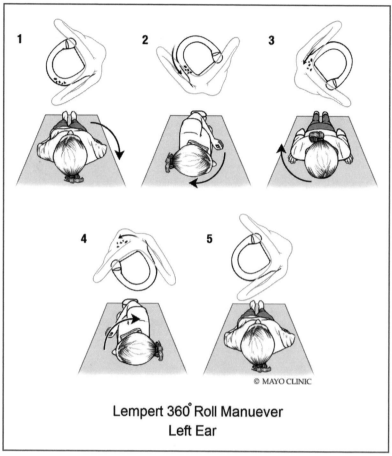

Lempert 360° Roll Manuever
Left Ear

B

FIGURE 5–28. *continued*

Gufoni (i.e., liberatory) Repositioning Maneuver for Geotropic Lateral Canal BPPV (Figure 5–29)

The procedure for the Gufoni repositioning maneuver (Figure 5–29A—left and B—right) (Asprella Libonati & Gufoni, 1999) is as follows:

1. The patient is asked to sit on the exam table with his or her legs hanging over the side, his or her upper arms close to the trunk, and his or her hands on their thighs.
2. The patient is rapidly maneuvered toward the healthy side, and the head is quickly rotated 45° downward.
3. The patient is held in this position for at least 90 s starting with when the sensation of vertigo stops.

4. The patient is brought back up into the sitting position.
5. The patient is instructed to sleep in the FPP the night of the CRP.

Apogeotropic HSC-BPPV

Apogeotropic HSC-BPPV is consistently reported as one of the rarest forms of BPPV and has been proposed to represent the presence of otolithic debris in the anterior (ampullar) arm near or attached to the cupula. This variant of BPPV generates a bidirectional apogeotropic nystagmus during the supine roll test, the mechanism of which is described earlier in this chapter. Apogeotropic HSC-BPPV has been shown in the literature to be more difficult to treat than geotropic HSC-BPPV

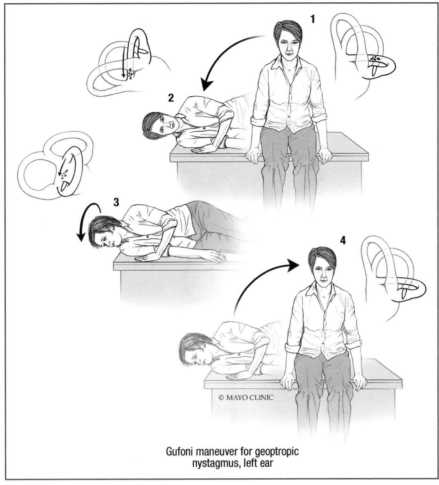

Gufoni maneuver for geoptropic
nystagmus, left ear

A

FIGURE 5–29. Illustration of the liberatory maneuver to treat left (**A**) and right (**B**) lateral semicircular canal BPPV when the observed nystagmus is geotropic. (Used with permission of Mayo Foundation for Medical Education and Research. All rights reserved.) *continues*

(White, Coale, Catalano, & Oas, 2005). This resistance to treatment may be due to the fact that the canaliths are located very close to the ampulla, providing an environment where they can easily adhere to the cupula and create cupulolithiasis. Reports have described three different forms of anterior canal HSC-BPPV. First, the particles can be freely moving in the anterior arm on the canal side of the cupula (see Figure 5–21). In order to treat this form of BPPV, the canaliths must be maneuvered out of the anterior arm into the posterior arm and then into the vestibule. The second variety again involves otolithic matter located on the canal side of the cupula, only the canaliths are attached to the cupula rather than freely moving (cupulolithiasis). In order to treat this form of BPPV, the debris must first be separated from the cupula and then transitioned into the posterior canal and finally the vestibule. The third type involves debris attached to the utricular side of the cupula (see Figure 5–22). In these cases, once the otolithic matter is detached from the cupula, there should be an immediate resolution (the particles migrate directly into the vestibule). Currently, there is no way to differentiate between the two types of cupulolithiasis during the assessment phase.

Once it has been confirmed that the patient has apogeotropic HSC-BPPV, the examiner must

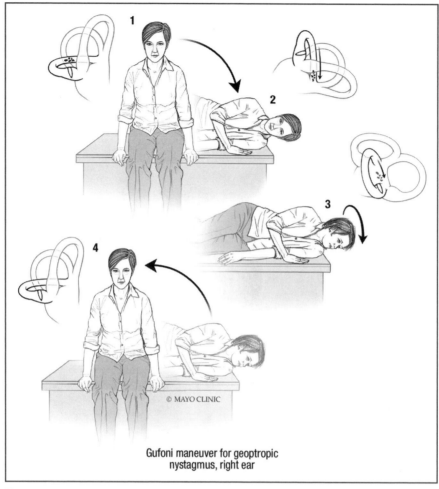

Gufoni maneuver for geoptropic
nystagmus, right ear

B

FIGURE 5–29. *continued*

determine which of the three variants is causing the symptoms. In an effort to differentiate between canalithiasis and cupulolithiasis, the clinician can perform what has been referred to in the United States literature as the "Gufoni" maneuver (Appiani, Catania, Gagliardi, & Cuiuli, 2005; Gufoni, Mastrosimone, & Di Nasso, 1998). This is a CRP designed to migrate freely moving canaliths from the canal side of the anterior (short) arm of the HSC into the posterior arm (Appiani et al., 2005; Gufoni et al., 1998). This has been termed the "conversion" stage of treatment for apogeotropic HSC-BPPV because the direction of the nystagmus "converts" from apogeotropic to geotropic once the canaliths have been relocated into the posterior arm. There have been several methods described regarding how to accomplish the conversion, yet at the time of this writing no consensus has been reached (Appiani et al., 2005; Casani et al., 2002). The Gufoni maneuver is one such method that has been shown to be successful in transitioning the debris from the anterior arm to the posterior arm of the HSC. Other methods that have been shown to facilitate the treatment of apogeotropic HSC-BPPV include head shaking and FPP (Oh et al., 2009; Vannucchi et al., 1997).

Gufoni Conversion Maneuver for Apogeotropic Lateral Canal BPPV

The conversion technique, also known as "the Gufoni for apogeotropic" (Figure 5–30) (Gufoni et al., 1998), is as follows:

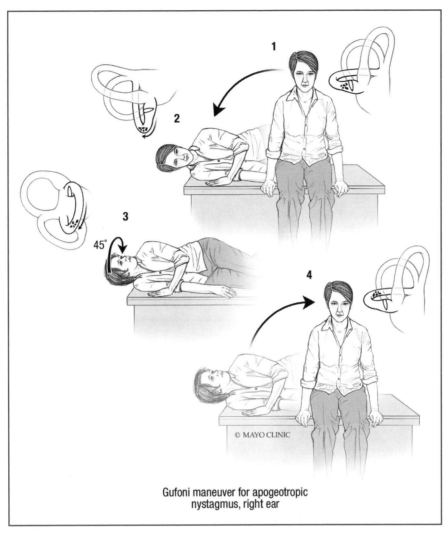

Gufoni maneuver for apogeotropic
nystagmus, right ear

A

FIGURE 5–30. A canalith repositioning procedure ("the Gufoni" for apogeo-tropic lateral canal BPPV) in a patient with right-sided (**A**) and left-sided (**B**) horizontal semicircular canal BPPV. This maneuver is used in cases where the observed nystagmus is apogeotropic and the canaliths are suspected of being located in the anterior arm of the horizontal canal. This maneuver can be used to convert apogeotropic BPPV into geotropic BPPV. (From Appiani et al., 2005; Used with permission of Mayo Foundation for Medical Education and Research. All rights reserved.) *continues*

1. The patient is positioned on the side of the exam table facing the examiner.
2. The patient is then briskly maneuvered into a side-lying position on the affected side. The patient is maintained in this position for 120 s starting once the nystagmus is no longer observable.

3. The patient's head is abruptly turned 45° upward and kept in this position for 120 s following the cessation of nystagmus.
4. The patient is returned to the sitting position for 10 to 15 min.
5. The patient is then positioned supine with the head angled upward 30° so that a supine roll

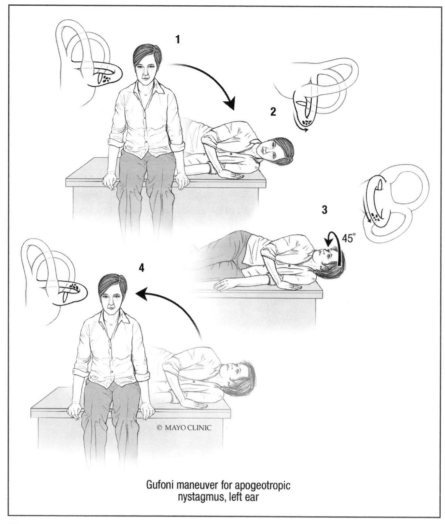

Gufoni maneuver for apogeotropic
nystagmus, left ear

B

FIGURE 5–30. *continued*

test can be undertaken to determine if the conversion was successful.

Following a conversion maneuver, the clinician can determine if it was successful by repeating the supine head-roll test. If lateral head turns generate a response that is geotropic, the conversion is considered successful and the clinician can perform the traditional HSC-BPPV treatments (e.g., roll CRP or Appiani). However, if the nystagmus continues to be apogeotropic, it can be assumed that the patient has a cupulolithiasis variant and the debris needs to be separated from the cupula (Casani, Giovanni, Bruno, & Luigi,

1997). Several procedures have been described in detail regarding how to detach the otolithic debris from the HSC cupula (Casani et al., 2011; Oh et al., 2009). One such method that has been suggested is head shaking. The patient is laid supine on an exam table with the head elevated approximately 30°. The patient's head is rotated back and forth with approximately 30° arc displacement at a frequency of 2 Hz for 15 s. Following this procedure, a Gufoni maneuver can be performed to move the particles from the anterior arm to the posterior arm, where a supine head-roll test can be performed to determine if the symptoms cease with head turns or if there has been a conversion from apogeotropic to geotropic nystagmus. Another method that has shown to detach the canaliths from the cupula is the FPP (Chiou et al., 2005; Vannucchi et al., 1997). When the FPP is indicated in cases of HSC cupulolithiasis, the patient is instructed to sleep on the side with the weaker response. If a supine head roll assessment is conducted following the FPP, a response manifesting geotropic nystagmus should be produced. Once the canaliths are detached, treatment can be accomplished by performing a liberatory or roll maneuver. Particles that detach from the utricular side of the cupula transition directly into the utricle, resolving the BPPV. The investigation of how to best treat apogeotropic nystagmus is still developing. Although this section provides the

background and description of some of the techniques employed, there are numerous other combinations and variations that have been reported in the literature. Figure 5–31 shows a flow chart that outlines how to use the methods described herein to treat apogeotropic HSC-BPPV.

Treatment of Anterior SCC-BPPV

The treatment of HSC-BPPV and PSC-BPPV is the subject of numerous studies; however, there is a paucity of data regarding the treatment of ASC-BPPV. One of the first canalith repositioning maneuvers proposed to treat ASC-BPPV was the "reverse Epley" (Honrubia et al., 1999). This pro-

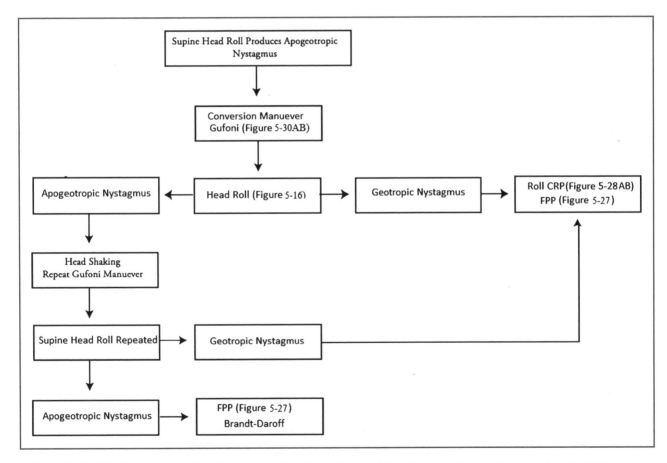

FIGURE 5–31. Algorithm for the treatment of horizontal canal BPPV where the canaliths are located in the anterior portion of the canal (apogeotropic nystagmus observed during the supine roll test). The patient sleeps on the side with the weaker response with the head oriented 45° toward the ground for 12 hours. Head-shaking maneuver: patient's head is moved back and forth 30° in the horizontal plane at a frequency of 2 Hz while the patient is supine with his or her head tilted 30° upward. FPP forced prolonged positioning; CRP canalith reposition procedure.

cedure consists of using the same method that is employed to treat PSC-BPPV, only the initial head position begins with the head turned toward the unaffected side rather than toward the affected ear. Following the article by Honrubia and colleagues, several other groups of investigators have described additional CRPs to treat ASC-BPPV based on the biomechanical properties (Crevits, 2004; Rahko, 2002). Kim, Shin, and Chung (2005) evaluated and treated 30 patients with ASC-BPPV. The maneuver is based on the concept that freely floating otoconia within the anterior canal should move away from the anterior canal cupula when the head is rotated away from the affected ear and then lowered at least 30° below the horizontal plane. Kim and colleagues reported that 96.7% of the patients in this group had complete resolution of their symptoms. In a certain percentage of patients presenting with ASC-BPPV, the response will be a down-beating nystagmus, but with a weak or even absent torsional component (Bertholon et al., 2002). Bertholon and colleagues suggested that this occurrence is due to the ASC being oriented primarily in the sagittal plane. In cases where there is little or no torsional component, identification of the affected side can be difficult. However, this method of treating anterior canal BPPV has largely been abandoned due to the studies supporting this approach using only small sample sizes (Korres, Riga, Balatsouras, & Sandris, 2008; Seok, Lee, Yoo, & Lee, 2008). Furthermore, when the anatomy of the canal system is examined, the head positions included in a "reverse" Epley should not be effective in clearing the debris from the anterior canal. Accordingly, the CRP for treatment of posterior canal BPPV that is described earlier in this chapter (see Figure 5–25) can be employed for treatment for anterior SCC canalithiasis (Jackson, Morgan, Fletcher, & Krueger, 2007). Lopez-Escamez and colleagues in 2006 reported that in their sample of 14 patients with anterior SCC canalithiasis, 11 had complete resolution of symptoms after one treatment using the same CRP as that applied to patients with posterior SCC.

Yacovino and colleagues (2009) proposed a therapeutic maneuver that is not dependent on identifying the impaired side.

Technique to Treat ASC-BPPV

The technique to treat ASC-BPPV (Figure 5–32), based on Yacovino et al. (2009), is as follows:

1. The patient is seated on a table facing the examiner.
2. A "deep" head-hanging maneuver is performed so that the head is brought to at least 30° (preferably 45°) below the horizontal plane for 2 min. Keep the patient in this position until there is a cessation of the vertigo and nystagmus.
3. The patient's head is lifted into a supine position bringing the chin to the chest.
4. The patient is brought into the sitting position.

Example of Counseling Following the Repositioning Maneuver

Below is an example of counseling following the repositioning maneuver. This form of counseling is used with the counseling material in Appendix B:

> Your balance testing was entirely normal with the one exception of the benign paroxysmal position vertigo (BPPV). We found it on one side only and we conducted the particle repositioning maneuver that we felt was appropriate to rid you of this problem. For 2 days, try not to do anything that would normally cause you to be dizzy. After 5 days, I would like you to call me at this telephone number and tell me, on a scale of 0 to 100, what percent better do you feel you are on that day compared to this day. Zero percent means that you feel no better on that day than you do today. One hundred percent means that the positional dizziness is completely gone.

Postmaneuver Restrictions

The use of postmaneuver restrictions following the treatment of BPPV has been examined by several groups (Massoud & Ireland, 1996; Roberts et al., 2005). The questions that are asked by investiga-

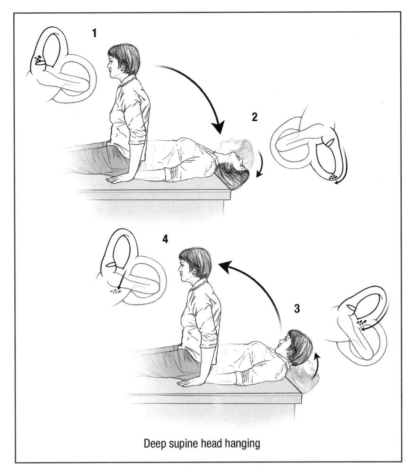

Deep supine head hanging

FIGURE 5–32. A canalith repositioning procedure to treat right and left anterior semicircular canal BPPV. (Adapted from Yacovino, Hain, & Gualtieri, 2009; Used with permission of Mayo Foundation for Medical Education and Research. All rights reserved.)

tors typically center on whether there is any benefit in having a patient keep their head in the upright position for 2 or 3 days following a treatment. The evidence appears to be converging on the decision that these posttreatment instructions are unnecessary (Massoud & Ireland, 1996; Nuti, Nati, & Passali, 2000). For example, in a study by Massoud and Ireland (1996), the investigators evaluated the recurrence rate of BPPV in two groups. Both groups were treated with a CRP or liberatory maneuver and asked to sleep upright for two nights and then sleep on the side of the unimpaired ear for five more nights. The second group was treated using the same methods as the first group but were not

given any posttreatment instructions. The success rate of the treatment procedures were documented at a follow-up appointment 1 week after the treatment. When the investigators compared the success rates between the two groups, there was no statistical difference. More recently, Nuti et al. (2000) examined the success rate of patients treated for BPPV at different time intervals (i.e., 20 minutes, 24 hours, and 7 days). Patients were not given any postmaneuver restrictions, and when reevaluated at 7 days, the vast majority of patients were asymptomatic. The conclusion reached by the investigators was that postmaneuver instructions and restrictions are unnecessary.

When Canaliths Repositioning Maneuvers Are Not Successful

Occasionally there are patients who are unable to be maneuvered through a CRP, or after repeated CRPs, the BPPV persists. In such instances, habituation exercises can be useful. First described by Brandt and Daroff (1980), this treatment for BPPV is able to be performed at home by the patient. The time course for resolution of BPPV using this technique has been reported to take longer than when a conventional CRP is used (Radtke, Neuhauser, von Brevern, & Lempert, 1999).

Brandt-Daroff Exercises for ASC-BPPV and PSC-BPPV

The Brandt-Daroff exercises for ASC-BPPV and PSC-BPPV are as follows:

1. The patient begins by sitting upright and turning his or her head 45° toward the healthy ear.
2. The patient is moved into the side-lying position on the side of the impaired ear keeping the head turned 45°.
3. The patient is kept in the side-lying position until the symptoms of vertigo subside.
4. The patient returns to the original sitting position and remains there for 30 s.
5. The patient turns their head in the opposite direction of step 1 (toward the impaired ear) and moves rapidly into the side-lying position toward the healthy ear.
6. This sequence of exercises is typically recommended to be performed three times (e.g., morning, noon, and night) per day with five repetitions until the vertigo is eliminated.

The Brandt-Daroff exercises can also be modified for BPPV affecting the horizontal SCC. Herdman and Tusa (2007) have described a modified Brandt-Daroff exercise where the same set of procedures as described above is followed. The modification relates to the fact that the head is kept facing forward (not turned 45°) when the patient is moved into the side-lying position. The exact mechanism that results in the Brandt-Daroff exercises resolving the symptoms of BPPV is currently unknown. There are three primary theories regarding how Brandt-Daroff exercises work (Herdman & Tusa, 2007). First, it has been suggested that the movement of endolymph causes the displaced otoconia to eventually dissolve. This may also be why BPPV often remediates without any treatment. Second, the central vestibular nervous system adapts and suppresses the erroneous responses being generated by the peripheral vestibular system. Third, the debris is disconnected from the cupula and moved into a part of the vestibular system where it can no longer generate aberrant responses.

Recurrent BPPV

A certain percentage of patients that are successfully treated for BPPV have a recurrence of the symptoms. Nunez, Cass, and Furman (2000) reported that in their population of patients who reported complete resolution after treatment, there was a recurrence rate of 26.8%. The course of action taken to address the patient with recurrent BPPV depends on a number of patient factors as well the accessibility of the clinician. The ideal method of treatment is to have the patient come back to undergo another assessment and CRP; however, there is a population of patients who continue to present with frequently recurring episodes of BPPV. In these instances, it is often disruptive for the patient to have to schedule an appointment for treatment each time a new instance of BPPV arises. Patients who have continually recurring BPPV should be referred to a physician specializing in dizziness. One alternative to having the patient come for treatment with each recurrence is to train the patient to conduct the canalith repositioning maneuver at home (Furman & Hain, 2004; Radtke et al., 2004; Tanimoto, Doi, Katata, & Nibu, 2005;).

Surgical Treatment for BPPV

There are instances where repeated canalith repositioning maneuvers or habituation exercises are unsuccessful in treating the positioning vertigo or the reoccurrence of symptoms. This can have a significant impact on a patient's quality of life and in rare cases, a surgical treatment may be considered for those patients with intractable BPPV. There are two primary surgical treatments that can be considered for these cases. First, it is possible to transect the posterior ampullary nerve innervating the posterior canal. This technique is referred to in the literature as a singular neurectomy. Second, the posterior semicircular canal can be plugged (i.e., posterior semicircular canal occlusion) (Leveque et al., 2007). These two techniques have been shown to be effective in controlling the symptoms associated with intractable BPPV and are accompanied by a low risk of postoperative hearing impairment (Agrawal & Parnes, 2001; Pournaras, Kos, & Guyot, 2008). These techniques, of course, should be recommended after all traditional rehabilitative approaches have been exhausted.

6

The Caloric Test

INTRODUCTION

The caloric examination is widely considered to be the most technically challenging subtest of the VNG examination, yet it is often the most informative. The primary advantage of caloric testing is the ability to stimulate each labyrinth separately. This ear-specific quantitative information coupled with the caloric tests' high sensitivity to common vestibular impairments continues to make it an important test in the balance clinic. The caloric test consists of two subtests (i.e., measurement of the caloric responses and fixation suppression), each of which evaluates distinctly different processes. If the responses are absent to the caloric irrigations, the ice water caloric test is commonly administered. This chapter describes each component of the caloric test and the role it plays in the VNG/ENG battery.

CALORIC STIMULATION OF THE VESTIBULAR SYSTEM

As is described in Chapter 1, the vestibular system is naturally sensitive to head movements; however, many quantitative vestibular assessments utilize nonphysiologic stimuli (e.g., acous-tic or thermal) to evoke calibrated responses from the end organs. With regard to the caloric test, it was Robert Barany in 1907 who first provided a description of how to do the caloric test, as well as the hypothesis that described the underlying mechanism of how it stimulated the inner ear of balance (Hood, 1989). When water, with a temperature above or below normal body temperature, is infused into the external auditory meatus, the temperature of the skin and tympanic membrane is either warmed or cooled. The lateral semicircular canal is sensitive to any temperature variations in the external auditory canal because of its close proximity to the middle ear space. Specifically, any change in temperature from normal body temperature is conducted through the middle ear space to the vestibule (Harrington, 1969). The physiologic mechanism underlying this test is that the temperature gradient induced by the irrigation results in a change in the specific gravity of the endolymph in the lateral semicircular canal on the side that is irrigated. The clever ability to unilaterally drive the firing rate above or below its baseline using a medium of different temperatures enables the clinician to generate asymmetries in the firing rates of the vestibular system and drive the VOR, as is discussed in Chapter 2. In Barany's original description of the caloric test, he noted that the test should be performed with the patient supine and the head elevated 30° (Figure 6–1A). When the head is oriented in this position, or if the

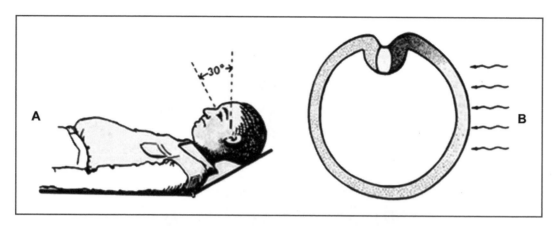

FIGURE 6–1. A. The 30° supine position for caloric testing that places the horizontal canals into a vertical position for maximal stimulation during caloric testing. **B.** An illustration of how endolymph rises during a warm caloric irrigation. (From Barber & Stockwell, 1976)

head is flexed 60° backward, the lateral semicircular canals are oriented vertically and placed in line with the gravity vector.

When the medium that has a temperature higher or lower than the body is introduced into the external auditory canal, the endolymph in the part of the lateral canal closest to the middle ear space is heated. When a fluid is heated, its density is lowered. A good example of this is when water is boiled. As the water is heated and begins to boil, it turns into steam and rises. So heat lowers the density of the water (makes it less heavy) and causes it to rise (Figure 6–1B). In the case of the caloric examination, the heat is diffused through the middle ear space and heats the endolymph in the portion of the lateral canal closest to the irrigation. As the heated endolymph rises, it is replaced by cooler (more dense) endolymph, which is in turn heated and its density lowered. This process of fluid motion, termed "convection current," goes on until the irrigation (stimulus) is terminated.

Introduction of a warm medium results in an excitatory response in the labyrinth on the side of the irrigation. As is described in Chapter 2, the cupula in the lateral semicircular canal has the same density as the surrounding endolymph, and the stereocilia that are embedded into the base of it are all oriented toward the utricle. Figure 6–2A illustrates what happens when we infuse a warm water stimulus into the external ear on the left side. As the endolymph near the middle ear space becomes lighter, it rises. This in turn pushes cupula toward the utricle, depolarizing the hair cells in the cristae, and increases the tonic-resting rate in the nerve above its baseline activity. This direction of movement of the cupula in the lateral semicircular canal has been termed "utriculopetal" and it mimics a head turn toward the irrigated ear (excitatory). With this type of response, a nystagmus is generated with fast phases beating toward the ear being irrigated.

In the case of a cool irrigation, the density of the endolymph is increased (becomes heavier) and it begins to sink where it is, and then it is replaced by lighter endolymph, again setting up a convection current, only this time in the opposite direction (Figure 6–2B). This type of endolymph movement deflects the cupula away from the utricle, which initiates a hyperpolarization (inhibitory) of the cells in the cristae on the irrigated side and a corresponding decrease in the firing rate of the vestibular nerve below its baseline-resting rate. The deflection of the cupula away from the utricle has been termed "uticulofugal" and mimics a head turn away from the stimulated side. The VOR response in this case is a nystagmus with the fast phase beating away from the irrigated ear. One easy way to remember the relationship between the temperature and the direction of the nystagmus is to employ the mnemonic "COWS":

Cold—Opposite   Warm—Same.

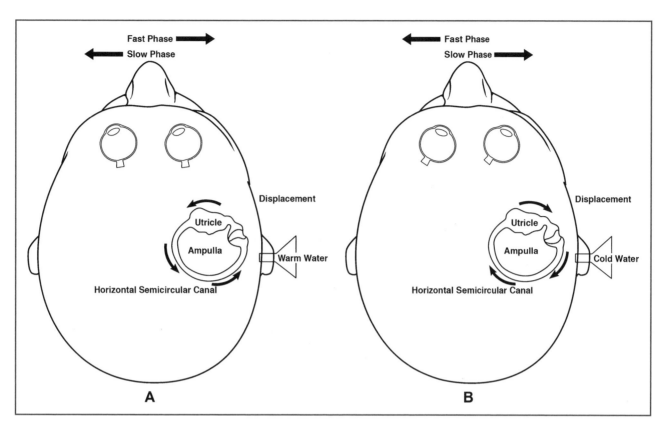

FIGURE 6–2. The movement of endolymph in the lateral semicircular canal and the associated eye movements following a warm (**A**) and cool (**B**) caloric irrigation.

For the most part, Barany's original hypothesis set forth in 1907 is correct; however, experiments following his initial explanations of the caloric effect have modified to some degree the theory regarding the exact mechanism. There is no question that the change in the density of the endolymph is a major contributor to the generation of the response. In an elegant series of experiments, Coats and Smith (1967) showed that the caloric response reverses when a patient is tested with their face pointing toward the ground (prone) versus lying on their back (supine). In the prone position, the lateral canals are also oriented vertically, only this time they are inverted with respect to the supine position described previously. If a medium of sufficient temperature is introduced into the external auditory meatus, the portion of the lateral canal nearest the middle ear space is heated. As in the supine position, the endolymph becomes lighter, starts to rise, and presses on the cupula. When the subject is in the prone position, an upward movement of the cupula bends it away from the utricle and the characteristics of the vestibular nystagmus are such that the fast phase beats away from the irrigated ear. Furthermore, when a cool irrigation is administered with the patient in the prone position, a nystagmus with the fast phase beating toward the irrigated ear can be observed. Coats and Smith (1967) reported this reversal of the caloric response in different head positions further confirming Barany's original hypothesis that the caloric response is dependent on gravity. The frequency of the caloric stimulus has been calculated to be approximately 0.003 Hz. Figure 6–3 shows a slow-phase velocity profile of a caloric response and illustrates the support for this assertion. The time course for the caloric induced nystagmus, beginning with the onset of the nystagmus to where it disappears, is approximately 140 s. The velocity profile of one caloric response

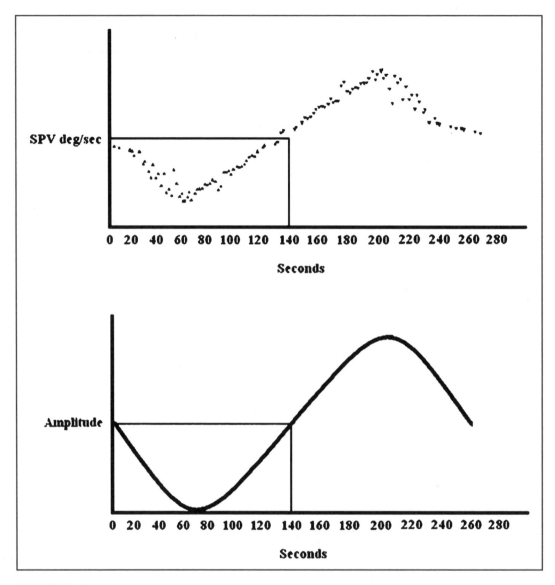

FIGURE 6–3. Illustration of a velocity profile of a caloric response showing the origin of the assertion that a caloric stimulus results in a response akin to a rotational frequency of 0.003 Hz. SPV, slow-phase velocity. (From McCaslin & Jacobson, 2009)

could represent a half cycle of a sine wave, and thus a full cycle would be twice as much (280 s). The reciprocal of 280 s is 0.004 Hz, which is very close to the reported 0.003 Hz. Coats and Smith (1967) also reported a difference in the amplitude of the response with head position. Specifically, the authors suggested that there is a second contributor to the caloric response that is not dependent on gravity. The authors proposed that this secondary component of transduction within the lateral canal system is associated with ther-

mal stimulation of the vestibular nerve itself. To further explore this concept, the origin of caloric stimulation warranted its own experiment on the Spacelab-I, which was a laboratory that traveled in the space shuttle's cargo bay. This allowed the caloric response to be evaluated in a weightless atmosphere. The idea was that if changing the weight of the endolymph is the only source of the caloric response, then in a zero gravity environment there should be an absent response. In fact, caloric nystagmus was elicited in space following an irrigation, proving that there are additional contributors to the response (e.g., firing rate of the nerve is increased when it is exposed to a temperature warmer or cooler than body temperature) (Scherer, Brandt, Clarke, Merbold, & Parker, 1986).

COMPONENTS OF THE CALORIC TEST

The primary advantage of the caloric test is the information it affords the clinician regarding the physiologic integrity of the right and left horizontal semicircular canals (HSCs) and superior vestibular nerves. The caloric test was originally described by Schmiederkam in the 1860s when he observed that following the irrigation of a patient's ear with water, he could evoke vestibular nystagmus. Barany (1907) is credited with being the first to employ the caloric test to make diagnostic statements regarding the vestibular system. This was later followed by Jung and Mittermaier (1939) describing how to quantify the nystagmus by measuring it via the corneoretinal potential, and plotting it for offline analysis. Today's contemporary caloric test consists of two primary components. First, following the irrigation of the external auditory canal with a caloric stimulus, vestibular nystagmus is generated. This peripherally driven response builds to a crescendo and then decays. The examiner typically performs an offline analysis and measures the peak amplitude of the reaction. Second, once the caloric response peaks in amplitude, a measure of vestibulo-ocular (VOR) reflex suppression is taken. Following the "peak" of the caloric response, the fixation-suppression test should be initiated. When a neurologically intact patient is instructed to fixate on a stationary target during the caloric response, the amplitude of the nystagmus attenuates. This phenomenon has been alternately termed "fixation suppression," "VOR suppression," or "VOR cancellation."

Occasionally, a patient is encountered where the conventional caloric irrigation does not produce a measurable response from the ear, and it is in these situations that the ice water test is administered (Proctor, 1992). The ice water test is most commonly used to determine if there is any residual function in the ear(s) that did not produce a response during the standard bithermal caloric examination. Ice water approaches a temperature near 10°C while the body maintains a temperature of approximately 37°C (a difference of 27°C), compared with the difference realized by the standard cool caloric irrigation (a difference of 7°C).

INSTRUMENTATION

Caloric Irrigators

At the time of this writing, there are two primary types of caloric irrigators available for the caloric test. Each of them has the ability to deliver a calibrated stimulus into the external auditory meatus. The most common irrigator at the moment is the air irrigator, followed by the water caloric irrigator. A third, less common, type of irrigator system known as a closed-loop water system was developed by Kenneth Brookler and Guenter Grams. Most irrigators sold today have a thermostat to control and monitor the temperature of the caloric stimulus, a flow meter to control the output of the medium, and a timer. In some instruments, the irrigator communicates with a computer that starts and stops the test, and records the caloric response as well.

Air Irrigators

While the caloric test has been around since the 1800s, the air irrigator was not commercially available until the mid-1900s (Coats, Herbert, & Atwood, 1976). Most air irrigators are composed of a similar set of components. First, air irrigators typically have an air pump enclosed in the system. Air can also be supplied from a wall source (e.g., larger, tertiary medical centers often have these). As the air is pumped through the system, it must be heated or cooled. In order to heat the air, Peltier thermoelectric devices are commonly used. These systems run electrical current through a junction between two different metals and, thereby, heat the air. The amount of heat that is produced depends on the voltage being applied. A thermistor housed in the delivery head samples the temperature of the air and adjusts the voltage to ensure that the air leaving the system is correct. When a cool caloric stimulus is desired, air irrigators often employ radiators. The air is passed through water-filled coils and cooled. Most air irrigators have a small reservoir that holds the water used in this process. The air is typically delivered to the external ear canal using a handset with a tube running through an otoscope specula (Figure 6–4).

Although air irrigators are by far the most widely used irrigation systems, they are not without controversy. Numerous reports exist citing the limitations of the caloric responses induced by air (e.g., less caloric capacity than water) (Bock & Zangemeister, 1978). For example, the air caloric has been reported to be extremely variable, unreliable, and incapable of generating sufficiently strong responses to measure with any degree of accuracy (Greven, Oosterveld, Rademakers, & Voorhoeve, 1979; Torok, 1979; Zangemeister & Bock, 1980). Reports such as these resulted in the air caloric test not being included in the ANSI standards (ANSI, 1999). Recommendations for the air caloric test were, however, published by the British Standards Association (BSA) in 1999.

A recent article by Zapala, Olsholt, and Lundy (2008) suggests that when carefully calibrated, air and water caloric tests elicit similar outcomes. The authors established a method for delivering air irrigations that generated caloric responses equivalent to those produced by water. The recommendations provided by this study and the BSA are presented in Table 6–1 and should be considered when establishing normative data for the caloric test.

Water Irrigators

Contemporary water irrigators routinely consist of two reservoirs that store the water for the warm and cool irrigations and a pumping system to deliver the water to the ear. The temperature of the water held in the "baths" is constantly monitored and kept at predetermined irrigation temperatures. Most systems have a foot switch, a hand switch, or both to trigger the transfer of water through the system. The trigger typically consists of a solenoid switch that begins and ends the flow of water based on the settings of a timer. Once the switch is activated, the irrigation is started and the pump begins to move the water from the reservoirs to the head of the delivery system (Figure 6–5). The volume of water being pushed through the system is regulated by a series of valves with settings to increase or decrease the flow rate. It is this elaborate system of valves and tubes that make using distilled water preferable to tap water. Tap water often contains traces of organic material that can accumulate over time and result in costly maintenance fees. Another important point is that

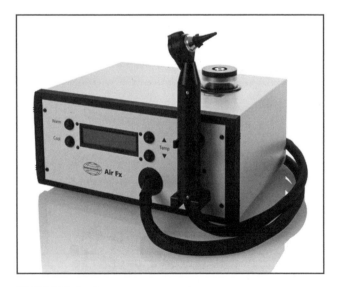

FIGURE 6–4. An example of an air irrigator is shown.

Table 6–1. Air Caloric Recommendations

	BSA (1999)	Zapala et al. (2008)
Temperature (°C)	50/24 (±0.4)	51/21
Duration (s)	60 (cool)	60 (warm)/70 (cool)
Volume (L)	8 (±0.5)	8

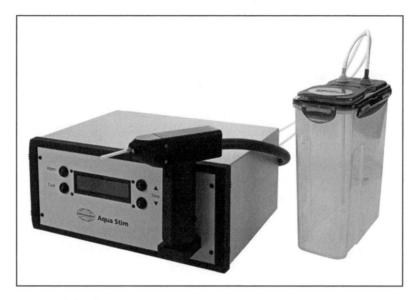

FIGURE 6–5. An example of a water irrigator is shown.

many water irrigators monitor and adjust the temperature at the level of the baths and not at the delivery head. The hoses that connect to the delivery head are often insulated in order to maintain the temperature of the water as it travels through the irrigator. An understanding of the workings of the irrigator the clinician is using is necessary to avoid pushing standing water that is not the correct temperature into the ear canal. There are some water irrigators that continually circulate the water through the delivery hose. These types of systems ensure that the clinician is ready to irrigate the ear at any point during the exam because the temperature of the water in the hose is continually the same as in the baths. If the irrigator does not continuously circulate the water, it may be necessary to "purge" or run one or two irrigations immediately before administering the caloric stimulus to the patient.

The ANSI and BSA have provided recommended parameters for water irrigations (Table 6–2). Both sets of recommended parameters generate robust caloric responses in the majority of patients, and currently there is no universal agreement on the duration of the stimulus or the flow rate. Each clinic should develop its own normative data or use normative values provided by studies employing similar stimulation techniques.

Table 6–2. Recommended Parameters for Water Irrigations

	BSA (1999)	*ANSI (1999)*
Temperature (°C)	44/30 (±0.4)	44/30 (±0.5)
Duration (s)	30	40 (±1)
Volume (ml)	250 (±10)	200 (±20)

PREPARATION FOR THE CALORIC TEST

One of the inherent limitations of the caloric test is that the responses are dependent on a multitude of factors, some of which the clinician cannot control. It is the examiner's responsibility to prepare for, and address controllable factors (e.g., blocked ear canal) and interpret uncontrollable factors (e.g., tympanic membrane perforation) correctly. In order to accomplish these tasks, the tester must have a thorough knowledge of the patient's medical history, a sense of the level of the patient's anxiety, and the current medications that the patient uses.

Inspection of Ear Canals

Prior to caloric testing, the clinician should take a thorough case history. An otoscopic inspection of the ear canal should be performed to identify any anatomic abnormalities (e.g., tympanic membrane perforations or mastoid bowls) for consideration during the analysis and interpretation of the responses. During the otoscopic examination, it is not uncommon for the clinician to discover debris in the ear canal. The most common form of debris that is encountered in the external auditory meatus (EAM) is cerumen. Prior to the caloric irrigation, earwax that significantly occludes the EAM should be removed. A blockage of the ear canal can impede the flow of the irrigation medium and alter the thermal properties of the stimulus being transferred to the lateral semicircular canal. The two most common techniques for removing debris from the EAM are through the use of a curette (Figure 6–6) or water irrigation. The irrigation method of clearing the canal is appropriate in cases where a water stimulus is being used to induce the caloric response. Clinics employing air caloric irrigators must be cautious

when water is used to clear the ear canal before the caloric test. When warm air is used as the caloric stimulus following a water irrigation, the residual irrigation fluid in the EAM is vaporized. Evaporation is a cooling process, and even though warm air is being delivered into the EAM, the evaporative cooling process produces a decrease in temperature in the EAM. This drop in temperature is radiated through the middle ear space to the vestibule and generates a nystagmus with the fast phase beating toward the nontest ear (Barin, 2008a), opposite the direction that a warm irrigation response normally beats. An otoscopic examination can also provide insight into the size and the shape of the ear canals. Occasionally, patients have extremely tortuous canals that can impede the flow of the air or water through the EAM and produce abnormally reduced caloric responses.

Immediately following the otoscopic examination, the patient should undergo immittance audiometry (tympanograms). The tympanogram provides the examiner with information regarding the status of the middle ear, as well as a volume measure of the external ear canal. This can be helpful in confirming that both labyrinths receive equivalent stimulation.

Instructions to Patient

Prior to irrigating the ear, the patient should be informed as to exactly what is going to happen during the caloric test. Patients have a higher tolerance for the procedure if they know what to expect and that any sensation experienced will not last long. It is often helpful to send information to the patient prior to the appointment detailing what tests will be performed and what they involve. In most clinics, the caloric test is the last part of the examination, and trust should be established by this point. It is not uncommon for a patient to be apprehensive before the caloric test. If a family member or friend accompanied them to the appointment, it can be helpful to have them stand next to the patient or hold their hand. A thorough case history and scores from the Hospital Anxiety and Depression Scale (HADS) (Zigmond & Snaith, 1983) can be helpful in predicting how a patient will react to either the irrigation or

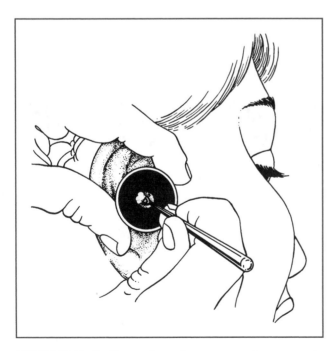

FIGURE 6–6. Illustration of curettage of cerumen is shown. (Illustration by Mary Dersch from Pender, 1992, with permission of Daniel Pender)

the sensation of motion during the response. In instances where the patient exhibits a high level of anxiety, the test can be modified accordingly (e.g., more time between irrigations). The following is an example of how the professional sets the expectations for a patient before the caloric examination is initiated:

> What I am trying to measure is what percent stronger one inner ear of balance is compared with the other. The only way we can do that is by changing the temperature of the fluid that is in the inner ear. To do this I am going to run some warm (cool) water in your outer ear for about 25 s. The water will be warmer or cooler than your body temperature. Warming your outer ear will change the temperature of the inner ear fluid by a fraction of a degree. This will make the inner ear fluid move a tiny bit, and that normally happens when you move your head. When you move your head, your eyes move. So, for about 1 min, I am going to fool your brain into "thinking" your head is moving when it isn't. That will make your eyes move and that is what I am measuring that will tell me how strong your inner ears of balance are. So you may feel like your head is moving a little bit. If you have that sensation, just know that it is short-lived. It will be important for you to keep your eyes open (for VNG; closed for ENG). I will be asking you some questions and watching your eyes for approximately a minute and a half after the water/air stops.

PROCEDURE FOR CONDUCTING THE ALTERNATING BINAURAL BITHERMAL CALORIC TEST (WATER AND AIR)

Preparation of the Patient

After the patient has been given instructions regarding the caloric test, the eye movement recording system should be calibrated (refer to Chapter 4 for a complete review of calibration). The BSA (1999), Committee on Hearing, Bioacoustics, and Biomechanics (CHABA, 1992), and ANSI (1999) standards all provide the recommendation that for ENG recordings, a recalibration should occur prior to each caloric irrigation; however, although this continual recalibration is necessary for ENG, it is not necessary for VNG. When VNG is employed as the recording technique, an initial calibration should be done prior to any testing. Because the video system tracks the pupils, there should be no need to recalibrate the system unless the goggles have been moved. It is often the case that patients ask to remove the goggles between irrigations or adjust them to increase comfort. In these instances, a recalibration of the VNG system is necessary; however, as discussed in Chapter 4, the recording of eye movements using ENG is more technically challenging because of the dynamic nature of the CRP. Specifically, the calibration procedure must be routinely performed throughout the entire test because the strength of the CRP changes over time and is increased by light (Jacobson & McCaslin, 2004). Several manufacturers of computerized VNG/ENG equipment enable the CRP value to be extracted from the calibration data. This allows the clinician to measure the CRP value and determine if the amplitude is sufficient to generate a clear recording (see Chapter 5 for a detailed explanation). Every effort should be made to ensure that the CRP is stabilized before each caloric is initiated.

The most common caloric test position is with the patient laying supine with their head ventroflexed 30°. This orientation aligns the HSCs in the vertical position where the convection current maximally deflects the HSC cupula. If water is being used as a caloric stimulus, a dental towel can be placed immediately under each ear to avoid getting the patient wet if water spills from the basin, and to give the examiner something upon which to rest the catch basin so that both hands are free. Before the caloric irrigation is delivered, visual fixation must be eliminated. If ENG is being used, the examiner should instruct the patient to close their eyes. ENG can be administered with eyes open if the test room is completely dark or if the patient wears goggles to occlude vision. Having an examination room that is completely devoid of light is rare and a potential risk for the examiner (e.g., falling or tripping). When utilizing VNG as the recording method, vision can be eliminated by placing a cover or shield over the front of the goggles. Any light source that is visible to the patient can be fixated on and thereby reduce the caloric responses. The examiner must also be knowledgeable about how much light can leak into the goggles that are being used.

Precaloric Search for Spontaneous Nystagmus

A search for spontaneous nystagmus (SN) should be performed before the first irrigation is administered and while the patient is in the caloric position (head ventroflexed 30°) (Figure 6–7). The patient's eye movements should be recorded in darkness while undergoing "alerting exercises." If any SN is observed over a 30-s period, its characteristics (e.g., nystagmus velocity and direction) are noted and documented for the final caloric analysis.

CALORIC TEST TECHNIQUE

Caloric Response

Following the precaloric search for SN, the clinician should position themselves at a point where he or she has ready access to the ear canal and it is clearly visible. Prior to beginning the irrigation, another set of instructions should be given and the recording system started. In order to reduce the anxiety of the patient, the examiner should provide an ongoing dialog describing exactly what is happening in the room. Below is an example of an instruction set that could be used immediately before delivering the irrigation:

> I am holding the tube that will run the water (air) into your ear. The water (air) may feel hot, but the ear is sensitive and it should not be painful. I am going to count to three and then the water (air) will begin to run into your ear. Try not to move or jerk your head away when the water (air) enters your ear. The water (air) will run into the ear for 25 s and we will record your eye movements for approximately 2 min afterward. Remember to keep your eyes open (closed if using ENG) and try not to blink too much. I am going to ask you some questions during the test and just do your best to answer them. Here we go . . .

If water is being used for stimulation, the irrigation will continue for 25 s (60 s for air). Immediately following the end of the irrigation, "alerting exercises" should ensue. Tasking consists of a set of questions (e.g., give me a boy's name that starts

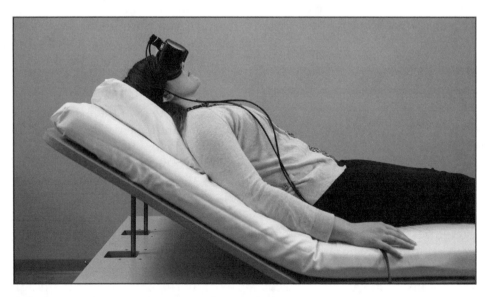

FIGURE 6–7. A patient prepared for caloric testing. Note that the patient is positioned with the head flexed forward approximately 30°.

with "A") that the patient must think about but can answer easily (a sample list is provided in Appendix D). The process of alerting the patient is critical to obtaining valid recordings for analysis. Patients that are not sufficiently alerted may produce caloric responses that are intermittent or are of insufficient amplitude for analysis. In fact, the process of simply focusing on an imaginary target has been shown to significantly reduce VOR responses (Barr, Schultheis, & Robinson, 1976; Jones, Berthoz, & Segal, 1984). The examiner should be prepared to change the task or speed of the questions if the patient is unable to respond quickly. Approximately 60 to 90 s after the irrigation is administered, the caloric response peaks and then begins to decline (i.e., the slope of the slow phase becomes less steep) (Figure 6–8).

Fixation Suppression

It is important that the fixation-suppression test be administered immediately after the peak caloric response is reached. This requires that the examiner continually monitor the ongoing caloric response in order to identify when the response reaches its maximum intensity. Depending on the system available and the mode of recording, different methods can be used to perform the test. If ENG is being used to record the response, the tester can simply have the patient open their eyes and fixate on a stationary target (Figure 6–9). If VNG is being used for the test, the same method as used for ENG can be used (i.e., lift the cover and fixate). Most contemporary VNG goggles have light sources inside the goggle system that can be activated during the recordings. The patient should fixate on the target for a period of at least 15 s, and the beginning of when the patient began to fixate on the target and when vision was once again denied should be marked on the recording (Figure 6–10). One must be careful not to do the fixation-suppression test too early. If fixation suppression is initiated during a point in the caloric reaction where the peak response occurs, the test will be subject to misinterpretation. To the author's knowledge, there is only one system that monitors the amplitude of the caloric response, identifies the peak, and then informs the clinician when it is appropriate to begin the fixation suppression test. According to Alpert (1974), the fixation-suppression test should be administered for both directions of nystagmus. In most instances, the clinician will evaluate a patient's fixation suppression during the response following the two warm irrigations (e.g., a fixation measure for right warm and left warm). One important technical note is that in order to compare fixation suppression between sides, the measurement should be taken at the point where the caloric responses have similar nystagmus intensity. For example, in cases where a warm irrigation is significantly

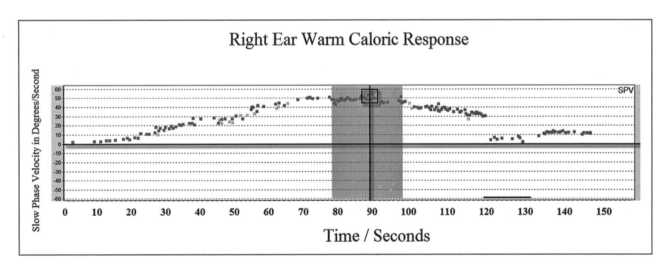

FIGURE 6–8. An example of a slow-phase-velocity profile of a warm caloric response delivered to the right ear. The dots represent the measured amplitude (in degrees per second) of the slow phase of each beat of nystagmus. The box indicates the peak of the caloric response.

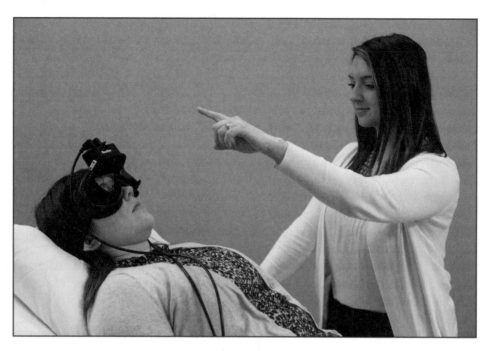

FIGURE 6–9. The fixation suppression test. The patient is asked to orient her gaze on the examiner's finger. This test is initiated immediately following the peak of the caloric response.

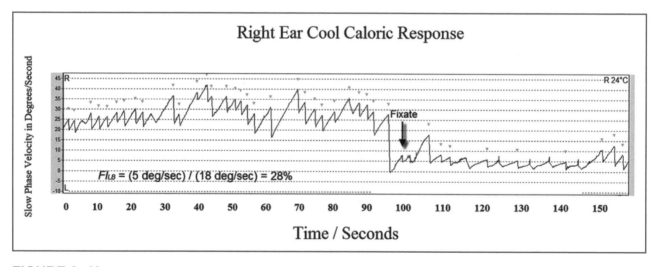

FIGURE 6–10. An example of fixation suppression during a caloric response.

larger than the other, it may be impossible to perform the suppression test at a point of equivalent nystagmus intensity. Similarly, in cases where there is a significant bilateral weakness (extremely small caloric responses bilaterally), there may be little or no nystagmus to suppress and the test in these cases the test is uninterpretable.

Ice Water Caloric Examination

When the caloric responses to standard bithermal stimuli are absent, the ice water test is employed to determine if there is any residual low-frequency function in the test ear(s). The ice water test is conducted with very cold water (i.e., 10°C).

Water this temperature can be obtained by placing sterile ice in a cup and then filling it with water (Figure 6–11).

To ensure patient cooperation the test should be explained in detail prior to the irrigation. The patient should be placed in the standard caloric position and then instructed to turn his or her head so that the test ear is facing upward. A 2-cc syringe can be used to draw water out of the basin. The examiner should then pull the pinna up and back to straighten the ear canal and then gently fill the ear canal with the water (Figure 6–12). After 20 s, the head should be turned so that the water runs out of the ear canal. The patient should then be provided alerting tasks and the eye movements recorded for at least 60 s. If nystagmus is recorded following the irrigation, and SN has been identified previously that beats in the same direction as the caloric response, the clinician needs to determine whether the response is the SN or a caloric-induced response. This can be accomplished by having the patient change from a supine (face

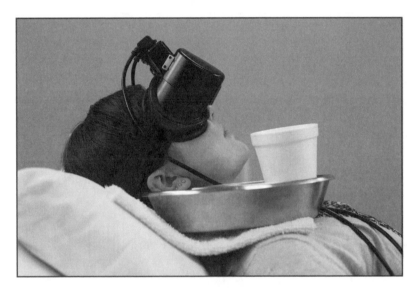

FIGURE 6–11. A patient prepared for the ice water test is shown.

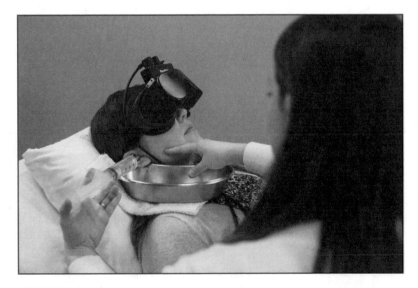

FIGURE 6–12. A patient being irrigated with 2 cc of ice water is shown.

up) to a prone position (face down) with the head hanging downward 30° (Figure 6–13). Each of these positions effectively places the lateral semicircular canals in a position that is parallel to the gravity vector. If the test ear has residual function, that is, if the observed response (nystagmus) is a reaction to the caloric irrigation, it should reverse direction. A change in the direction of the response with a change in the position of the patient suggests that the irrigated ear has some degree of function.

Procedure

The procedure for the ice water caloric examination is as follows:

1. Irrigate the ear using ice water (i.e., 10°C).
2. After 20 s, turn the patient's head and drain the water out of the ear canal. The patient's head should be in the primary caloric position.
3. Record the patient's eye movements while looking for caloric-induced nystagmus with

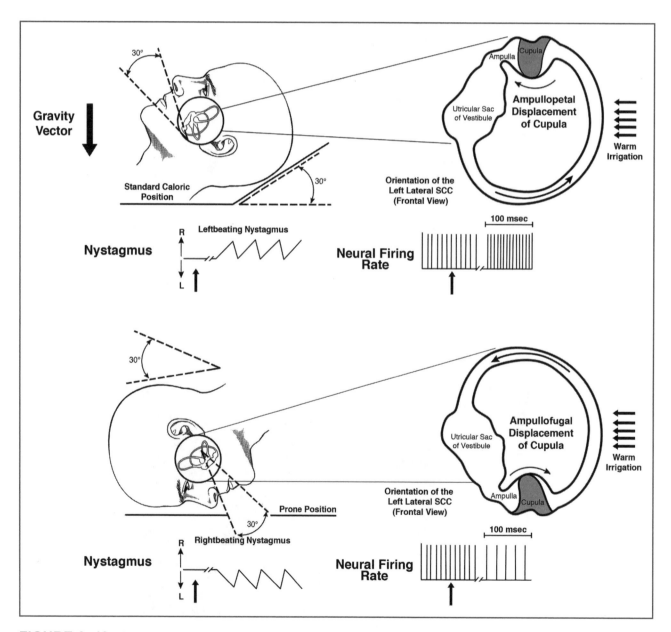

FIGURE 6–13. Caloric response in two different head positions. *Top:* Supine with the head flexed forward 30° (primary caloric position). *Bottom:* Prone with the head hanging downward 30°. (Adapted from Barin, 2009)

vision denied for 40 s. Alerting should be performed for the duration of the recording.

4. Next, move the patient into the prone position (face down) with the head hanging downward 30°. Record the eye movements again with vision denied and mental alerting for another 40 s. Record any change in the nystagmus.

5. The patient should be returned to the primary caloric position.

ANALYSIS OF CALORIC RESPONSES

It has been reported that the velocity of the slow phase component of nystagmus taken at the peak of the caloric response is the most useful variable to quantify the reaction (ANSI, 1999; Jacobson, Newman, & Peterson, 1993). According to Jacobson et al. (1993), slow-phase velocity (SPV) of the caloric response can be reported as an average of one of the following four techniques:

1. During the peak of the caloric response, the three beats of nystagmus with the greatest SPV

2. An average of the SPV of all the beats of nystagmus collected during a 5-s period

3. An average of the SPV of all the beats of nystagmus collected during a 10-s period

4. Ten beats obtained at the peak of the caloric response (no time interval specified)

The velocity profile of the caloric response has a characteristic shape when the SPV is plotted on the ordinate and time in seconds on the abscissa. Most commercial VNG systems have either a manual or automatic option for identifying and measuring the velocity of each beat of nystagmus. Once the irrigation begins, most systems are triggered to start recording. The velocity profile of the caloric response begins to increase in amplitude approximately 20 s following the onset of the irrigation. The response reaches its peak amplitude at approximately 60 to 90 s and then begins to decline. The envelope of this response reflects the heat entering and leaving the lateral semicircular canal. In most instances, the caloric response is immeasurable at 3 min. When interpreting the caloric test, a series of analyses can be performed that can answer several questions regarding the status of the peripheral vestibular system and the associated central connections. The questions related to these analyses are given in Table 6–3.

Most systems for recording nystagmus plot all four caloric responses on the display simultaneously

Table 6–3. Measurement Parameters and Questions Regarding the Peripheral Vestibular System

Measurement Parameters	Questions
Unilateral weakness	Are there interaural (left versus right ear) differences in slow-phase velocity nystagmus?
Directional preponderance	Is there a bias in the direction of the responses (e.g., is right-beating nystagmus always larger than left-beating nystagmus)?
Fixation index	Can the central nervous system appropriately exert control over the vestibular nuclei and reduce amplitude of the caloric nystagmus with visual fixation?
Hypofunction	Is the total of all four caloric responses abnormally low?
Hyperfunction	Is the total of all four caloric responses abnormally high?

so that each can be compared with the other. The SPV plots of the caloric response have been termed "pods" because of their lenticular shape (Figure 6–14). Although many computerized recording systems automatically perform the analysis outlined in this section, it is important for the clinician to understand what the equations are and how they are used. In this section, the variables and measurement parameters used to analyze caloric responses are discussed. The following is how each of the caloric responses is represented in the analysis section (Table 6–4).

Calculation of Total Caloric Response

In order to ensure that the final interpretation of the caloric responses is accurate, the clinician must first determine the sum of the total peak SPV of all four irrigations. When the total peak SPV of the four caloric responses (LW, RW, LC, and RC) is extremely low (e.g., below the 95% lower limit for normal patients), the calculations of traditional caloric parameters is not applicable. In other words, when it is determined that the patient demonstrates significantly reduced responses bilaterally, the clinician should not perform any additional analysis (e.g., unilateral

weakness or directional preponderance measures). This is because very small changes in small caloric responses can result in large changes in the traditional symmetry formulas increasing the likelihood of misinterpretation. To calculate the total caloric response, the peak SPV for each caloric response needs to be assigned and then entered into the following equation:

$$\text{Total caloric response} = RW + LW + RC + LC$$

To determine if a bilateral weakness is present, the clinician must have a set criterion. Several studies of minimum caloric strength have been reported with various conclusions. Barber and Stockwell (1980) suggested that if a patient's total

Table 6–4. Caloric Responses

Caloric Response
Left warm (LW)
Right warm (RW)
Left cool (LC)
Right cool (RC)

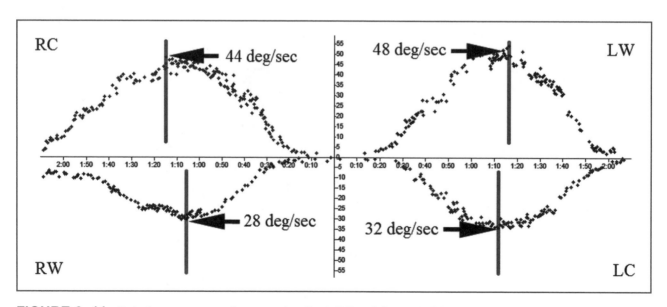

FIGURE 6–14. Caloric responses of a normal patient. RC = right cool; RW = right warm; LW = left warm; LC = left cool.

caloric response is <30° per second, a bilateral weakness exists. Jacobson and Newman (1993) have suggested a total caloric response of <22° per second before a patient is considered to have significant bilateral hypofunction. The British Standards Association (1999) operationally defines a bilateral weakness as an examination where each of the four irrigations is <8° per second. Barin (2008a) has suggested incorporating elements from both the Barber and Stockwell (1980) and Jacobson and Newman (1993) to calculate bilateral weakness. Barin (2008a) requires that the total response for both temperatures from each ear be less than 12° per second (Table 6–5). An example of a patient with a bilateral weakness is presented in Figure 6–15.

Calculation of Hyperactive Responses

The total caloric response can also be used to determine if the caloric reactions are too large. Caloric responses that exceed the upper limits of normal are classified as hyperactive. The reported criterion varies from maximum SPVs greater than 40° per second to 80° per second. In the classic text by Barber and Stockwell (1980), a response was qualified as hyperactive if the responses to warm irrigations exceeded 80° per second and cool responses exceeded 50° per second. Jacobson et al. (1993) suggest using the following criterion for defining hyperactive caloric-induced nystagmus (Table 6–6).

Table 6–5. Criteria for Bilateral Weakness

Criterion	Response (degrees/second)
Total right ear peak response (RW + RC)	<12
Total left ear peak response (LW + LC)	<12

Source: From Barin (2008a).

Table 6–6. Criteria for Hyperactive Responses

Criterion	Response (degrees/second)
Total cool peak response (LC + RC)	>99
Total warm peak response (LW + RW)	>146
Total peak response (LC + RC + LW + RW)	>221

Source: From Jacobson et al. (1993).

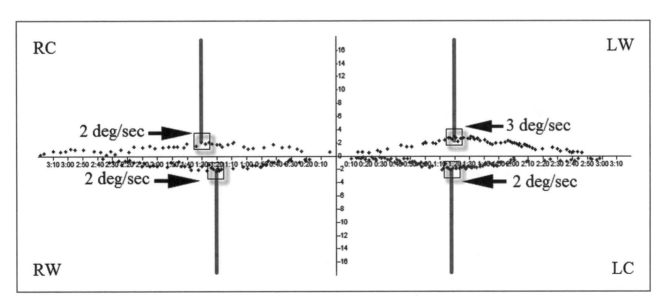

FIGURE 6–15. Caloric responses of a patient with a significant bilateral vestibular system weakness. Total slow phase velocity = 9° per second. RC = right cool; RW = right warm; LW = left warm; LC = left cool.

Calculation to Determine Symmetry of Function (i.e., Unilateral Weakness)

If the patient does not demonstrate a bilateral weakness, then it is appropriate to continue with further analysis of the caloric responses. The following calculation first proposed by Jongkees and Philipszoon (1964) is designed to compare the difference in caloric responses from the right ear with those from the left ear. The numerator contains the total left ear peak SPV minus the total right ear peak SPV and the denominator is the total peak SPV of all responses summed. This final value is multiplied by 100 to yield a percentage difference. This percentage has been termed a "unilateral weakness" and expresses to what degree the caloric responses from the two ears are different. A positive symmetry value indicates that the left ear is weaker than the right, and a negative number indicates that the right ear is weaker than the left. A unilateral weakness of 100% indicates that there was no measurable caloric response from one of the ears, and a unilateral weakness of 0% indicates that the responses from the two ears were perfectly symmetric (i.e., both ears had the same total SPV for warm and cool caloric responses). When a unilateral weakness is reported it refers to the ear that is weaker (e.g., a right unilateral weakness would be a symmetry measure with a negative number).

The percentage of unilateral weakness is calculated as follows:

$$\text{Unilateral weakness (\%)} = \frac{(LW + LC) - (RW + RC)}{(RC + RW + LC + LW)} \times 100$$

Directional Preponderance

When the standard bithermal caloric test is administered, there are two responses that produce right-beating nystagmus (i.e., right warm and left cool) and two responses that produce left-beating nystagmus (i.e., left warm and right cool). In normal individuals, all four of these responses should be approximately equal in amplitude; however, in some instances a patient demon-strates responses that are stronger in one direction than the other. This phenomenon was originally described by Fitzgerald and Hallpike (1942) and is known as a directional preponderance (DP). According to the equation, a positive number is totaled when the caloric responses that produce right-beating nystagmus are stronger than those producing left-beating nystagmus. A negative DP is calculated when the left-beating responses are stronger than right-beating responses, and a value of 0 indicates that they are equal. A DP is conventionally reported in terms of the direction in which the nystagmus is strongest (e.g., if the number is positive, then the patient is reported as having a DP to the right). There are two primary conditions that contribute to the finding of a significant DP. The first, and by far the most common, is the presence of a pre-existing nystagmus that is present with vision denied. The second type is uncommon and has been reported in the literature by Halmagyi et al. (2000) as a "gain asymmetry." Both types of DP must be accounted for in the analysis of the caloric data in order for the clinician to accurately interpret the responses.

The equation for calculating the DP percentage is as follows:

$$\text{Directional preponderance (\%)} = \frac{(RW + LC) - (LW + RC)}{(LC + LW + RC + RW)} \times 100$$

Fixation Suppression

The fixation index (FI) is a ratio of nystagmus before and after a patient fixates on a target. Demanez and Ledoux (1970) described this calculation as an assessment of the inhibitory interaction that occurs between the midline cerebellum and the vestibular nuclei. The FI should be calculated once for each direction of nystagmus generated by the caloric response (e.g., right warm and left warm). The process for analyzing the FI consists of the following steps:

1. Identify a 5-s time period just before fixation occurs.

2. Identify a 5-s period after fixation ends.
3. Identify and measure three beats of representative nystagmus in each of the 5-s time periods. If there is no visible nystagmus, its intensity should be qualified 0.
4. Calculate the FI percentage.

The FI percentage is calculated as follows:

$$FI\ (\%) = \frac{SPV\ eyes\ open}{SPV\ eyes\ closed} \times 100$$

Monothermal Warm Caloric Screening Test

The Jongkees and Philipszoon (1964) equation can be adapted to provide a symmetry measure for two warm caloric responses called the monothermal warm screening test (MWST). This screening test of caloric function not only reduces the amount of time required for testing but also can be useful in cases where a patient is unable to continue the test after two irrigations. Although the use of two cool irrigations has been reported on as a potential screening measure, it is beyond the scope of this book to discuss them. The MWST was first described by Barber, Wright, and Demanuele, (1971), and its performance as a screening measure has since been described in various ways by a number of different groups (Enticott, Dowell, & O'Leary, 2003; Jacobson, Calder, Shepherd, Rupp, & Newman, 1995; Jacobson & Means, 1985; Murnane, Akin, Lynn, & Cyr, 2009). The MWST has been shown to demonstrate a high sensitivity and high specificity for predicting the outcome of the bithermal test if a simple set of rules are followed. Jacobson and Means (1985) presented a set of criteria for when it is appropriate to use the MWST (Table 6–7).

Monothermal warm is calculated as follows:

$$Monothermal\ warm = \frac{RW - LW}{RW + LW} \times 100$$

INTERPRETATION OF CALORIC RESPONSES

Unilateral Weakness

In the author's clinic, a significant unilateral weakness is operationally defined as an interaural difference in peak SPV of >22% (Mayo Clinic-Rochester normative data criterion). A significant right unilateral weakness is illustrated in Figure 6–16. The physiologic mechanism of a unilateral weakness stems from an asymmetry in the neural input entering the two vestibular nuclei from the peripheral vestibular system following caloric stimulation. The asymmetry in neural drive to the VOR sets up a situation where the intensity of the caloric-induced nystagmus is larger from the intact side and smaller from the impaired side. Once the responses exceed a difference of greater than 22%, they fall outside the criterion of normal (two standard deviations from a normal mean caloric response) and a patient

Table 6–7. Criteria for When to Perform the Monothermal Warm Caloric Screening Test (MWST)

No abnormalities identified during any subtests leading up to the caloric examination.
An MWST can be performed only if each of the warm irrigations exceeds 11° per second.
It is understood that an alternate binaural bithermal caloric examination is performed if the difference between sides exceeds the critical upper limits (i.e., 25% for Jacobson and Means [1985] or 10% for Murnane et al. [2009]).
The fixation suppression test is performed during each warm caloric response.

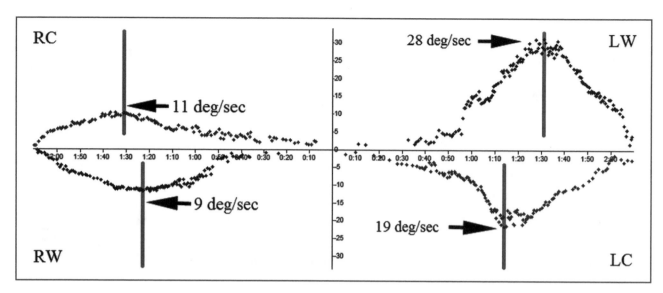

FIGURE 6–16. Caloric responses of a patient with a significant unilateral vestibular system impairment on the right side. RC = right cool; RW = right warm; LW = left warm; LC = left cool.

can be said to have significant peripheral vestibular system impairment. In the case of the caloric examination, "peripheral" refers to structures distal to the vestibular nuclei. This includes the lateral semicircular canal, the superior portion of the vestibular nerve, and the root entry zone of the superior vestibular nerve. In most instances, when a unilateral weakness is identified it can be tracked back to an impairment in one or more of these structures; however, while the caloric test provides lateralizing information (i.e., it can identify the impaired side), localization between the lateral semicircular canal, superior portion of the eighth cranial nerve, and root entry zone is not possible.

Calculation of caloric weakness for the responses illustrated in Figure 6–14:

$$\text{Unilateral weakness (\%)} =$$

$$\frac{(28 + 19) - (9 + 11)}{(11 + 9 + 19 + 28)} \times 100$$

$$= 40\% \text{ right caloric weakness}$$

According to Barber and Stockwell (1980) a unilateral weakness without significant spontaneous nystagmus (>6° per second) is the most common abnormality encountered during VNG

testing. These patients often present with symptoms such as the following:

1. Quick head movements that create disorientation
2. Complaints of drifting one way or the other when walking and bumping into people walking next to them
3. A clear event of severe vertigo that may have initiated a visit to the emergency room
4. Hearing loss and ringing in one ear

Once the alternate binaural bithermal test is completed and the unilateral weakness is identified, the examiner should confirm that it is a "true weakness" and not due to some technical error or artifact. During the interpretation of the responses the clinician must be confident that the patient was appropriately alerted during each of the caloric tests and that the irrigations were equivalent. Issues related to confirming that the caloric responses are valid are briefly covered in the "Technical Tips for Caloric Testing" section of this chapter. Once any artifacts or examiner errors have been ruled out, it is safe to document that the patient has unilateral vestibular system impairment on the weak side.

Summary: Unilateral Weakness Abnormalities

The criterion for unilateral weakness abnormalities is >22% asymmetry between the right and left-side maximum slow-component velocity (based on Mayo Clinic-Rochester normative data). The location of impairment is the unilateral labyrinth, superior portion of the superior vestibular nerve, or root entry zone. It is important to rule out as the cause improper irrigations, lack of alertness, and medications.

Interpretation of Directional Preponderance

The clinical utility of the DP has been debated because of the initial article containing the equation by Jongkees and Phillipzoon (1964). To date, there are two commonly accepted variants of DP (Barin, 2008a). The first variant is observed in patients with a significant degree of SN and is by far the more common. The second type of DP was detailed in a report by Halmagyi, Cremer, Anderson, Murofushi, and Curthoys (2000) and occurs in the absence of SN. The authors have termed this type of DP as "gain asymmetry." The following two sections describe how each type of DP should be approached during analysis and the necessary measures that should be taken to account for it in the final interpretation.

Directional Preponderance in the Presence of Spontaneous Nystagmus

When a unilateral weakness is identified along with significant SN, the analysis becomes more challenging. Spontaneous nystagmus with the slow phase beating toward the side with the impairment is often a sign that the impairment is acute. The very presence of SN implies that compensation mechanisms have not yet equilibrated the neural activity arriving at the vestibular nuclei (one peripheral system is producing more neural input than the other and aberrantly driving the VOR). Patients who have incurred a loss of peripheral vestibular function typically complain of vertigo and/or severe unsteadiness. What is important to account for when interpreting caloric test results from a patient with SN is the effect that the SN has on the peak amplitude of the caloric reaction. Given that peripherally generated SN is direction fixed, caloric responses that generate nystagmus beating in the same direction as the SN are larger (response sums with the SN) than those responses beating in the direction opposite the SN (Fitzgerald & Hallpike, 1942). If the SN is of sufficient amplitude, a significant DP is observed. In the pretest section of this chapter, the technique for searching for pre-existing nystagmus is described. If a significant SN (>6° per second) is identified prior to the caloric examination, it needs to be accounted for during the analysis of the caloric responses. In other words, the examiner must document the amplitude of the SPV of the SN and correct for it in order to provide a true representation of the status of the patient's peripheral vestibular function. The effect of SN on the caloric profile can be described in terms of what happens relative to the recording "baseline." In most instances (not all), a patient with no SN will have a "baseline" near 0. When a caloric stimulus is administered to a patient with no SN, a response emerges at approximately 20 s causing a shift in the baseline activity (either up or down). A patient with a pre-existing SN does not have a starting baseline of 0. Because nystagmus (spontaneous) is present prior to the stimulus being delivered, the system registers this response and the starting baseline is shifted up or down relative to the direction and amplitude of the SN. This concept is illustrated in Figure 6–17.

Calculation of the directional preponderance for the responses illustrated in Figure 6–17:

$$DP\,(\%) = \frac{(\text{Total RB}) - (\text{Total LB})}{(\text{Total RB}) + (\text{Total LB})}$$

$$= \frac{(0) - (38)}{(0 + 38)} \times 100 = 100\%\ DP\ \text{to the left}$$

SN should always be accounted for in the final analysis of the caloric responses. Traditionally, the influence of SN on caloric is corrected for by adding or subtracting it from the peak response of the reactions. When SN is identified, its amplitude (in

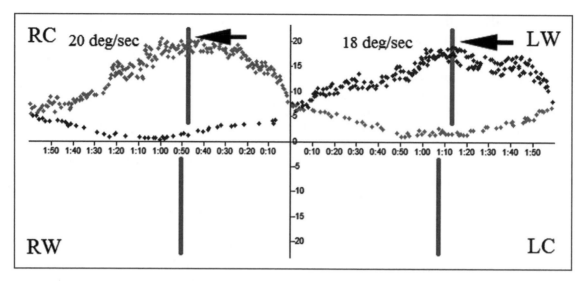

FIGURE 6–17. An example of a significant directional preponderance in a patient with left-beating spontaneous nystagmus. Note that the baseline is shifted 7° to the left (i.e., expressed with respect to the direction of spontaneous nystagmus fast phases). Peak SPV peak slow phase velocity; RC = right cool; RW = right warm; LW = left warm; LC = left cool.

degrees per second) should be calculated by measuring five representative beats over a 20-s period and averaging them. Once the velocity of the SN is calculated, it must be either subtracted or added to each caloric response. The reason for this is that a right-beating SN sums with the response generated by a right warm caloric (right-beating nystagmus) and subtracts from a right cool (left-beating nystagmus). In this way, the SN biases the caloric responses with nystagmus that beats in the same direction. The corrections presented in Table 6–8 can be performed to address the influence of SN and normalize the caloric results. It is noteworthy that some commercially available systems allow the tester to move the baseline up or down during the analysis portion of the caloric profile in order to account for SN (Figure 6–18).

Calculation of the directional preponderance for the baseline adjusted (7° to the left) responses illustrated in Figure 6–18:

$$DP\ (\%) = \frac{(Total\ RB) - (Total\ LB)}{(Total\ RB) + (Total\ LB)}$$

$$= \frac{(14 - 24)}{(14 + 24)} \times 100 = 26\%\ DP\ to\ the\ left$$

Correction for Directional Preponderance When There Is a Gain Asymmetry

Step 1 — Calculate the average baseline asymmetry (BL_{avg}):

$$AVG_{BL} = \frac{(RW_{BL} + LW_{BL} + RC_{BL} + LC_{BL})}{4}$$

A DP resulting from a gain asymmetry creates a dilemma in the final analysis of the caloric data (Figure 6–19). This is because there is no preexisting SN value to subtract or add to the caloric responses. In order to correct the caloric responses in cases of gain asymmetry, an examination of the baseline from each of the caloric responses should be recorded. This can be done by measuring the nystagmus in the first 10 to 15 s of the recording (Barin, 2008a). A baseline average (BLavg) can then be calculated using a fraction where the numerator is the sum of the baseline values from each caloric response divided by total number of caloric response administered (i.e., 4). This BLavg value effectively controls for the effect of gain asymmetry and allows the clinician to accurately interpret the caloric response without any central influence.

It is noteworthy that the following formula for calculating gain asymmetry can also be applied

Table 6–8. Correction for Directional Preponderance for Direction-Fixed Spontaneous Nystagmus (*SN*)

Direction of SN	Caloric Response	Correction
Right-beating SN (degrees/second)	Peak right warm (RW)	RW − SN degrees/second = CPR
	Peak left warm (LW)	LW + SN degrees/second = CPR
	Peak right cool (RC)	RC + SN degrees/second = CPR
	Peak left cool (LC)	LC − SN degrees/second = CPR
Left-beating SN (degrees/second)	Peak right warm (RW)	RW + SN degrees/second = CPR
	Peak left warm (LW)	LW − SN degrees/second = CPR
	Peak right cool (RC)	RC − SN degrees/second = CPR
	Peak left cool (LC)	LC + SN degrees/second = CPR

CPR = corrected peak response.

Note. Once the caloric responses have been corrected for, the SN for the corrected values should be entered into the formula for calculating unilateral weakness and recalculated.

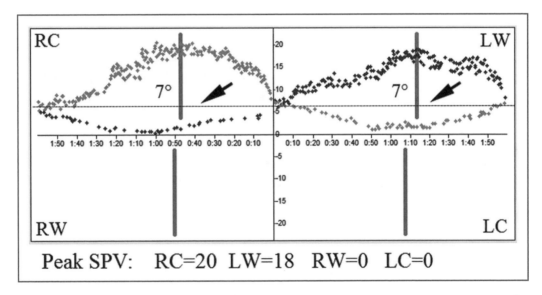

Peak SPV: RC=20 LW=18 RW=0 LC=0

FIGURE 6–18. An example of how the baseline can be moved (*arrows*) to adjust for the spontaneous nystagmus. Baseline average is shifted 7° to the left (corrected for in the accompanying equation). Note how the value of the directional preponderance is reduced following this adjustment. RC = right cool; RW = right warm; LW = left warm; LC = left cool.

to cases where the baseline has been shifted due to the presence of SN (Barin, 2008a).

Procedure to correct for a directional preponderance in the presence of a gain asymmetry:

Step 2—Correct (subtract) AVG_{BL} from each caloric response (Table 6–9).

Step 3—Once the caloric responses have been corrected for, the corrected peak responses should be entered into the gain asymmetry formula (Barin & Stockwell, 2002).

$$\text{Gain Asymmetry (\%)} = \frac{\text{CPR RB} - \text{CPR LB}}{\text{CPR RB} + \text{CPR LB}} \times 100$$

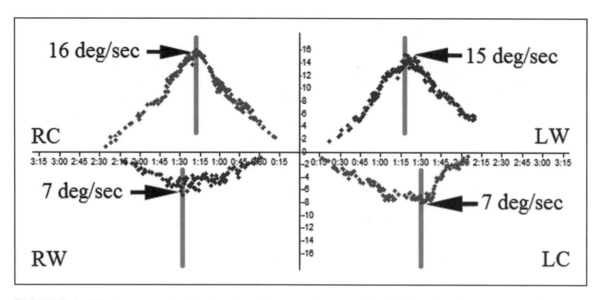

FIGURE 6–19. An example of a directional preponderance with significant gain asymmetry (*arrows*). Note that the baseline is approximately 0. RC = right cool; RW = right warm; LW = left warm; LC = left cool. CPR = corrected peak response.

Table 6–9. Correction for Directional Preponderance When There Is a Gain Asymmetry

Baseline Average (AVG$_{BL}$)	Caloric Response	Correction
Gain Asymmetry	Peak right warm (RW)	RW − AVG$_{BL}$ = CPR
	Peak left warm (LW)	LW − AVG$_{BL}$ = CPR
	Peak right cool (RC)	RC − AVG$_{BL}$ = CPR
	Peak left cool (LC)	LC − AVG$_{BL}$ = CPR
Adjustment for Baseline Shift		
CPR RB = −RW CPR − LC CPR		
CPR LB = RC CPR + LW CPR		

CPR = corrected peak response.

SUMMARY: SIGNIFICANCE OF A DIRECTIONAL PREPONDERANCE

The criterion for a DP is >28% asymmetry between the left-beating and right-beating maximum SPV (based on Vanderbilt normative data). The mechanisms of impairment are interaction of caloric induced nystagmus with SN and enhanced dynamic gain of the vestibular nucleus on the impaired side. It is conventional to report baseline shift in the direction of the higher intensity slow phase. In contrast, a gain asymmetry is reported in the direction of the higher intensity fast phases. To avoid misidentifying the cause of DP, it is important to rule out improper irrigations.

Interpretation of VOR Fixation Suppression

The percentage that the VOR is attenuated during the caloric response that is considered normal varies in the literature (Coats, Herbert, & Atwood,

1976). In the author's clinic, patients are considered to have normal fixation suppression if they are able to suppress the caloric response by at least 60% with visual fixation. The neural structures underlying VOR fixation suppression are fairly well described. Fixation suppression has been reported to be largely governed by the cerebellar flocculus, which is a structure known to regulate the VOR. Takemori and Cohen (1974) reported that localized lesions in the flocculus of animals results in impairments in fixation suppression; however, the cerebellum does not appear to be the only contributor to fixation suppression. It has also been reported that there is a strong relationship between fixation suppression and the smooth pursuit system (see Chapter 1 for a review of smooth pursuit). Halmagyi and Gresty (1979), among others, have reported that individuals manifesting impaired fixation suppression commonly have impaired smooth pursuit performance (Alpert, 1974; Kato, Kimura, Aoyagi, Mizukoshi, & Kawasaki, 1977). Because of the diffuse nature of the fixation-suppression circuit, the exact pathways and structures driving fixation suppression are currently unknown. In fact, it has been suggested by Tomlinson and Robinson (1981) that a separate system known as "vestibular cancellation" exists to override vestibular input and reduces nystagmus intensity when required. The gaze-holding system, smooth pursuit system, and the fixation suppression systems all interact, and often when impairments are seen in one they are observed in

the others. Consequently, it is not uncommon for patients with impaired VOR fixation suppression to have impaired pursuit or gaze-evoked nystagmus. An example of impaired VOR fixation during the caloric examination is displayed in Figure 6–20.

Summary: Fixation-Suppression Abnormalities

The criteria for fixation-suppression abnormalities are as follows:

1. VOR fixation suppression is abnormal if it does not attenuate the caloric nystagmus by at least 60% (i.e., a fixation index of 40%) (based on Vanderbilt upper limits).
2. Fixation index
   a. 0% = complete suppression of the caloric nystagmus
   b. 1% to 100% = partial suppression of the caloric nystagmus
   c. >100% = an enhancement in the caloric nystagmus

Impairment in VOR fixation suppression implicates the neural substrate governing the visual–vestibular interaction (e.g., pursuit system and gaze-holding network). The inferior olives as well as the cerebellar flocculus and/or fiber connections between the vestibular nuclei and the

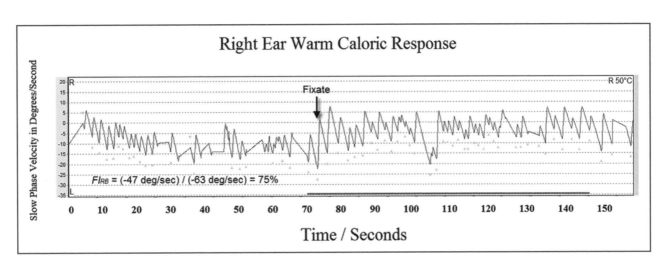

FIGURE 6–20. An example of abnormal fixation suppression during a caloric response.

flocculus must be intact to suppress the VOR. In the presence of impaired VOR fixation suppression there are often accompanying oculomotor signs of brainstem and/or cerebellar disease (e.g., impaired saccades, down-beating nystagmus, saccadic pursuit). Unilaterally impaired VOR fixation suppression suggests that the lesion is focal (e.g., vascular or tumor). To avoid misidentifying the causes of fixation-suppression abnormalities, it is important to rule out medications (some can impair the cerebellum).

Ice Water Caloric Test

The ice water caloric test is routinely reserved for situations where the ABBT test produces no measurable caloric response(s), or if caloric testing must be performed at the bedside. Interpre-

tation of the ice water test can be complex when SN is present. In cases where the ice water test is being employed to determine if there is any residual function in a severe unilateral weakness, the examiner must have a good measure of any SN in the supine position. This is because SN typically beats in the direction of the healthy ear. When a cold stimulus is infused into the impaired ear, if there is any residual function the caloric nystagmus beats toward the healthy ear (in the same direction as the SN); thus, the challenge for the clinician is to determine whether any change in the ongoing nystagmus is due to the caloric response or something else (e.g., alerting). As described in the technique section of the ice water test, the mechanism for elucidating the change in the characteristics of the SN is from the caloric stimulation or from placing the patient in the prone position. Figure 6–21 illustrates the nystagmus profile for

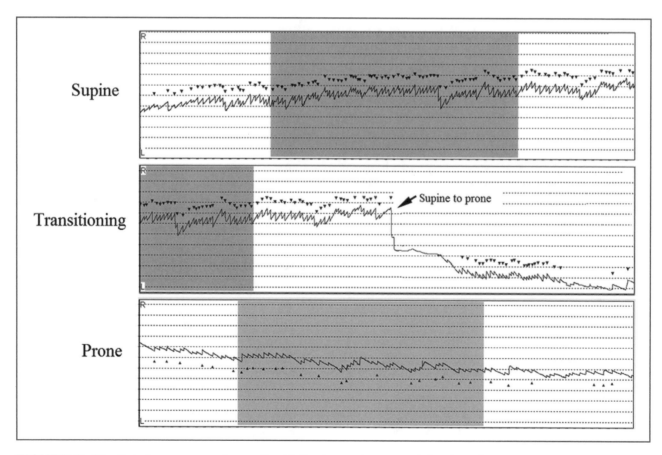

FIGURE 6–21. Caloric responses in a patient following an ice water irrigation of the right ear. The patient has a left-beating spontaneous nystagmus in the supine position that changes to right-beating nystagmus upon transitioning to the prone position.

a patient with SN who had a positive response when he was transitioned from the supine to the prone position. Table 6–10 illustrates the process of interpreting the ice water caloric test.

Summary: Bilaterally Hypoactive Caloric Responses

The criterion for bilaterally hypoactive caloric responses is less than 12° per second total SPV for both the right and left ears (each ear must demonstrate at least 12° per second for warm and cool irrigations) (Figure 6–22). The location of impairment is the labyrinth, superior portion of the vestibular nerve, or root entry zone. To avoid misidentifying the cause, it is important to rule out improper irrigations, middle ear pathology, medications, and saccadic defect.

Interpretation of Hyperactive Responses

There is a substantial body of literature reporting the characteristics of hyperactive caloric responses and their origin. The majority of the work converges on the role of the inhibitory connections between the cerebellum and the vestibular nuclei (Dow, 1938). Specifically, when the situation requires, the cerebellum (i.e., nodulus) can inhibit the VOR (Fernández, Alzate, & Lindsay, 1960; Fredrickson & Fernández, 1964). In cases where a patient has an impairment of the nodulus, the inhibitory influence over the vestibular centers is diminished and the vestibular nuclei assume a higher level of activity. Figure 6–23 illustrates the caloric responses and magnetic resonance imaging in a patient with "hyperactive" caloric responses. Examiners who encounter patients with hyperactive responses must interpret them with caution, as factors other than central nervous system disease have been reported to produce abnormally large caloric responses. For instance, patients who have undergone a mastoidectomy or are extremely anxious can produce larger responses (Figure 6–24). Nonorganic and psychological factors must be accounted for before qualifying a patient as having a cerebellar impairment.

Summary: Hyperactive Responses

The criteria for hyperactive responses are as follows:

1. Total cool peak response (LC + RC) is >99° per second
2. Total warm peak response (LW + RW) is >146° per second
3. Total peak response (LC + RC + LW + RW) is >221° per second

The location of impairment is the cerebellum (flocculonodular lobe). There is: (a) decreased inhibitory influence on the vestibular nucleus, (b) impaired cerebellar control on the pontine saccade center, and (c) control for nonorganic and psychological contributions.

Table 6–10. Position and Response Following an Ice Water Irrigation of the Right Ear

Supine	Prone/Sitting, Head Tilted	Interpretation
Left-beating nystagmus	Right-beating nystagmus	Positive canal response
Left-beating nystagmus	No nystagmus	Positive canal response
Left-beating nystagmus	Left-beating nystagmus	Negative canal response
Right-beating nystagmus	Any condition	Negative canal response
No nystagmus	Any condition	Negative canal response

Source: Adapted from Proctor (1992).

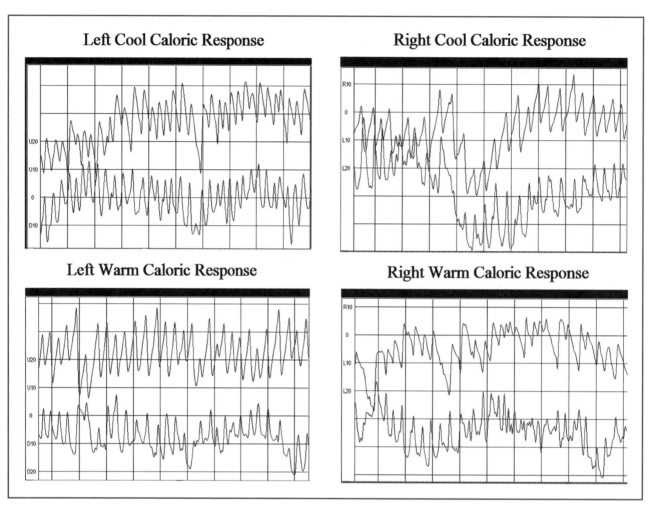

FIGURE 6–22. Example of "hyperactive" caloric responses. Note the vertical nystagmus in addition to the horizontal nystagmus.

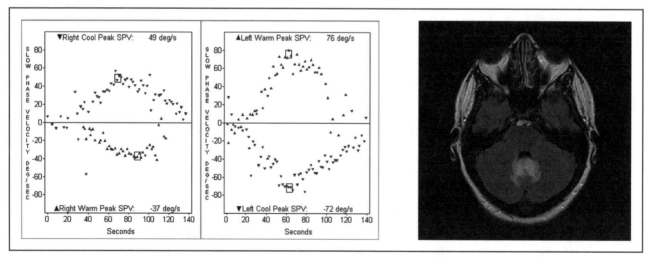

FIGURE 6–23. Caloric pods and a magnetic resonance image with increased enhancement in the midline posterior to the fourth ventricle. Surgical pathology showed this to represent a cerebellar glioma.

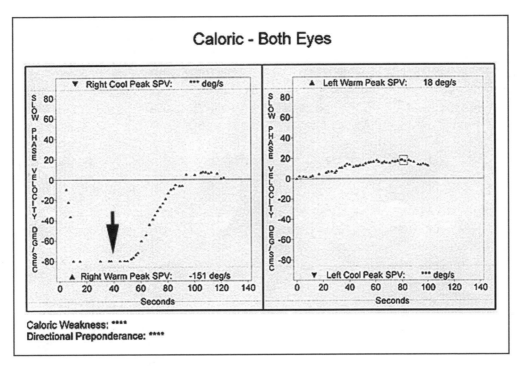

FIGURE 6–24. An example of a caloric response from an ear with a mastoidectomy.

TECHNICAL TIPS FOR CALORIC TESTING

Alerting Tasks

It is well documented that it is necessary to alert patients whenever caloric testing is done in the absence of fixation (Jacobson & Newman, 1993). Alerting during vestibular testing is used to provide the cortex with a consistent level of stimulation to reduce the variability in the fast phases of the vestibular nystagmus (Barin, 2009). The level of cortical activation (i.e., how attentive the patient is) can act as an uncontrolled variable that influences the nystagmus intensity during the test and potentially result in an erroneous result. Although the exact neural mechanism of the "tasking effect" is not completely understood, it is known that cortical structures provide inhibitory input to the vestibular system at the level of the brainstem. When the cortex is challenged with the tasking exercise, the inhibitory control that the cortex maintains over the brainstem reflex is disrupted and the caloric response emerges. There are a number of studies that have reported on the effects of different tasks as they relate to tasking during the caloric response (e.g., Davis & Mann, 1987; Kileny, McCabe, & Ryu., 1980). It has been shown that the alerting challenges that provide the most stable and robust caloric responses are those that require the patient to recall items. This can be as simple as engaging the patient in conversation about their past life or providing names of states or people starting with a particular letter. It is the responsibility of the clinician to be monitoring both the difficulty of the alerting task for the patient as well as the corresponding caloric response. Often, an indication that a task may be too difficult is when there is an observed decrease in the amplitude of the nystagmus each time the patient is attempting to respond.

Interstimulus Interval for Caloric Irrigations

It is not advisable to begin a caloric test immediately following a previous caloric until it has been confirmed that there is no residual response.

According to ANSI, the next caloric should begin 5 minutes following the prior irrigation or when the nystagmus from the previous caloric has been abolished (ANSI, 2009). It is noteworthy that while in the majority of patients the caloric response is abolished in approximately 3 minutes, the author has observed patients where the caloric response has extended far beyond this time. Accordingly, a test to determine if there is any residual nystagmus (vision denied with tasking) should always be performed in the caloric position prior to initiating the next caloric. Findings from a report by Beattie and Koester (1992) suggest that starting the irrigation immediately after the cessation of nystagmus from the previous irrigation will not negatively influence the caloric response.

The absence of any nystagmus following a caloric irrigation may not completely ensure that the labyrinths have equilibrated. Specifically, it has been suggested that there may be an existing variability in the residual temperature gradient across the labyrinth following caloric irrigations (Barin, 2009). For example, in the case of an extremely intense caloric reaction, the temperature in the labyrinth may take over 10 minutes to return to its baseline level (Barnes, 1995). Studies have shown that there is variability between patients and even between irrigations. The current recommendation by the BSA standard committee is to wait a minimum of 7 minutes between the start of the initial irrigation and consecutive one. They do include the caveat that if there is caloric-induced nystagmus present prior to the beginning of the second caloric more time should be provided in order for the response to dissipate (BSA, 2010).

Order of Irrigations

With regard to the order of irrigations, the author suggests beginning with a warm irrigation in the patient with a normal exam up to the point of caloric testing (allowing for monothermal analysis). Second, irrigate with one temperature and then the other (e.g., RW–LW–RC–LC). Third, if the patient has significant hearing loss, irrigate the ear with the poorer hearing first. This is in line with the ANSI and British standards recommendations that warm irrigations are to be performed first followed by cool irrigations (ANSI, 2009; BSA, 2010).

The ANSI standard requires the right ear to be irrigated first for both warm and cool irrigations, whereas the BSA does not specify an ear to start with. Interestingly, there is currently little convincing evidence that starting with cool temperature irrigations will produce erroneous results in the overall test and may actually provide more accurate results (Noaksson et al., 1998). Warm irrigations produce an excitatory response in the end-organ being tested and are often larger in amplitude than their cool counterpart. In patients that have severe motion intolerance it may be advisable to begin with cool irrigations.

Drugs

With regard to drugs, make sure that the medications that the patient is currently taking are documented in the report and that their effect on the caloric response is accounted for (see Chapter 4 for a detailed account of medication effects). Medications can result in both abnormal hyperactive responses as well as abnormal bilateral vestibular weakness

Age

With the renewed interest in vestibular disorders in pediatric patients, clinicians are challenged with how young of a patient can be tested. Reports in the literature have described responses in children as young as 4 years old; however, the developmental age and cooperation of the patient are more important in this demographic than the chronological age (Melagrana, D'Agostino, Pasquale, & Taborelli, 1996). Our clinic employs the rule that if a child can perform a conditioned play audiometry (CPA) evaluation, then they should be able to complete a caloric test that is valid.

Tympanic Membrane Perforation

In cases where a tympanic membrane perforation has been identified prior to the caloric test during otoscopy, testing is still possible. One consideration is the medium used to deliver the caloric stimulus. Air is the stimulus of choice because water, in the case of a tympanic membrane perforation, is contraindicated. In cases where air is being used as the stimulus, a nystagmus that beats in a paradoxical direction can be encountered in patients with tympanic membrane perforations. The mechanism for this is again related to the process of evaporation. When a warm-air stimulus is infused into an ear canal with a tympanic membrane perforation, the warm air enters the middle ear space that has a moist mucosal lining. Once the warm air encounters the wet tissue, evaporative cooling occurs and the temperature in the middle ear space decreases below body temperature. This drop in temperature is transferred to the HSC and creates a caloric response analogous to irrigating with a cool stimulus. These responses are often very robust in patients with large perforations because the irrigation is being directly delivered to the labyrinth, rather than having to pass through an intact tympanic membrane. When one (or two) tympanic membrane is not intact, it is not appropriate calculate asymmetry or directional preponderance because the premise for quantitatively comparing ears is based on the idea that the patients physiology is the same on both side. The information that can be obtained from a caloric response from an ear with a perforated eardrum is simply whether there is measurable peripheral vestibular function or not.

When One Caloric Response Is significantly Stronger or Weaker

When one caloric response is significantly weaker than the other three, it is typically the result of a poor irrigation or inadequate tasking (Figure 6–25A). When one caloric response is significantly stronger than the other three, it is often the first irrigation performed. This has been suggested to be a result of hyperalertness (Figure 6–25B). The process for resolving the invalid caloric response is as follows:

1. Repeat the outlying irrigation (weakest or strongest).
2. If the repeated response continues to be the same, repeat the other temperature in the same ear as the outlier.
3. If the responses continue to be the same, the patient may need to be brought back for another appointment at a later date. It is not recommended that more than six irrigations be performed consecutively (Barin, 2008a).

Temperature Effect

The temperature effect (Figure 6–26) refers to the effect when one irrigation temperature produces significantly different amplitude responses than the other. This is typically due to poor calibration of the stimulus (e.g., temperature or flow). This effect does not influence the calculations of unilateral weakness or DP, and thus in most instances, does not change the outcome of the test; however, every effort should be made to have a calibrated system that generates equivalent responses for warm and cool irrigations.

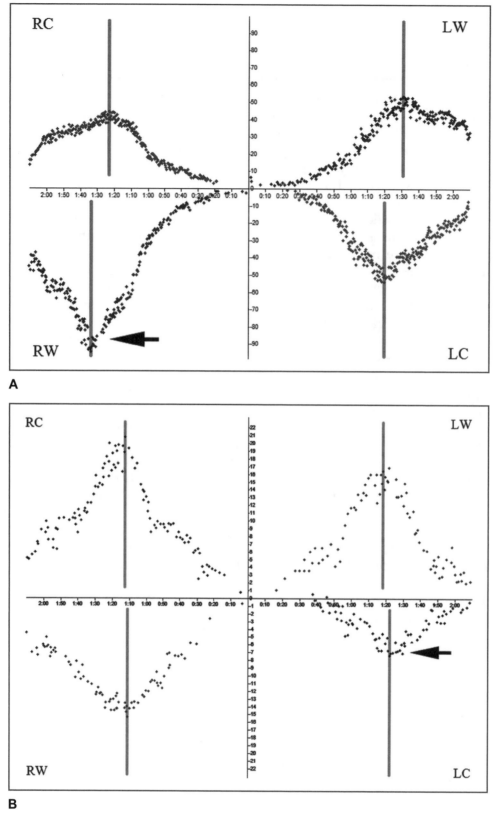

FIGURE 6–25. Two sets of caloric responses that are interpretable and need to be repeated. **A.** A set of caloric responses where one is significantly stronger than the other three. **B.** A set of caloric responses with one response significantly weaker than the other three. The arrow indicates the response that is significantly different than the other three. RC = right cool; RW = right warm; LW = left warm; LC = left cool.

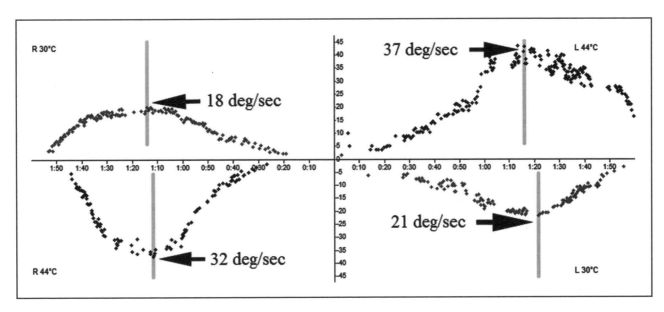

FIGURE 6–26. An example of the "temperature effect" for the binaural bithermal caloric test. Note that the warm responses are significantly stronger than the cool responses.

||| 7 |||

Common Vestibular Disorders: Clinical Presentation

INTRODUCTION

Disorders of both the peripheral and central vestibular system can cause dizziness and vertigo. In some instances, these are not exclusive and a patient may present with abnormalities in both systems. For the clinician that is performing the VNG it is important to be able to provide the ordering provider with useful information that will help with the patient's differential diagnosis. During a VNG examination, the provider administering the tests has an excellent opportunity to take a comprehensive case history that can be matched to the test findings. The VNG test results (e.g., caloric findings, positional testing, and ocular motor testing) along with imaging and a thorough physical examination can provide localizing information in order for the team to provide an accurate diagnosis and most appropriate approach to management.

One of the key elements that the clinician should be able to provide the team following completion of the VNG is supporting evidence as to whether the patient's disorder is peripheral, central, or psychiatric. As discussed in Chapter 3, there are key pieces of information that the examiner can obtain during the VNG that will help build a case for the patients underlying disorder(s). For example, if a patient complains of episodic external rotary vertigo (i.e., room- spinning dizziness) accompanied by nausea and vomiting lasting hours, there is a good chance that this may represent a unilateral peripheral vestibular disorder. Conversely, a patient may complain of a slowly worsening unsteadiness that is continuously present and accompanied by gait ataxia and diplopia, which would be more suggestive of a central disorder (e.g., cerebellar degeneration).

When trying to determine which disorder or disorders a patient may have, it is helpful to have criteria to match the presenting symptoms against. When one looks in the literature, there are several criteria for every disorder that are published by either independent laboratories or national organizations (e.g., American Academy of Otolaryngology Head and Neck Surgery). The Bárány Society is an organization that has begun to work towards developing internationally agreed upon criteria for disorders that have a main symptom of dizziness and vertigo (http://www.baranysociety .nl/). Beginning in 2006, the society held its initial meeting of the Classification Committee. This committee's charge was to develop a structured approach to developing an international criteria for vestibular and balance disorders. This set of criteria is referred to as the International Classification of Vestibular Disorders (ICVD) (Bisdorff, Staab, & Newman-Toker, 2015). The following sections will address the major disorders associated with vertigo and dizziness and, when possible, provide the criteria set forth in the ICVD. The exception will be benign paroxysmal positional vertigo, which is addressed in detail in Chapter 5 of this text.

COMMON DISORDERS CAUSING DIZZINESS

Vestibular Neuritis

Background

It is common for the clinician evaluating dizzy patients to see those who report having an acute episode of rotary vertigo (e.g., room spinning) accompanied by nausea that is then followed by unsteadiness and a leaning or veering to one side when ambulating. When these patients are found to be clear of any neurologic signs such as dysarthria, dysphagia, numbness, or weakness, it is often the case the patient is presenting with a syndrome referred to as vestibular neuritis (VN). VN has been reported to be the third most commonly reported cause of vertigo related to peripheral impairment following benign paroxysmal positional vertigo and Ménière's disease (Brandt, Dieterich, & Strupp, 2005). Sekitani and colleagues (1993) have reported that the incidence of VN is approximately 3.5/100,000. The most common age of patients presenting with VN range from 30 to 60 years of age (Strupp & Brandt, 2013).

Clinical Presentation

The key presenting features of VN are a spontaneous episode of sustained external rotary vertigo and imbalance. During the physical examination an acute patient will demonstrate horizontal spontaneous nystagmus with a slight torsional component (see Chapter 2 for full review of spontaneous nystagmus). This episode is often accompanied by nausea and vomiting and the patient may have a wide-based gait with a slow cadence. In neurologically intact patients, the vertigo will typically decrease over a few days. However, it is often the case that even after the perceptions of vertigo has subsided, patients will report symptoms of dizziness that is provoked with head/body movements and describe a sense of generalized unsteadiness. These symptoms can last for months or even years following the initial event. In neurologically intact individual, full recovery will usually occur in 1 to 2 weeks.

Pathophysiology

Although there is not a firm consensus regarding the cause of VN, reports have the disorder to be a result of inflammation of the vestibular nerve stemming as a result of a viral attack on one or both of the branches (i.e., inferior or superior) of the vestibular nerve (Baloh, 2003). Support for a viral origin of the condition is based on histopathology and the fact that when queried about their symptoms, patients describe a clear prodrome (e.g., fever and nausea) prior to the primary event. The histopathological evidence has shown that the herpes simplex virus (HSV I) was present in the vestibular ganglia in approximately two-thirds of human autopsies. Furthermore, these studies showed that there were significant degenerative changes in the peripheral vestibular nerve fibers in patients with VN that are similar to the pathological changes observed in other nerves of patients that have a history of similar viral disorders (e.g., shingles, measles) (Baloh, Ishiyama, Wackym, & Honrubia, 1996). Evidence from animal models supports HSV I as a likely cause of VN. In 1993, Hirata and colleagues used a mouse model where the investigators inoculated the HSV I into the ear. After a latent period, the mice manifested symptoms that are associated with VN. Additionally, when the vestibular nerves of these animals were studied, it was found that HSV-1 antigens were present in the vestibular ganglion. Based on vestibular laboratory testing (e.g., caloric and head impulse testing), when a patient suffers from VN the nerve branch/s typically maintain some level of function. That is, there is more often than not some level of measurable function suggesting only partial paresis of the nerve. The branch of the vestibular nerve that has been reported to be the most vulnerable to VN is the superior portion which supplies the horizontal anterior semicircular canals as well as the utricle (Fetter & Dichgans, 1996). Goeble and colleagues (2001) have reported that this increased susceptibility of the superior branch of the vestibular nerve to VN is due to the fact that the distal portion of the nerve is longer and travels through a longer (7 times longer) and more narrow bony channel. Accordingly, the arterioles that provide the blood supply to the superior vestibular nerve must travel through these same small bony channels, predisposing the nerve to more compression, and subsequently ischemia, when the nerve becomes inflamed and swells.

Findings on Laboratory Testing

With recent advances in tests of vestibular function, it is now possible to identify which branch of the vestibular nerve is impaired. Using the diagnostic patterns that are provided by the video head impulse testing (vHIT), caloric testing, and vestibular evoked myogenic potentials (VEMPs), it is now possible to localize the branch of the nerve that is impaired (Figure 7–1).

Treatment

A customized physical therapy program is the treatment of choice to drive central nervous system compensation and reduce symptoms in the neurologically intact patient suffering from an acute VN. Treatment should begin as early as possible in the course of the disease. It may be that in the early course of unilateral VN, the patient may only be able to tolerate short periods of therapy because the exercises may exacerbate the symptoms. However, these should be repeated as much as is possible, which is determined by the therapist. A significant decrease in symptoms of VN when enrolled early on in a vestibular rehabilitation program should occur within 6 weeks. This can vary depending on the patient's age, level of activity, and medical comorbid conditions (e.g., neurological disorders or visual impairments). Medications such as Valium or Meclizine are often

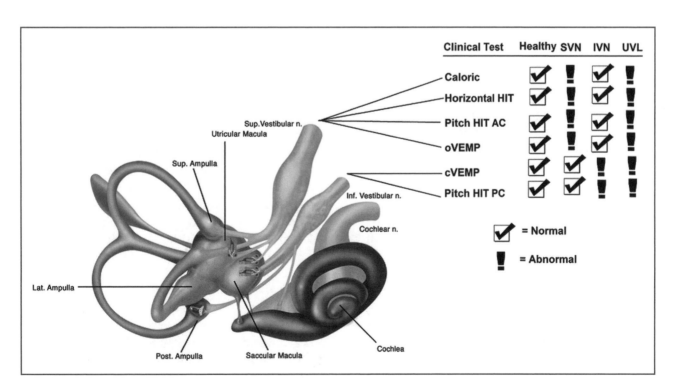

FIGURE 7–1. Summary of the patterns of abnormality that are frequently observed. SVN = superior vestibular nerve; IVN = inferior vestibular nerve; and UVL = complete unilateral vestibular loss.

used to reduce symptoms in the early stages of VN but should be discontinued as soon as is reasonably possible. These medications act as vestibular suppressants and can delay the patient's recovery.

Ménière's Disease

Background

Ménière's disease (MD) is an inner ear disorder that is multifactorial in origin and most likely represents a combination of genetic predispositions and exposures to certain environmental factors. In 1861, Prosper Ménière presented a case of a young girl that suffered from vertigo and hearing loss to the French Academy of Medicine. At that time it was assumed that vertigo was always a manifestation of impairment in the brain (cerebral) and not the peripheral vestibular system. The treatments for vertigo during this period were rudimentary (e.g., bleeding) and Ménière's position was that inner ear involvement should be considered in patients with symptoms of vertigo (Baloh & Honrubia, 2001). The incidence of Ménière's disease has been estimated to be 15/100,000 persons in the United States (Wladislavosky-Waserman, Facer, Mokri, & Kurland, 1984). The average age of when symptoms are first reported is between 40 and 60 years of age and is most commonly unilateral (Kitahara, 1991; Paparella & Mancini 1985). According to Balkany and colleagues (1980), the rate of patients diagnosed with the disorder in one ear, and who go on to develop MD in the other ear, can be anywhere from 2% to 78%.

Clinical Presentation

The clinical presentation of patients with Ménière's disease is widely varied among patients. It is important to note that there is no definitive diagnostic test or set of features acquired during the case history that can identify the underlying cause of the constellation of symptoms that are Ménière's disease clinical syndrome that is comprised of spontaneous episodes of unilateral fluctuating sensorineural hearing loss, external rotary vertigo, aural fullness, and tinnitus. In many patients, there is a predictable progression of symptoms. Spells of vertigo are commonly pre-

ceded by a sense of aural fullness, an increase in the severity of the tinnitus, and decreased hearing acuity. Following these three aural symptoms, a severe episode of external rotary vertigo will occur with a duration of 2 to 3 hours and is typically accompanied by nausea and vomiting. Other symptoms associated with MD are the sudden unexplained falls that have been associated with otolithic dysfunction. In 1963, Tumarkin described events where patients felt as thought the floor dropped out from under them, or they had the distinct feeling of being pushed to the floor. These attacks were subsequently referred to as otolithic crises of Tumarkin. It has been estimated that up to 6% of patients diagnosed with MD will suffer from drop attacks (Baloh & Honrubia, 1990).

Patients will often report that they may have small episodes that present with cochlear symptoms, but no vertigo between the severe episodes. The frequency of severe attacks is more common early on in the course of the disease, and it has been reported that almost half of patients do not experience vertiginous episodes after 2 years (Silverstein, Smouha, & Jones,, 1989). What is both frustrating to the clinician and the patient is that in many instances, there is no clear trigger and the symptoms do not follow the traditional progression as described above. This is most likely due to the fact there are a number of phenotypes of MD. Patients who have been diagnosed with MD often have other comorbidities such as migraine, allergies, and autoimmune diseases that complicate the physician's ability, in some cases, to find an effective treatment early on in the disease. This fact, coupled with the inability of the patient to know when an attack will occur, leads to significantly decreased quality of life and depression and anxiety (Anderson & Harris, 2001; Filipo et al., 1988). The Bárány Society has published guidelines for making a diagnosis of Ménière's disease (Lopez-Escamez et al., 2015).

Definite MD

1. Two or more spontaneous episodes of vertigo, each lasting 20 minutes to 12 hours
2. Audiometrically documented low to medium frequency
3. Sensorineural hearing loss in one ear, defining the affected ear on at least one occasion

before, during, or after one of the episodes of vertigo

4. Fluctuating aural symptoms (hearing, tinnitus, or fullness) in the affected ear that is not better accounted for by another vestibular diagnosis.

Probable MD

1. Two or more episodes of vertigo or dizziness, each lasting 20 minutes to 24 hours
2. Fluctuating aural symptoms (hearing, tinnitus, or fullness) in the affected ear that is not better accounted for by another vestibular diagnosis

Pathophysiology

The most commonly reported pathological basis for Ménière's disease has been endolymphatic hydrops (EH) (Schuknecht & Igarashi, 1964). Endolymph is the fluid in the inner ear that is potassium-enriched that has been proposed to be either inadequately resorbed or is produced in excessive quantities in patients with MD (See Chapter 2 for review of endolymph). Animal models of EH have been developed and have shown that when the endolymphatic sac is surgically ablated in animals, they develop evidence of hydrops that is similar to findings reported in the temporal bones of humans with the disorder (Kimura, 1967). The effects of EH have been reported to manifest most commonly in the pars inferior of the labyrinth (i.e., saccule and cochlea) (Schuknecht & Igarashi, 1964). Cochlear EH will demonstrate a bowing of Resiner's membrane into the scala vestibuli, whereas saccular hydrops is grades by the degree of membrane distention toward the stapes footplate. The latter may be an explanation for the symptom of dizziness that is experienced when pressure translates the stapes footplate (i.e., Hennebert's sign). This accumulation of endolymph in the vestibular organs and cochlear duct, however, does not explain all clinical features MD. The evidence that the accumulation of endolymph in the vestibular organs and cochlear duct is responsible for the all the symptoms associated with MD is still weak. This is because EH in humans has only been documented postmortem, and the determination of whether the patient was hydropic during the time of their symptoms can be debated. Additionally, animal studies have shown that when the volume of endolymph is increased, cochlear thresholds do not significantly change (Salt & Rask-Andersen, 2004). Accordingly, the exact mechanism underlying EH remains unknown. Recently, advances in imaging techniques have made it possible to view the inner ear membranous structures. These studies have provided some insight into some of the structural abnormalities that may predispose an individual to develop MD. For example, Mark (1994) reported that gadolinium-enhanced imaging was capable of seeing inflammation of the endolymphatic sac in patients diagnosed with MD. Additionally, Albers, Van Weissenbruch, and Casselman, (1994) reported that patients with DM have significantly smaller endolymph drainage systems.

Other mechanisms that affect inner ear homeostasis and may result in symptoms associated with MD. Research has shown that autoimmune processes may play a role in those patients with bilateral Ménière's patients. Specifically, antibodies against Heat Shock proteins found in the inner ear have been found to increase in patients with autoimmune disease. Rauch, San Martin, Moscicki, and Bloch, (1995) reported that half of patients with bilateral Ménière's disease had elevated antibodies. Viral infections that attack that endolymphatic sac and duct have been suggested to be related to the onset of MD (Gacek & Gacek, 2002). Underlying vascular mechanisms may play a role to the extent that they cut off perfusion to the endolymphatic sac resulting in damage (Lee & Kimura, 1992). One such mechanism may be that there is a common vascular physiological component common to patients with migraine and Ménière's disease. Patients that suffer from migraines have been shown to have increased prevalence of MD (Radtke et al., 2002).

Common Findings on the Laboratory Testing

When using laboratory testing to assist in the diagnosis of Ménière's disease, there is no one specific abnormality or set of abnormalities that can establish or rule out a diagnosis of the disorder (Table 7–1). Audiometric thresholds, caloric weakness, and cervical vestibular-evoked myogenic

Table 7–1. Common Findings on the Laboratory Testing—Ménière's Disease

Test	Possible Common Findings
Caloric	Caloric paresis on the affected side
Cervical Vestibular Evoked Myogenic Potentials	Significant amplitude asymmetry (weaker on the ipsilesional side)
Ocular Vestibular Evoked Myogenic Potential	Significant amplitude asymmetry (weaker on the ipsilesional side)
Video Head Impulse testing	Often normal in the presence of abnormal caloric responses (McCaslin, Rivas, Jacobson, & Bennett, 2015)
Ocular motor testing	Common to see spontaneous nystagmus *Acute*—spontaneous nystagmus will beat toward the unaffected ear (fast phase) *Recovery nystagmus*—spontaneous nystagmus will beat toward the affected ear (See Chapter 2 for review)
Audiometry	Low-frequency fluctuating sensorineural hearing loss early in the course of the disease.

potentials have been shown to correlate best with the progression of the disease (Benson, McCaslin, Shepard, & McPherson, 2019). Although electrocochleography (ECochG) has been widely used to assist with the diagnosis of Ménière's disease, there is still discussion in the literature regarding the tests exact specificity and sensitivity. This may be related to the fact that there are a number of disorders (besides endolymphatic hydrops) that can lead a patient to meet the diagnostic criteria.

Treatment

The management of Ménière's disease involves decreasing patient symptoms using medical regimens such as altering diet, medical, and surgical treatments. When patients are queried about their symptoms, it is the spontaneous episodes of external rotatory vertigo that that are most debilitating to them. In this regard, the initial front-line treatments are centered on controlling the spells of vertigo. Once the symptoms of vertigo have been extinguished, the clinician can then work to mitigate the aural symptoms of fullness, fluctuating hearing, and tinnitus. The front-line medical regimens that are centered on decreasing the episodes of vertigo are those that have been suggested to reduce the severity of endolymphatic hydrops (e.g., low sodium diet and diuretic) (Figure 7–2). Recommendations for a low-salt diet are typically given to the patient, and to not add any additional salt in cooking, limiting sodium intake to 1500 to 2000 milligrams (mg) per day, and drinking 6 to 8 glasses of fresh water each day. If a patient is taking a prescription diuretic, then it is often suggested that he or she include certain foods in their diets, such as apricots (dried), artichokes, bananas, peaches (dried), broccoli, or orange juice in order to maintain healthy potassium levels.

Vestibular Migraine

Background

It has been long understood that there is a relationship between migraine and vertigo, and both are common disorders in the adult population. There are a number of terms that are used in the literature to describe migraines that have

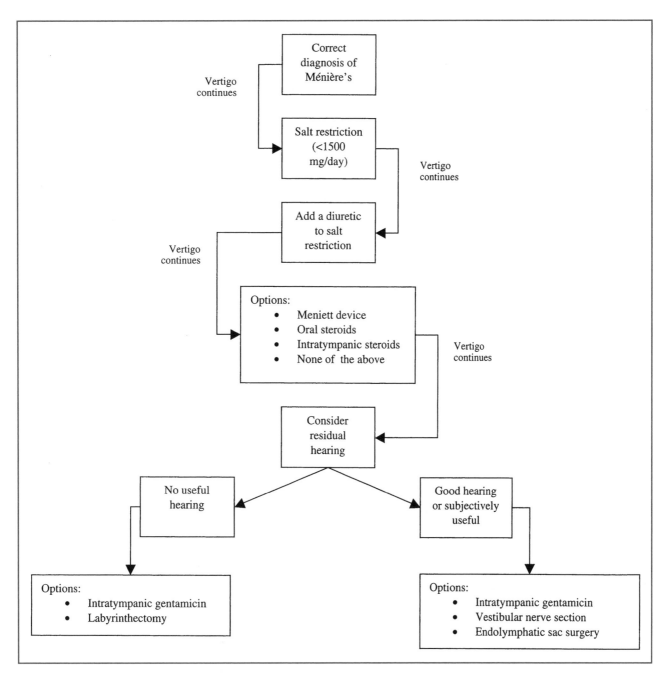

FIGURE 7–2. Algorithm for the management of Ménière's disease (Neff & Wiet, 2016).

dizziness associated with them. Some of these include migrainous vertigo, vestibular migraine, migraine-related dizziness, migraine-associated dizziness. It has been estimated that 16% of adults have migraine headaches and 23% have dizziness during their lifetime (Kroenke & Price, 1993; Rasmussen, Jensen, & Olesen 1991). Recent epidemiological studies have provided compelling evidence

that these two common symptoms are related to one another. That is, well-controlled experimental studies have shown that there is a greater than chance probability that the two are associated. For example, Neuhauser, Leopold, von Brevern, Arnold, and Lempert, 2001 placed the prevalence of migraine in a sample of 200 patients seen in a dizzy clinic at 1.6 times greater than a control group. These investigators have also reported that migrainous vertigo (MV) affects 1% of the adult populations with a female-to-male predominance (Furman, Marcus, & Balaban, 2013). Kayan and Hood (1984) reported that patients with migraine headache were significantly more likely to report accompanying vestibular symptoms than patients with tension headache. In a population-based study investigating the link between migraine and vestibular symptoms, it was found that migraine patients suffering from vertigo will have an accompanying headache more often than patients who do not have migraine (odd ratio 8) (Neuhauser et al., 2006). The challenge for the clinician seeing the dizzy patient with migraine is to determine whether the headache is causing the dizziness or whether the two are occurring independently of each other.

Clinical Presentation

Although MV can be by patients of any age, investigators have reported that the age of onset is typically between 30 to 60 years of age. (Cass et al., 1997). According to Furman and Whitney (2016), the headaches will occur approximately 8 years before the onset of the symptoms of dizziness. The symptoms that are associated with MV are can be quite varied and are typically either spontaneous, provoked by head/body motion, or positional (Bisdorff et al., 2015). In the instance of positional vertigo, the characteristics are different than benign paroxysmal positional vertigo (BPPV). BPPV will only last seconds (see Chapter 5 for full review); however, in the MV patient, the nystagmus will continue as long as the head is in the provocative position. Care should be taken not to confuse this with cupulolithiasis, and when positional nystagmus is present, patients should be asked to describe their symptoms. It is noteworthy that 40% to 70% of patients with MV may report positional vertigo, but it does not occur with every spell (von Brevern, Schmidt, Schönfeld, Lempert, & Clark, 2005). Individuals with MV will also report symptoms of light-headedness, visual vertigo (symptoms exacerbated my motion-rich environments), swimming sensation, a rocking or internal rocking sensation, and motion sickness.

MV usually occurs in spells that can last anywhere from seconds to days, with an upward limit of 72 hours. Some patients will report that it may take them a week to fully recover (Versino et al., 2003).

The temporal relationship of MV and the headache is also highly variable. The headache can precede, follow, or occur simultaneously with the symptoms of dizziness. Interestingly, there are patients that will report that they do not always experience the symptoms together. In fact, it has been reported that as many as one third of patients never have the headache and vertiginous symptoms occurring at the same time (Cutrer & Baloh, 1992).

In a subset of patients with MV, there are reported auditory symptoms. Although the vertigo is typically described as the most disabling features, fluctuating hearing loss and changes in the severity of the tinnitus have also been described by patients with MV (Cass et al., 1997). According to Johnson (1998), in the majority of patients with MV, the only mild decreases in hearing acuity that occur are not progressive. There are patients with MV, however, that do present with fluctuating sensorineural hearing loss and headache. In these cases, it can be difficult to determine whether the patient's primary diagnosis is Ménière's disease or MV (Shepard, 2006).

A careful case history is key in determining if there are any precipitants that may be triggering an episode. Women that are undergoing hormonal changes or other well-known triggers for headaches, such as poor sleep quality, stress, hot showers, specific food/beverages, changes in weather, or sensory stimuli (e.g., fluorescent lights) should be documented. Triggers are highly specific to each patient, and patient diaries can be extremely helpful to the clinician in determining what (if any) are the offending triggers. Lempert et al. (2012), in conjunction with the Bárány Society, have provided diagnostic criteria. These criteria are summarized below.

Definite Vestibular Migraine:

1. At least five episodes with vestibular symptoms of moderate or severe intensity, lasting 5 minutes to 72 hours

2. Current or previous history of migraine with or without aura according to the International Classification of Headache Disorders (ICHD)
3. One or more migraine features with at least 50% of the vestibular episodes
   a. Headache with at least two of the following characteristics: one sided location, pulsating quality, moderate or severe pain intensity, aggravation by routine physical activity
   b. Photophobia and phonophobia
   c. Visual aura
4. Not better accounted for by another vestibular or ICHD diagnosis

Probable Vestibular Migraine:

1. At least five episodes with vestibular symptoms of moderate or severe intensity, lasting 5 minutes to 72 hours
2. Only one of the criteria two and three for vestibular migraine is fulfilled (migraine history or migraine features during the episode)
3. Not better accounted for by another vestibular or ICHD diagnosis

Pathophysiology

To date, the exact mechanisms underlying MV are still not completely understood. There have been a number of hypotheses set forth in the literature. One such hypothesis is that MV may be related to a vasospasm of the internal auditory artery (IAA). This artery supplies the organs of hearing and balance, and a sudden constriction of the IAA mediated by migraine mechanisms would potentially produce audio-vestibular symptoms during an attack. Furthermore, it may also explain the common link between BPPV and migraine. Another theory, and one that is related to migraine aura, is the concept of a spreading depression across the cortex. The concept is that if the areas of the cortex (or brainstem) that receive vestibular input (posterior insula or temporo-parietal junction) are stimulated, then it would reason that there may be manifest vestibular symptoms (Fasold et al., 2002). Other hypotheses that may trigger vestibular symptoms in patients MV are related to the release of various neuropeptides (calcitonin-gene,

serotonin, dopamine). It has been suggested that these protein-like molecules may trigger activation of vestibular neurons and result in abnormal activation of the trigeminovascular system (Furman, Marcus, & Balaban, 2003).

Common Findings on the Laboratory Testing

When evaluating the patient with MV in the vestibular laboratory, it is important to remember that there is one finding that is specific to the disorder. However, there are a number of vestibular test findings that have been reported in the literature patients with MV. These abnormalities include, but are not limited to, an isolated directional preponderance on rotational testing, spontaneous nystagmus, significant unilateral peripheral vestibular paresis, and abnormal vestibular-evoked myogenic potentials. Maione in 2006 reported that 20% of patients with MV presented with an unexplained sensorineural hearing loss. Table 7–2 summarizes some of the commonly reported vestibular laboratory test abnormalities reported in the literature.

Treatment

In patients with MV, when possible, a team approach should be taken where the team is led by a physician knowledgeable in MV. When forming the management strategy for the patient with MV, it is common to include otolaryngologists, physical therapists, psychologists, nutritionists, and neurologists. Once the primary coordinating physician has a comprehensive picture of the patients overall health, he or she can recruit experts from other disciplines to address any specific medical comorbidities that may be contributing to or causing the attacks. Depending on the frequency, duration, and severity of patient's attacks, the treatment approach will be either abortive, preventative, or a combination of the two. Nonpharmaceutical approaches to MV such as sleep hygiene, avoidance of dietary triggers, and routine exercise have been firmly established in the literature as frontline measures to reduce the severity and frequency of the symptoms.

Table 7–2. Common Findings on the Laboratory Testing—Vestibular Migraine

Test	Common Clinical Findings (migraine only)
Caloric	Unilaterally reduced caloric responses have been reported to occur in patients with MV with a prevalence ranging from 8% (Dieterich and Brandt, 1999) to 60% (Olsson, 1991).
Cervical Vestibular Evoked Myogenic Potentials	Significant amplitude asymmetry
Ocular Vestibular Evoked Myogenic Potential	Significant amplitude asymmetry
Video Head Impulse Testing	Often normal
Ocular motor testing	May show increased difficulty with pursuit and optokinetic testing (reported in 26% of patients) (Dieterich & Brandt, 1999) Pathologic nystagmus observed in 70% of patients when patient was experiencing an attack. Could appear as central or peripheral pattern (von Brevern et al., 2005).
Rotational Chair	Isolated directional preponderance (20% of patients (Dieterich & Brandt, 1999)

Although there is still paucity in the literature regarding which medications are most effective as a prophylaxis for MV, triptans are a common therapeutic approach (e.g., Imitrex), as is propranolol, and carbonic anhydrase inhibitors (e.g., acetazolamide). Patients should be counseled on the possible side effects of such medications (e.g., orthostatic hypotension or weight gain). Key to adjusting the dosage of such medication is a careful logging by the patient of their attacks. It has been suggested that after a period of three months, a successful response to treatment would be a 50% or greater decrease in the frequency of the episodes. The pharmaceutical approach to treating an acute patient will typically involve the use a combination of triptans and vestibular suppressant medications (e.g., meclizine) and antinausea agents (Baloh & Kerber, 2011).

Finally, in some cases of MV, it is appropriate to consider vestibular rehabilitation (Alghadir & Anwer, 2018). MV patients often complain of motion or visual sensitivity, which can be addressed through certain forms of physical therapy (e.g., habituation). They may also present with persistent vestibulo-ocular deficits or with symptoms of unsteadiness, which can also be alleviated through therapy. Finally, there are recent reports that show that in patients with MV, a physical therapy program can reduce the level of anxiety, severity of headache symptoms, self-reported handicap as it relates to dizziness (Sugaya, Arai, & Goto, 2017).

Superior Canal Dehiscence

Background

Superior semicircular canal dehiscence syndrome (SCDS) was a disorder characterized by vestibular and auditory manifestations that was first described by Minor, Solomon, Zinreich, & Zee in 1998. The organs of the inner ear are encased in bone (i.e., otic capsule), with only two points of increased compliance, or windows, that facilitate the transmission of sound from the middle ear space into the inner ear (i.e., oval and round windows). There are those patients that will present with a "third mobile window" located at the eminence of the superior canal (Figure 7–3). In many cases, the dehiscence can occur when a cholesteatoma, or an infectious disease (syphilis), erodes the bone of the superior canal. Superior canal dehiscence has also been associated with physical trauma that may have causes a temporal bone fractures or a fistula involving the round or oval windows. Some people are simply born with a congenital malformation of the bone overlying the SSC. Regardless of the cause, of a third mobile window, patients can present with a similar constellation of auditory and vestibular symptoms. Correctly identifying SCD in the clinic is best when a multidisciplinary approach incorporating audiology and otolaryngology is taken.

Pathophysiology

The pathophysiological mechanism of SCDS is centered around the concept that the third window in the superior canal makes the canal abnormally responsive to sound and pressure stimuli. That is, whereas normally the superior canal is tightly encased in bone, the third mobile window allows acoustic energy to be shunted up through the canal and through the dehiscence. One of the keys to initially describing this disorder was the observation that when a patients subjected symptoms were provoked using sound or pressure, there were noted corresponding eye movements (i.e., nystagmus) that would accompany them. Specifically, the eye movements were shown to align with the plane of the superior canal and have properties that would be expected from the vestibulo-ocular reflex of the superior canal (i.e., nystagmus with upward, counterclockwise slow phases) (Minor et al., 2001).

Clinical Presentation

Patients that have been confirmed to have SCD will often present with oscillopsia that is provoked by changes in intracranial pressure, such as when they perform a Valsalva maneuver, when they are subjected to loud sounds (Tullio phenomenon), and when variations in pressure in the external ear canal are encountered (Hennebert sign) (Minor et al., 2001).

It is not uncommon for the professional seeing patients in an otologic center to encounter patients with an unusual sensitivity to loud

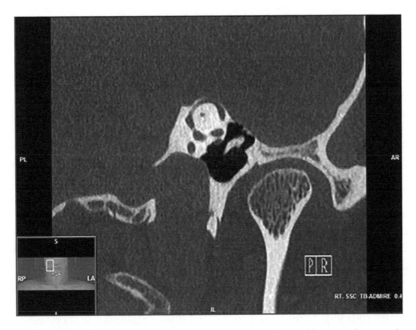

FIGURE 7–3. Example of a CT scan in a patient with superior semicircular canal dehiscence.

sounds. However, although there can be any a number of reasons for these reported symptoms (e.g., psychological issues or recruitment due to sensorineural hearing loss), there are some key features of SCD that can help the clinician with the differential diagnosis. When a careful case history is taken, patients with SCD will often report pulsating tinnitus, hyperacusis, and autophony. Specifically, patients may report that they can hear self-generated sounds including breathing, their heartbeat, and their eyes moving. One common symptom is that patients will report that the impact of the feet during walking or running is bothersome. In some, they will avoid singing or speaking at a normal conversational level because it will exacerbate their symptoms.

The high-resolution temporal bone CT is the gold standard for the identification of SCD. There are specific protocols with parameters that are important in ensuring that the SCD is accurately identified and the size characterized. In order to maximize the specificity and sensitivity of an SCD, a .5 mm collimated helical CT scan has been recommended (Belden, Weg, Minor, & Zinreich, 2003). There is convincing data that shows the size of the SCD is related to patient symptoms and the degree of air-bone gap (ABG) on the audiogram. Using computerized tomography (CT) to confirm the SCD in their study participants, Yuen, Boeddinghaus, Eikelboom, and Atlas (2009) showed that 100% of patients with dehiscence larger than 3 mm had a significant ABG.

Common Findings on the Laboratory Testing

In patients where an SCD is suspected because of their reported symptoms, there are a number of factors that should be carefully examined when doing a routine hearing test. One such factor is to measure the lowest bone conduction threshold possible. Due to the pathophysiological mechanism of SCD, patients with the disorder may manifest bone conduction thresholds during audiometry that are less than 0 nHL (Brantberg et al., 2001). Therefore, in patients with SCD, it is possible to have an air-bone gap that is usually greatest at the lower frequencies (250 to 1000 Hz) with normal air conduction thresholds (Figure 7–4).

Normal acoustic reflexes and tympanograms can be helpful in further confirming the presence of a third window in these cases where there are symptoms suggesting and SCD along with the presence of a significant air-bone gap.

Using immittance measures can help ensure that the air-bone gap on audiometry due to superior canal dehiscence from an air-bone gap due to middle ear pathology is correctly differentiated. Additionally, when the Weber tuning fork test (512 Hz) is performed in patients with a unilateral SCD, they will localize it to the affected side. Interestingly, when the tuning fork is struck and placed on the lateral round bony prominence of the affected patient's ankle, the patient will hear the tuning fork and it will lateralize to the affected ear.

The most sensitive vestibular laboratory test for SCD is the vestibular-evoked myogenic potential (VEMP) (Table 7–3). VEMPs are evoked potentials that are short-latency electromyographic (EMG) potentials generated by the otoliths (i.e., saccule or utricle). These responses are typically recorded either from the sternocleidomastoid muscle (SCM) (i.e., cervical VEMP), or the contralateral inferior oblique muscle (i.e., ocular VEMP). Patients with confirmed SCD have larger amplitude and lower threshold responses in the affected ear/s (Brantberg, Bergenius, & Tribukait, 1999).

Arts and colleagues in 2008 reported that it is possible to record an ECochG with an elevated SP/AP ratio in patients with confirmed SCD. Although the elevated SP/AP ratio is typically associated Ménière's disease, this is the initial observation that describes this pattern of findings in patients with superior semicircular canal dehiscence. The authors evaluated the ECochG results of 11 patients (15 ears) with confirmed SCD using vestibular evoked myogenic potentials and high resolution temporal bone computed tomography. Of the 15 ears, 14 were shown to demonstrate an elevated SP/AP ratio (>0.40). From this data, the investigators concluded that the SP/AP ratio is a highly sensitive measure to identify SSCD.

Treatment

In many patients, simply understanding the cause of the symptoms is adequate. However, when the symptoms are disabling, the definitive treatment

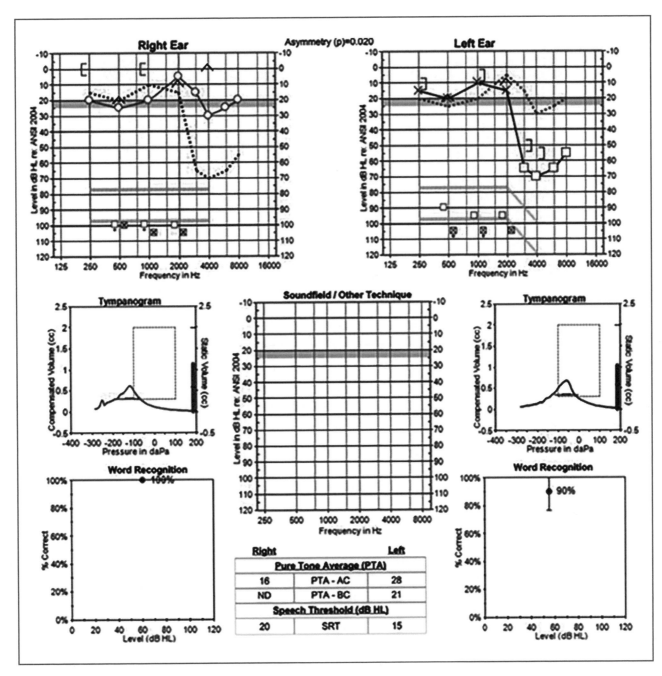

FIGURE 7–4. Example of an audiogram from a patient with confirmed superior semicircular canal dehiscence.

is surgical. This involves either plugging or resurfacing the dehiscence. To gain access to the bony defect, either a middle cranial fossa or transmastoid approach is taken. The dehiscence can be plugged with fascia and bone chips or the surgeon can place a roof over the abnormality (i.e., resurfacing) using fascia and a bone graft. This procedure spares the canal lumen of the canal maintains its function. Minor 2005 reported that when the two procedures were compared, the canal plugging reduced symptoms to a greater degree than resurfacing. Following surgery, the air-bone gap is typically closed and VEMP thresholds return to normal (Limb, Carey, Srireddy, & Minor, 2006).

Table 7–3. Common Findings on the Laboratory Testing—Superior Canal Dehiscence

Test	Common Clinical Findings
Caloric	Typically normal amplitude and symmetrical responses
Cervical Vestibular Evoked Myogenic Potentials	Significantly reduced threshold and increased amplitude in the affected ear
Ocular Vestibular Evoked Myogenic Potential	Significantly reduced threshold and increased amplitude in the affected ear
Video Head Impulse testing	Normal
Ocular motor testing	Normal
Audiometry	Air-bone gap in the presence of normal tympanograms and acoustic reflexes
Electrocochleography (EcochG)	Elevated SP/AP ratio (>0.40)

Persistent Postural Perceptual Dizziness

Background

The clinician seeing dizzy patients inevitably encounters patients who complain not of vertigo, but of a constant dizziness or "rocking." These patients may also have normal results on quantitative assessments of vestibular system impairment and neuroimaging. This pattern of symptoms and findings on quantitative assessments can be suggestive of an anxiety disorder. It is now known that there is a strong relationship between anxiety and dizziness (Ruckenstein & Staab, 2009). In fact, McKenna, Hallam, and Hinchcliffe (1991) reported that approximately 64% of dizzy patients seen in an audiology clinic also had an associated anxiety disorder. In line with these findings, Furman and Jacob (2001) found that the prevalence of psychiatric disorders in dizzy patients is higher than that found in the general population. In an article by Odman and Maire (2008), 80% to 93% of patients with chronic dizziness had a psychiatric disorder contributing significantly to their symptoms. When patients suffering from dizziness and anxiety are compared with patients with either dizziness or anxiety alone, they remain symptomatic for longer periods of time, have poorer treatment outcomes, and report increased handicap. In order to begin the process of correctly identifying and treating these patients, Staab and Ruckenstein (2005) have worked to replace the vague terms "space and motion discomfort" and "phobic postural vertigo" with the term persistent postural perceptual dizziness (PPPD).

Clinical Presentation

PPPD is defined using both the results of a neurotological examination and the presence of a specific set of physical symptoms. The physical symptoms include the persistent sensation (greater than 3 months) of non-vertiginous dizziness that may include lightheadedness, heavy headedness, or a feeling of imbalance that is not apparent to others (Staab & Ruckenstein, 2007). Other complaints, such as a hypersensitivity to motion, and worsening of symptoms in complex visual environments are also suggestive of PPPD (Figure 7–5). Interestingly, the term anxiety is purposefully excluded from the core definition of PPPD in order to avoid the premature assumption that the patient's dizziness is due to a psychi-

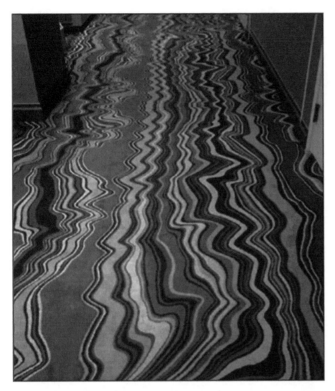

FIGURE 7–5. Example of a patterned floor that would commonly exacerbate symptoms in a patient diagnosed with PPPD.

atric disorder. The primary age range of patients presenting with PPPD is 40 to 50 years with the majority being female. PPPD occurs in patients with and without otological (e.g., neuritis) or neurological disease (e.g., migraine). In this regard, Staab and Ruckenstein (2005) have devised a classification system consisting of three patterns of illness.

The determination of whether a person has PPPD or not is based on several factors, which include a case history, self-report measures of anxiety/depression, dizziness handicap, and results of quantitative balance function testing (e.g., ENG/VNG). One instrument that has been employed to screen for the presence of anxiety and depression is the Hospital Anxiety and Depression Scale (HADS). The HADS is a 14-item self-report scale developed to detect anxiety and depression in a medical outpatient clinic (Zigmond & Snaith, 1983). The HADS has been reported to be a reliable measure for screening current states of anxiety and depression. The anxiety and depression

subscales each consist of seven items, and each item is assigned a score from 0 to 3 points. For each of the subscales, a score of 11 or greater is associated with the presence of clinically significant anxiety or depression (Zigmond & Snaith, 1983) (Table 7–4).

Persistent Postural-Perceptual Dizziness (3PD)—Bárány Society Diagnostic Criteria (Staab et al., 2017).

1. One or more symptoms of dizziness, unsteadiness
   a. or non-spinning vertigo on most days for at least 3 months
      ■ Symptoms last for prolonged (hours-long) periods of time, buy may wax and wane in severity.
      ■ Symptoms need not be present continuously throughout the entire day
2. Persistent symptoms occur without specific provocation, but are exacerbated by three factors: (1) upright posture, (2) active or passive motion without regard to direction or position, and (3) exposure to moving visual stimuli or complex visual patterns.
3. The disorder is triggered by events that cause vertigo, unsteadiness, dizziness, or problems with balance, including acute, episodic or chronic vestibular syndromes, other neurological or medical illnesses, and psychological distress.

   When triggered by an acute or episodic precipitant, symptoms settle into the pattern of criterion "a" as the precipitant resolves, but may occur intermittently at first, and then consolidate into a persistent course.
4. When triggered by a chronic precipitant, symptoms may develop slowly at first and worsen gradually.
5. Symptoms cause significant distress or functional impairment.
6. Symptoms are not better accounted for by another disease or disorder.

Pathophysiology

Although the pathophysiology of PPPD is not yet completely understood, investigations leveraging

Table 7–4. Hospital Anxiety and Depression Scale (HADS) Scoring

Question Number	Item Answers A	B	C	D	Item Score
1					
3					
5					
7					
9					
11					
13					
Anxiety Score (sum from odd-numbered questions)					
2					
4					
6					
8					
10					
12					
14					
Depression Score (sum from even-numbered questions)					
Total Score (Anxiety + Depression)					

Modified from Staab (2008).

new imaging techniques have begun to provide insight into underlying mechanisms of the disorder. With the recent development of an international criterion by the Barany Society, research is now able to be accomplished in a coordinated manner. At the time of this writing, there are numerous laboratories from around the world investigating the underlying physiological mechanisms that contribute to this debilitating condition. It is currently accepted that the disorder develops following a trigger that evokes an abnormal physiological response from the patient. This is followed by a number of key characteristics that will become persistent, which include a stiffening of postural control, an overreliance on visual input, and an interruption in the brain's ability to properly manage postural control, and the accurate processing of spatial information. When an individual is struck by an attack of vertigo or dizziness, the natural response is to stiffen their posture and shorten their stride length. Once the episode has passed and the symptoms resolved, the individual will typically return to their normal baseline strategies. Patients that go on to develop PPPD following an episode with vestibular symptoms are often characterized by developing a heightened sense of vigilance regarding their balance and an increase in their anxiety. They will also begin to develop an overreliance on the visual sense (i.e., visual dependence), regardless of the environment. It has become clear that there are people who have a predisposition (i.e., genetic) to developing PPPD. This includes patients that have higher innate personality traits of neuroticism (i.e., chronic worriers) and anxiety (i.e., susceptible to higher levels of anxiety when stressed). Recent work in neuroimaging is beginning to elucidate the cortical processes that may be facilitating the development of PPPD in certain patients (Van Ombergen, Heine, & Jillings, 2017). When the processing of the cortical networks of patients with PPPD is examined using imaging, the level of neural activity and the strength of the connections are more robust in the visual areas, as compared to the vestibular areas and areas responsible for space-motion input. This would be in line with the reported behavioral manifestation of PPPD patients over relying on visual input, regardless of the environment they find themselves navigating (e.g., motion-rich environments) and the continued use of inappropriate postural control strategies.

Common Findings on the Laboratory Testing

There is no one pattern of findings on vestibular laboratory testing that is diagnostic for PPPD. In cases where patients may have experienced a vestibular crisis prior to the onset of their chronic symptoms it is not uncommon for he or she to present with a caloric weakness or abnormalities during VEMP testing. One laboratory test that is beginning to show promise in identifying patients with PPPD is computerized dynamic posturography (CDP). It has recently been reported that patients with PPPD will have lower scores when compared to their normal counterparts on conditions 2–6 (Sohsten, Bittar, & Staab, 2016). Furthermore, the PPPD group when compared to a group of patients with a compensated vestibular deficit did poorer on conditions 2–3. The CDP pattern of performing worse on earlier conditions (1–3) compared to later conditions (4–6) is atypical in most patients and almost never observed in normal patients. The authors recommended that although the pattern of postural sway observed in patients with PPPD may be in line with what was once termed a malingering pattern, care should be taken in interpretation of postural control when PPPD is suspected.

Treatment

Once a diagnosis of PPPD has been made, treatment should begin with a thorough explanation about the nature of the disorder. When possible and appropriate, family members should be brought back and included in the counseling session. Patient education should start with informing the patient that what they are suffering from has a formal name and it is a common disorder that is in fact chronic. If patient education material is available, it is best to counsel them while using it as a guide. Topics covered should include informing the patient that PPPD is a specific set of symptoms, that it may or may not be related to another condition, that it can be treated, and that "it is not all in their head." From this point, it is helpful to walk through the criterion of PPPD and then provide an overview regarding what treatments are available.

It has been shown that for patients with PPPD, vestibular and rehabilitation therapy is efficacious. Depending on the co-morbidities of the patient, the therapy program may vary. In patients without vestibular deficits, therapy is most often targeted at reducing the sensitivity to visual stimuli that exacerbate the patient's symptoms. The most provocative situations (e.g. motion-rich environments, complex visual environments, and visually focused tasks) should be evaluated during the therapy appointment and the program customized accordingly. These therapy programs designed around habituation have been shown to have positive long-term outcomes (Thompson, Goetting, Staab, & Shepard, 2015). One important factor to consider when prescribing a therapy program is to inform the patient that he or she should avoid being too aggressive with the exercises early on but rather to slowly increase the intensity.

Physical therapy, in combination with a pharmaceutical approach, has been shown to provide good patient outcomes (Thompson et al., 2015). Unfortunately, at the time of this writing, there is currently a lack of large-scale, randomized, controlled trials of medications or other treatments for PPPD. However, there is some support in the literature for the use of selective serotonin reuptake inhibitors (SSRI) and serotonin-norepinephrine reuptake inhibitors (SNRI) (Staab, 2012). It has been noted in the literature that the response to these medications in the patient with PPPD will depend to some degree on the underlying psychiatric co-morbidities. For example, SSRIs were shown to significantly reduce patients' chronic symptoms of dizziness (Staab, Ruckenstein, & Amsterdam, 2004). Studies using serotonin-norepinephrine reuptake inhibitors (SNRIs) have reported similar findings (Horii et al., 2004; Staab, 2011).

Recent work has shown that cognitive-behavioral therapy (CBT) may be efficacious for patients with PPPD. CBT is a form of psychotherapy that was initially designed to treat patients suffering from depression. However, over the years the role of CBT has been expanded to treat other disorders such as anxiety and post-traumatic stress. Edelman, Mahoney, and Cremer, (2012) reported their results from a closely controlled trial that evaluated the effect of three sessions of CBT on 41 patients diagnosed with chronic subjective dizziness. The authors reported that following three sessions of CBT, 75% of patients reported a significant decrease in symptoms. When this same group was evaluated 1 to 6 months following treatment, their symptoms continued to be improved suggesting that CBT may offer a long-lasting solution to symptom reduction. (Mahoney, Edelman, & Cremer, 2013). Accordingly, CBT and VBRT are complementary treatments that, in appropriate cases, can be used together.

Appendix

A

Dizziness Questionnaire

Dizziness Questionnaire: Characteristics of Dizziness

IS YOUR DIZZINESSS ASSOCIATED WITH ANY OF THE FOLLOWING SENSATIONS? PLEASE READ THE ENTIRE LIST FIRST. THEN CIRCLE YES OR NO TO DESCRIBE YOUR FEELINGS MOST ACCURATELY.

Yes No   1. Lightheadedness or swimming sensation in the head.

Yes No   2. Blacking out or loss of consciousness.

Yes No   3. Tendency to fall.

Yes No   4. Objects spinning or turning around you.

Yes No   5. Sensation that you are turning or spinning inside, with outside objects remaining stationary.

Yes No   6. Loss of balance when walking in the light: Veering to the Right? Left?

Yes No   7. Loss of balance when walking in the dark: Veering to the Right? Left?

Yes No   8. Headache.

Yes No   9. Nausea.

Yes No   10. Vomiting.

Yes No   11. Pressure in the head.

Yes No   12. Tingling in the fingers or toes.

Yes No   13. Tingling around the mouth.

Dizziness Questionnaire: Associated Ear Symptoms

DO YOU HAVE ANY OF THE FOLLOWING SYMPTOMS? PLEASE CIRCLE YES OR NO AND CIRCLE THE EAR INVOLVED, IF APPLICABLE.

Yes No	1. Dizziness. Describe dizziness.	
	_____	
Yes No	2. Difficulty in hearing?	Both Ears Right Left
Yes No	3. Does your hearing change with dizziness? If so, how?	
	_____	
Yes No	4. Do you have noise in your ears?	Both Ears Right Left
Yes No	5. Does noise change with dizziness? If so, how?	
	_____	
Yes No	6. Do you have fullness or stuffiness in your ears?	Both Ears Right Left
Yes No	7. Do you have pain in your ears?	Both Ears Right Left
Yes No	8. Do you have a discharge from your ears?	Both Ears Right Left

Dizziness Questionnaire: Associated Neurologic Symptoms

HAVE YOU EXPERIENCED ANY OF THE FOLLOWING SYMPTOMS? PLEASE CIRCLE YES OR NO AND CIRCLE IF CONSTANT OR IN EPISODES.

Yes No	1. Double vision	Constant In Episodes
Yes No	2. Blurred vision	Constant In Episodes
Yes No	3. Blindness	Constant In Episodes
Yes No	4. Numbness of the face or extremities	Constant In Episodes
Yes No	5. Weakness in the arms or legs	Constant In Episodes
Yes No	6. Confusion or loss of consciousness	Constant In Episodes
Yes No	7. Difficulty with speech	Constant In Episodes
Yes No	8. Difficulty with swallowing	Constant In Episodes
Yes No	9. Pain in the neck or shoulders	Constant In Episodes

Dizziness Questionnaire: Past Medical History, Family History, Social History

Yes No   1. Did you have a history of earaches or ear infections as a child?

Yes No   2. Did you ever injure your head? When? _____

Yes No   3. Were you ever unconscious? When? _____

Yes No   4. Did you suffer from motion sickness before age 12? _____

Yes No   5. Have you suffered from motion sickness in the last 10 years? _____

Yes No   6. Do you now take any medications regularly? What?

_____

Yes No   7. Have you taken medication in the past for dizziness? Which ones?

_____

_____

Yes No   8. Do you have a past medical history of: Diabetes? Heart disease?

Yes No   9. Do you have a family history of: Ear disease? Neurologic disease?
Migraine headache?

Yes No   10. Do you use tobacco in any form? What kind? _____ How much? _____

Yes No   11. Does caffeine affect your dizziness? How? _____

_____

Yes No   12. Does alcohol affect your dizziness? How? _____

_____

Dizziness Questionnaire: Time Course and Aggravating Factors

1. When did your dizziness first occur? _____

2. How often do you become dizzy? _____

3. If dizziness occurs in attacks, how long does an attack last? _____

Yes No   4. Do you have any warning that dizziness is about to start?

Yes No   5. Does dizziness occur at any particular time of the day or night?

Yes No   6. Are you completely free of dizziness between attacks?

Yes No   7. Does change of position make you dizzy? Which movements?

Yes No   8. Do you become dizzy when rolling over in bed?   To the right?   To the left?

Yes No   9. Do you know of any possible cause for your dizziness? What?

_____

Yes No   10. Do you know of anything that will:

                    a. Stop your dizziness or make it better? _____

                    _____

                    b. Make your dizziness worse? _____

                    _____

Yes No   11. Do you become dizzy when you bend your head forward?

Yes No   Backward?

Yes No   12. Do you become dizzy when you cough?

Yes No   When you sneeze?

Yes No   When you have a bowel movement?

           13. Can any of the following make your dizziness worse or start an attack?

Yes No   Fatigue

Yes No   Exertion

Yes No   Hunger

Yes No   Menstrual period

Yes No   Stress

Yes No   Emotional upset

Yes No   Alcohol

Yes No   14. Do you have any allergies? What? _____

                    _____

Source: From Furman, Cass, & Whitney (2010).

Appendix

III B III

Understanding Dizziness[1]

[1]Used with permission of Mayo Foundation for Medical Education and Research. All rights reserved.

MAYO
CLINIC

Dizziness

Understanding Dizziness

Feeling lightheaded or woozy is a common complaint. Every year, more than 2 million people tell their doctors something like, "I feel dizzy."

It probably surprises most of those people to learn that dizziness is a symptom of a different problem. By itself, dizziness isn't a disorder.

This material describes how your body works to stay in balance and what happens when you feel dizzy. It also explains how your condition is examined and which treatment options may help you.

How Your Body Stays in Balance

Throughout the day, your brain manages a constant flow of information. It uses messages from your eyes, muscles, tendons, and inner ears to help you stay in balance. This is true when you when you move and when you are standing, seated and lying down.

Your balance also depends on these issues:

- You need to have enough blood to reach all parts of your body.

- Your heart has to pump well enough to keep a strong supply of blood going to your brain.

- Your blood vessels have to keep a steady blood pressure.

- You need to be well hydrated.

Some dizziness and balance issues happen due to problems in your inner ear. However, problems in various parts of your body could lead to dizziness or feeling out of balance. (See Figure 1.) In addition, medications could cause you to become dizzy. Heart problems, such as abnormal heart rhythm, could do it too.

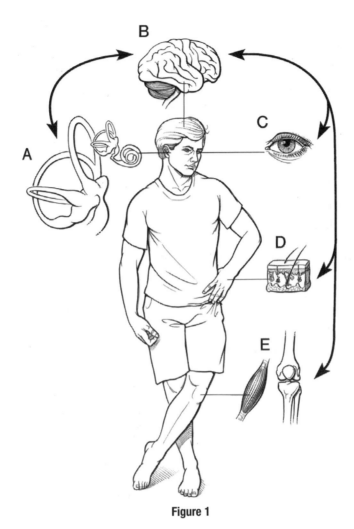

Figure 1

A. The inner ear contains your primary hearing structure, the cochlea, and your primary balance structure, the vestibular labyrinth.

B. The brain relays information to and from the eyes, skin, joints and muscles to the inner ear's vestibular labyrinth.

C. The eyes record the body's position and surroundings.

D. When you touch things, sensors in your skin send information about your environment to your brain.

E. Muscles and joints report bodily movement to the brain.

Conditions Called "Dizziness"

There are three sensations that people often call "dizziness."

- **Dizziness** is being lightheaded or woozy. Some people say that it feels like they are floating or ready to faint or pass out.

- **Vertigo** is the sensation that your surroundings are moving while your body and head are still. Some people say it feels like the room is spinning or slowly rotating. Or it feels like the room is rocking or tilting.

  These sensations can happen within your head with the room is still. And, it's possible that these sensations can happen in your head and in your room (or a larger environment) at the same time.

  Benign paroxysmal positional vertigo (BPPV) is a type of vertigo. This is a disorder of the inner ear. With BPPV, you feel dizzy very suddenly when you move your head up and down, or, for example, when you turn over in bed. These symptoms usually go away within a few minutes. Special exercises and positions can reduce BPPV symptoms.

- **Unsteadiness** is the sensation that you have to touch something to stay in balance when you are walking. If it is difficult to stand without falling, that's a more severe type of unsteadiness. (Unsteadiness is also called imbalance.)

Common Balance Problems

Dizziness has many causes. Your treatment depends on the type of dizziness or balance problem you have. Below are brief descriptions of these problems.

Common problems

Inner ear problems, such as BPPV or vestibular neuronitis, usually are treated with medications to improve the symptoms.

If this is your diagnosis, your health care provider may also suggest vestibular and balance therapy. If advised, you should return to your normal activities. Vestibular and balance therapy can help your brain get used to, or compensate for, certain inner ear problems. But if you are not active, it may take longer to recover from dizziness and other balance problems.

Uncommon problems

- **Meniere's disease.** Meniere's disease is a disorder of the inner ear that causes sudden episodes of vertigo. The episodes of vertigo may happen hours, months or even years apart. Meniere's disease also causes hearing loss that comes and goes, ringing in the ear (called tinnitus), and sometimes a feeling of fullness or pressure in your ear. In many cases, Meniere's disease affects only one ear. The cause is not known.

   Treatment may include following a special diet and taking medications to relieve most symptoms. If symptoms of Meniere's disease are severe, your health care provider may advise surgery.

- **Bilateral inner ear dysfunction.** If tests show that you have problems with balance that affect both ears, it is called bilateral inner ear dysfunction. If this is causing your dizziness, you need to rely on your vision and muscle responses to keep your balance. You have to use great caution when you swim under water, walk in the dark or walk on unfamiliar surfaces. Vestibular and balance therapy can help if you are diagnosed with this condition.

Other possible causes of dizziness

- **Migraine headaches.** Migraines can cause people to be sensitive to motion and dizziness.
- **Vestibular neuritis.** This inflammatory disorder may damage the inner ear.
- **Psychiatric conditions, such as anxiety.** People with psychiatric conditions may experience dizziness or lightheadedness.
- **Problems with the central nervous system (CNS).** Stroke and tumors can produce symptoms of dizziness, unsteadiness or even vertigo. These conditions are rarely found to be the cause of most cases of dizziness. But your health care provider may want to rule them out.

Diagnosing and Treating Your Condition

Describing your dizziness

The way that you describe your problem can have a direct impact on your diagnosis and treatment.

Because problems of dizziness and balance can have many different causes, your health care provider will talk to you about your complete medical and psychiatric history.

- A physical examination includes a check of your eyes and ears.
- A neurologic exam checks how you walk and maintain your balance. It also checks to see how the major nerves of your central nervous system are working. This is a simple, painless exam.

Your health care provider likely will also order many tests. Your provider will give you more information about them at that time.

Before your tests

You may feel dizzy or sick to your stomach (nauseous) during some tests. **Follow the directions on your patient preparation information to get ready for each test or exam.**

Tests you may have

Hearing test

Different parts of your inner ear affect your hearing and balance. A hearing test checks the part of your inner ear that helps you hear. Problems with hearing often are related to balance problems.

Vestibular evoked myogenic potentials (VEMP) test

This test collects information about two inner-ear areas that help you balance. To do the test, you lie on your back. The person who tests you puts electrodes on the sides of your neck and under your eyes. He or she asks you to lift your head and turn it to the right or left. Sounds are sent to each ear through small earphones placed in your ears. The electrodes pick up signals from the neck and eye area to see if they are working properly.

Videonystagmography (VNG) or Electronystagmography (ENG)

Your eyes and eye muscles work with your inner ear to control your balance. This test collects information about the messages that your inner ear sends to your eyes.

During the test, a video camera or electrodes around your eyes record your eye movements while:

- You stare at a moving spot or a light.

- You lie on a bed in different positions, such as on your right or left side.

- The person who tests you puts water or air into your outer ear canals. The water (or air) will be warmer or cooler than your body temperature.

You may feel dizzy during some parts of the test, especially the last part. This is normal. That usually lasts only two or three minutes.

Posturography

This test can show which parts of your balance system you use most. You stand in your bare feet on a special platform. You try to keep your balance in different situations while the platform moves. For example, you try to balance with your eyes open. Then you try to balance with your eyes closed.

Many people are nervous that they will fall during this test. Fear can affect whether you are able to do the test. **The staff member who helps you with this test takes steps to help keep you safe.** For example, you may wear a safety harness over your clothes to keep you from falling.

Rotary-chair test

This test checks the part of your inner ear that helps with balance. You sit in a chair that a computer controls. The computer moves the chair very slowly in a full circle. It also moves the chair back and forth in a very small arc at faster speeds. The testing room is dark. However, you have a microphone on the chair so you can talk to the person who tests you. A camera in the room lets that person watch you.

Other tests

Your health care provider may suggest other tests for you such as an MRI, a CT scan, blood tests, or heart tests. "MRI" refers to magnetic resonance imaging. "CT" refers to computed tomography. Ask for more information if other tests are set up for you.

Treatment

Your treatment will depend on the type of balance problem you have.

Many patients are referred to other health care providers for some aspects of their treatment. Some of the other care providers work in neurology, psychiatry and physical medicine and rehabilitation.

Common treatments for balance and dizziness include medical care, physical therapy and other activities, counseling, and medication. Rarely, surgery may be needed.

When to Get Emergency Care

Dizziness and vertigo do not usually signal a serious condition. **But if you have any of the following conditions, you should get medical care right away.**

These conditions may signal a serious problem, such as a stroke, brain tumor or aneurysm, or heart disease.

- A new, different or severe headache.
- Blurred or double vision.
- Hearing loss.
- Speech problems.
- Weakness in your arm(s) or leg(s).
- Loss of consciousness.
- Problems walking.
- Numbness or tingling anywhere on the body.
- Chest pain or a fast or slow heart rate.

For More Information

If you have questions after you read this material, talk to your health care provider.

Appendix

III C III

Pediatric Literature for Vestibular Testing

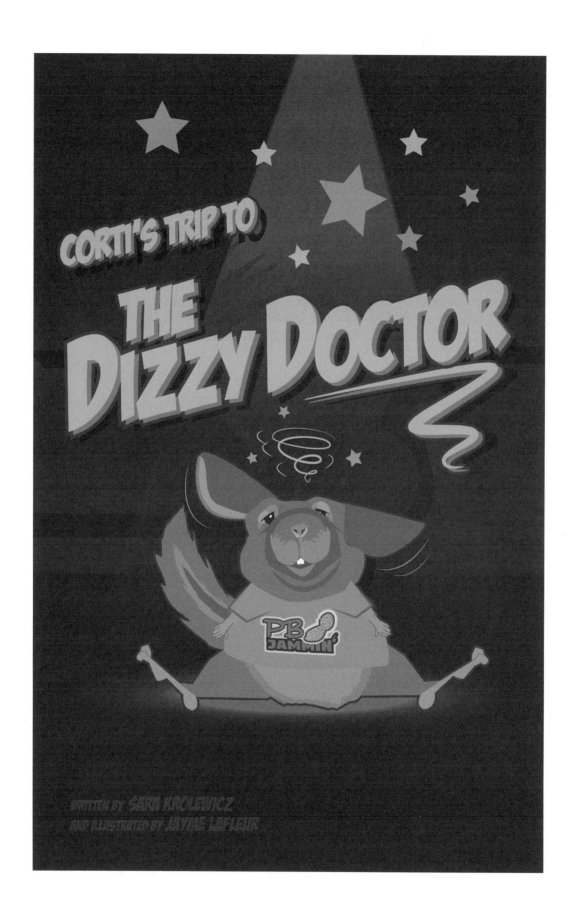

CORTI'S TRIP TO

THE DIZZY DOCTOR

WRITTEN BY SARA KROLEWICZ
AND ILLUSTRATED BY JAYME LAFLEUR

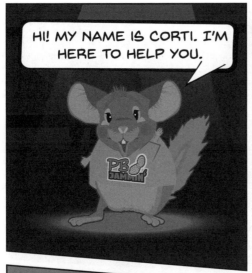

HI! MY NAME IS CORTI. I'M HERE TO HELP YOU.

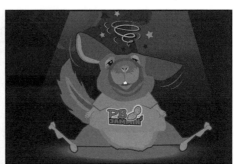

SOMETIMES, I DON'T FEEL GOOD AND HAVE TO GO TO THE DIZZY DOCTOR. BUT THAT'S OKAY. THE DIZZY DOCTOR IS A SPECIAL DOCTOR THAT TESTS EARS TO CHECK FOR DIZZINESS AND UNBALANCE.

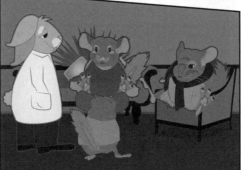

SHE SAYS WE ARE GOING TO PLAY GAMES, BUT THAT EACH ONE IS A TEST TO SEE HOW MY EARS ARE WORKING.

THE FIRST GAME IS FUNNY...I HAVE TO SIT IN A VERY BIG CHAIR THAT MOVES! THE DOCTOR SAYS SHE WILL TEST MY EARS' SIGNALS -- BUT BY WATCHING MY EYES!

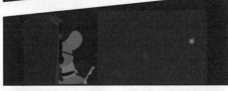

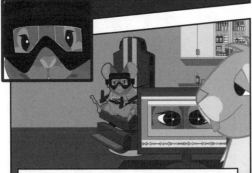

THEN THE DIZZY DOCTOR PUTS SOME GOGGLES WITH CAMERAS ON ME AND MAKES MY EYES LOOK HUGE ON THE COMPUTER.

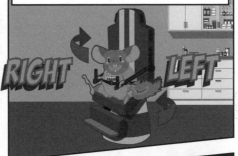

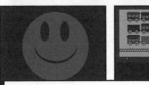
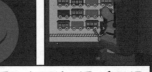

I GET TO LOOK AT SOME PICTURES. PICTURES OF SMILES, PICTURES OF TRAINS, PICTURES OF ALL KINDS OF COOL THINGS.

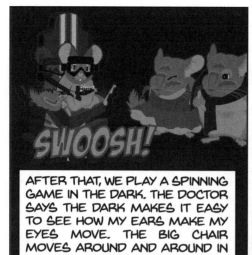

AFTER THAT, WE PLAY A SPINNING GAME IN THE DARK. THE DOCTOR SAYS THE DARK MAKES IT EASY TO SEE HOW MY EARS MAKE MY EYES MOVE. THE BIG CHAIR MOVES AROUND AND AROUND IN CIRCLES.

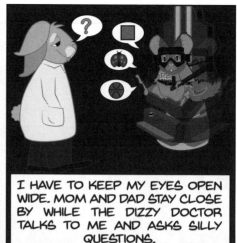

I HAVE TO KEEP MY EYES OPEN WIDE. MOM AND DAD STAY CLOSE BY WHILE THE DIZZY DOCTOR TALKS TO ME AND ASKS SILLY QUESTIONS.

I GET A LITTLE TIRED OF THE GAME AS WE SPIN AND SPIN, BUT THEN THE DOCTOR IS THERE WITH A LIGHT IN THE DARK FOR ME TO STARE AT AS I GO ROUND!

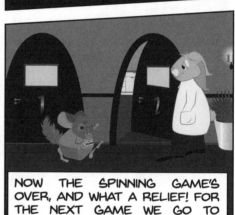

NOW THE SPINNING GAME'S OVER, AND WHAT A RELIEF! FOR THE NEXT GAME WE GO TO ANOTHER ROOM...

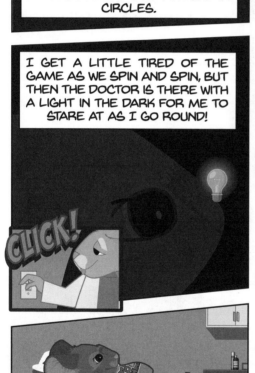

THERE'S ANOTHER BIG CHAIR, BUT THIS ONE JUST SITS STILL. IT ONLY LEANS BACKWARDS SO I CAN LAY BACK LIKE IN BED!

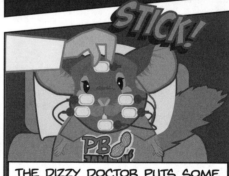
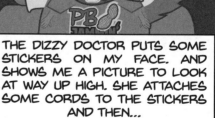

THE DIZZY DOCTOR PUTS SOME STICKERS ON MY FACE. AND SHOWS ME A PICTURE TO LOOK AT WAY UP HIGH. SHE ATTACHES SOME CORDS TO THE STICKERS AND THEN...

I LOOK UP TO THE SKY AND HEAR A BIG THUMP! AND THUMP, THUMP, THUMP, THUMP.

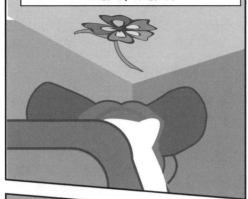

NOW THAT THAT'S DONE, I CAN SHOW HOW STRONG I AM! SOME MORE THUMPS GO BY, WHILE I HOLD UP MY HEAD.

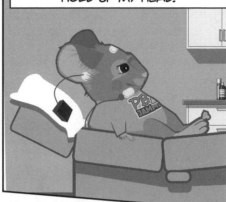

AFTER THE THUMP GAME, THE STICKERS ARE GONE AND DIZZY DOCTOR SAYS MORE GOGGLES WILL COME.

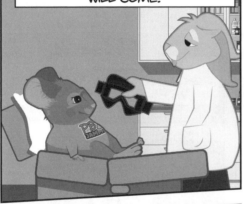

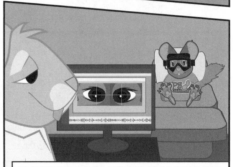

THESE GOGGLES MAKE MY EYES LOOK BIG WITH CAMERAS JUST LIKE BEFORE. AND NOW WE PLAY SIMON SAYS!

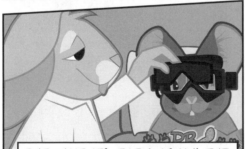

BUT WAIT ITS DARK AGAIN! THE DIZZY DOCTOR SAYS THE CAMERA GOGGLES NEED DARK TO MAKE MY EYES BRIGHTER -- MY EYES ARE HOW SHE CAN TELL MY EARS ARE WORKING.

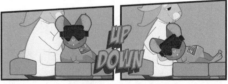
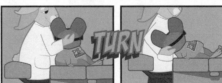

SHE TALKS ABOUT WINNING. I SHOW HER I'LL WIN AND DO ALL SIMON SAYS! SIMON SAYS LAY DOWN! SIMON SAYS SIT UP! WE DO THIS ONE TWICE.

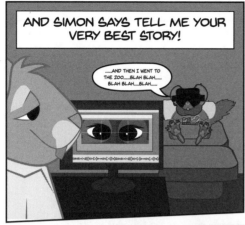

AND SIMON SAYS TELL ME YOUR VERY BEST STORY!

.....AND THEN I WENT TO THE ZOO.....BLAH BLAH..... BLAH BLAH.....BLAH.....

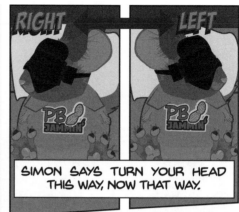

RIGHT LEFT

SIMON SAYS TURN YOUR HEAD THIS WAY, NOW THAT WAY.

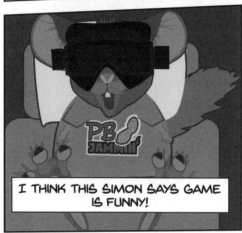

I THINK THIS SIMON SAYS GAME IS FUNNY!

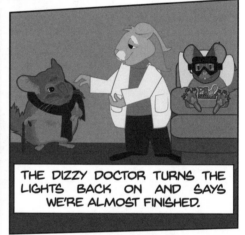

THE DIZZY DOCTOR TURNS THE LIGHTS BACK ON AND SAYS WE'RE ALMOST FINISHED.

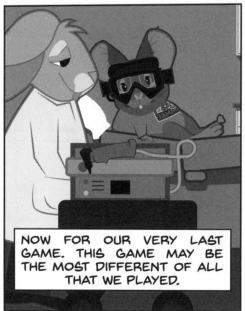

NOW FOR OUR VERY LAST GAME. THIS GAME MAY BE THE MOST DIFFERENT OF ALL THAT WE PLAYED.

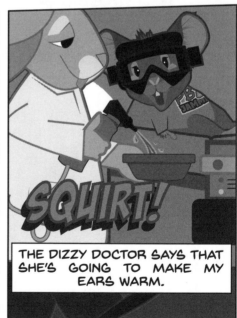

SQUIRT!

THE DIZZY DOCTOR SAYS THAT SHE'S GOING TO MAKE MY EARS WARM.

VERY WARM WATER LIKE BATH TIME AT HOME, STRAIGHT INTO MY EARS. THIS MAKES ME FEEL DIZZY.

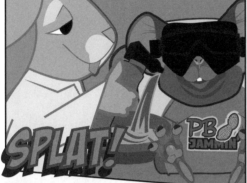

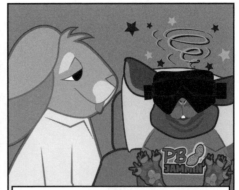

BUT DIZZY DOCTOR IS THERE AND ASKS FOR A STORY! I TELL HER ALL OF MY FAVORITE THINGS DETERMINED TO TELL THE VERY BEST STORY.

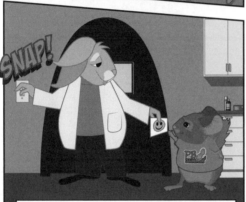

AFTER EACH EAR, SHE TURNS ON THE LIGHTS AND I GET A SURPRISE!

THE DIZZY DOCTOR TELLS MOM AND DAD HOW BRAVE I'VE BEEN AND HOW MY EARS WORK.

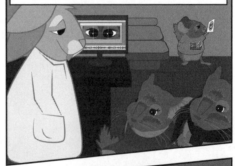

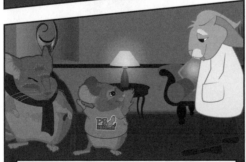

WHILE MOM AND DAD TALK, I THINK THIS TRIP WAS PRETTY GOOD AFTER ALL! WE PLAYED LOTS OF FUN GAMES THAT TESTED MY EARS.

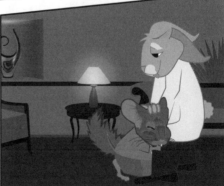

NOW WHEN I FEEL LESS THAN MY BEST, I KNOW THE DIZZY DOCTOR IS THERE TO HELP ME OUT!

Copyright © 2017 Jayme LaFleur

For information on how to obtain a copy of *Corti's Trip to the Dizzy Doctor* send an e-mail to lafleurjayme@gmail.com

Appendix

D

Example Alerting Tasks for Vestibular Testing

Count . . .

by 3s to 100.

by 4s to 100.

backward by 2s from 100.

backward by 2s from 99.

Name . . .

a woman's name for each letter of the alphabet.

a man's name for each letter of the alphabet.

a city, state, or country for each letter of the alphabet.

an animal for each letter of the alphabet.

something you buy in a grocery store for each letter of the alphabet.

all the U.S. presidents you can recall.

pieces of furniture.

items of clothing.

professional sports or players.

types of flowers or trees.

all the holidays you can recall.

all the colors you can think of.

all the colleges and/or universities.

TV shows/movies (or shows from your childhood).

directions from your house to the _____ clinic.

famous entertainers, musicians, or movie stars.

fruits and/or vegetables.

towns or cities in home state.

For patients that are difficult to task

Name the first names of immediate family and relatives.

Recite a recipe.

Explain what is happening in a television series he or she is watching.

Describe how you would repair a car.

Talk about their hobbies.

Appendix

E

Reliability and Localizing Value of VNG Findings

Test	Abnormality	Reliability[a]	Localization[b] Peripheral Vestibular	CNS	Comment
Gaze	Horizontal nystagmus (follows Alexander's law)	+++	+++	0	
	Bilateral gaze nystagmus, eyes open	+++	0	+++	
	Bilateral gaze nystagmus, eyes closed	++	0	+++	
	Unilateral gaze nystagmus, eyes open	+++	++	++	
	Unilateral gaze nystagmus, eyes closed	+	0	+	
	Rebound nystagmus	+++	0	+++	Cerebellar system lesion
	Periodic alternating nystagmus	+++	0	+++	Usually posterior fossa lesion
	Up-beating nystagmus	+++	0	+++	Lesion, drug induced
	Down-beating nystagmus	+++	0	+++	Lower medullary lesion
	Pendular nystagmus	+++	0	+++	Usually congenital nystagmus

Test	Abnormality	Reliability[a]	Localization[b] Peripheral Vestibular	CNS	Comment
Gaze *continued*	Square wave movements	++	0	+++	Overalert patient, occasionally cerebellar system lesion
	Internuclear ophthalmoplegia	+++	0	+++	Medial longitudinal fasciculus lesion
Saccade	Ocular dysmetria	+++	0	+++	Cerebellar system lesion
	Saccadic slowing	+++	0	+++	Saccadic system (supranuclear) lesion
	Internuclear ophthalmoplegia	+++	0	+++	Medial longitudinal fasciculus lesion
Tracking	Saccadic pursuit	+++	0	+++	
	Disorganized pursuit	+++	0	+++	
	Disconjugate pursuit	+++	0	+++	
Optokinetic	Asymmetry	+++	0	+++	Supratentorial, brainstem lesion
	Declining response to increasing stimulus speeds	+++	0	+++	Usually brainstem lesion
	Inversion	+++	0	+++	Usually congenital nystagmus
Positional	Direction-fixed nystagmus, eyes open	+++	0	+++	
	Direction-changing nystagmus, eyes open	+++	0	+++	
	Direction-fixed nystagmus, eyes closed	++	++	+	
	Direction-changing nystagmus, eyes closed	++	+	++	If apogeotropic, probably CNS lesion (except PAN II)
	Direction-changing nystagmus, single head position	+++	0	+++	
Dix-Hallpike maneuver	Unilateral benign paroxysmal type positioning nystagmus	+++	++	+	Usually undermost ear lesion
	Bilateral benign paroxysmal type positioning nystagmus	+++	++	++	Both ears, CNS lesion
	All other nystagmus	++	+	++	

Test	Abnormality	Reliability[a]	Localization[b] Peripheral Vestibular	CNS	Comment
Caloric	Unilateral weakness	+++	+++	+	Almost always weak ear lesion
	Directional preponderance	+	+	++	Localization uncertain
	Bilateral weakness	+++	++	+	Both ears, CNS lesion
	Hyperactive response	+	0	+++	Overalert patient, cerebellovestibular disease
	Failure of fixation suppression	+++	0	+++	
	Premature caloric reversal	++	0	+++	
	Caloric inversion	+++	0	+++	Brainstem lesion
	Caloric perversion	+++	0	+++	Brainstem lesion

[a]+++ A "hard" finding, nearly always denotes a lesion; ++ an "intermediate" finding, usually denotes a lesion; + a "soft" finding, sometimes denotes a lesion.

[b]+++ Nearly always denotes the indicated site of lesion; ++ usually denotes the indicated site of lesion; + sometimes denotes the indicated site of lesion; 0 almost never denotes the indicated site of lesion.

Source: From Barber & Stockwell (1980b).

References

Agarwal, Y., Carey, J. P., Della Santina, C. C., Schubert, M. C., & Minor, L. B. (2009). Disorders of balance and vestibular function in U.S. adults: Data from the National Health and Nutrition Examination Survey, 2001–2004. *Archives of Internal Medicine, 169,* 938–944.

Agrawal S. K., & Parnes L. S. (2001). Human experience with canal plugging. *Annals of New York Academy of Sciences, 942,* 300–305.

Albers, F. W., Van Weissenbruch, R., & Casselman, J. W. (1994). 3DFT-magnetic resonance imaging of the inner ear in Ménière's disease. *Acta Otolaryngologica, 114,* 595–600.

Alghadir, A., & Anwer, S. (2018). Effects of vestibular rehabilitation in the management of a vestibular migraine: A review. *Frontiers in Neurology, 9,* 1–9.

Alpert, J. N. (1974). Failure of fixation suppression: A pathologic effect of vision on caloric nystagmus. *Neurology, 24,* 891–896.

American Academy of Otolaryngology-Head and Neck Surgery Committee on Hearing and Equilibrium. (1995). Committee on hearing and equilibrium guidelines for the diagnosis and evaluation of therapy in Meniere's disease. *Otolaryngology-Head and Neck Surgery, 113,* 181–185.

American National Standards Institute. (1999). Procedures for testing basic vestibular function. *American National Standards Institute,* BSR S3.45-200, revision of ANSI S3.45.

Anderson, J. P. & Harris, J. P. (2001). Impact of Meniere's disease on quality of life. *Otology and Neurotology, 22*(6), 888–894.

ANSI. (2009). Procedures for testing basic vestibular function. *American National Standards Institute,* ANSI/ASA S3.45-2009 (Revision of ANSI S3.45-1999).

Appiani, G. C., Catania, G., Gagliardi, M., & Cuiuli, G. (2005). Repositioning maneuver for the treatment of the apogeotropic variant of horizontal canal benign paroxysmal positional vertigo. *Otology and Neurotology, 26,* 257–860.

Arts, H. A., Adams, M. E., Telian, S. A., El-Kashlan, H., & Kileny, P. R. (2008). Reversible electrocochleographic abnormalities in superior canal dehiscence. *Otology and Neurotology, 30*(1), 79–86.

Asprella Libonati, G., & Gufoni, M. (1999). Vertigine parossistica da CSL: manovre di barbecue ed altre varianti. In *XVI Giornate Italiane di Otoneurologia. Revisione critica di venti anni di vertigine parossistica posizionale benigna* (VPPB), (pp. 321–336). Milano, Italy: CSS Formenti [Google Scholar].

Asprella Libonati, G. (2005). Diagnostic and treatment strategy of lateral semicircular canal canalolithiasis. *Acta Otolaryngologica Italica, 25,* 277–283.

Balkany, T. J., Sires, B., & Arenberg, I. K. (1980). Bilateral aspects of Ménière's disease: An underestimated clinical entity. *Otolaryngology Clinics of North America, 13*(4), 603–609.

Baloh, R. W. (1998a). Vertigo. *Lancet, 352,* 1841–1846.

Baloh, R. W. (1998b). *Dizziness, hearing loss, and tinnitus.* Philadelphia, PA: Davis.

Baloh, R. W. (2003). Clinical practice. Vestibular neuritis. *New England Journal of Medicine, 348,* 1027–1032.

Baloh, R. W., & Furman, J. M. (1989). Modern vestibular function testing. *Western Journal of Medicine, 150,* 59–67.

Baloh, R. W., & Honrubia, V. (1990). *Clinical neurophysiology of the vestibular system* (2nd ed.). New York, NY: Oxford University Press.

Baloh, R. W., & Honrubia, V. (2001). *Clinical neurophysiology of the vestibular system* (3rd ed.). New York, NY: Oxford University Press.

Baloh, R. W., Honrubia, V., & Jacobson, K. (1987). Benign positional vertigo: Clinical and oculographic features in 240 cases. *Neurology, 37,* 371–378.

Baloh, R. W., Ishiyama, A., Wackym, P. A., & Honrubia, V. (1996). Vestibular neuritis: Clinical pathological correlation. *Otolaryngology-Head and Neck Surgery, 114,* 586–592.

Baloh, R. W., & Kerber, K. A. (2011). *Clinical neurophysiology of the vestibular system* (4th ed.). New York, NY: Oxford University Press.

Baloh, R. W., Konrad, H. R., Dirks, D., & Honrubia, V. (1976). Cerebellar-pontine angle tumors. Results of quantitative vestibulo-ocular testing. *Archives of Neurology, 33,* 507–512.

Baloh, R. W., & Spooner, J. W. (1981). Downbeat nystagmus: A type of central vestibular nystagmus. *Neurology, 31,* 304–310.

Baloh, R. W., Yee, R. D., & Honrubia, V. (1980). Optokinetic nystagmus and parietal lobe lesions. *Annals of Neurology, 7,* 269–276.

Barany, R. (1907). *Physiologie und Pathologie des Bogengapparates beim Menshen.* Vienna, Austria: Deuticke.

Barber, H. O., & Stockwell C. W. (1976). *Manual of electronystagmography.* St. Louis, MO: Mosby.

Barber, H. O., & Stockwell, C. W. (1980). *Manual of electronystagmography* (2nd ed.). St. Louis, MO: Mosby.

Barber, H. O., & Wright, G. (1973). Positional nystagmus in normals. *Advances in Oto-Rhino-Laryngology, 19,* 276–283.

Barber, H. O., Wright, G., & Demanuele, F. (1971). The hot caloric test as a clinical screening device. *Archives of Otolaryngology, 94*(4), 335–337.

Barin, K. (2008a). Interpretation and usefulness of caloric testing. In G. P. Jacobson & N. T. Shepard (Eds.), *Balance function assessment and management* (pp. 230–252). San Diego, CA: Plural Publishing.

Barin, K. (2008b). Interpretation of static position testing in VNG/ENG. In *Insights in Practice for Clinical Audiology,* May, pp. 1–6.

Barin, K. (2009). Neurophysiology of the vestibular system. In J. Katz, L. Medwetsky, & R. Burkhart (Eds.), *Handbook of clinical audiology* (6th ed., pp. 431–466). Philadelphia, PA: Lippincott Williams & Wilkins.

Barin, K., & Durrant, J. D. (2000). Applied physiology of the vestibular system. In R. F. Canalis, & P. R. Lambert (Eds.), *The ear: Comprehensive otology* (pp. 113–140). Philadelphia, PA: Lippincott Williams & Wilkins.

Barin, K., & Stockwell, C. W. (2002). Directional preponderance revisited. In *Insights in practice* (pp. 1–6). Denmark: Otometrics.

Barnes, G. (1995). Adaptation in the oculomotor response to caloric irrigation and the merits of bi-

thermal stimulation. *British Journal of Audiology, 29*(2), 95–106.

Barr, C. C., Schultheis, L. W., & Robinson, D. A. (1976). Voluntary, non-visual control of the human vestibuloocular reflex. *Acta Otolaryngolica, 81,* 365–375.

Beattie, R. C., & Koester, C. K. (1992). Effects of interstimulus interval on slow phase velocity to ipsilateral warm air caloric stimulation in normal subjects. *Journal of the American Academy of Audiology, 3,* 297–302.

Belden, C. J., Weg, N., Minor, L. B., & Zinreich, S. J. (2003). CT evaluation of bone dehiscence of the superior semicircular canal as a cause of sound- and/or pressure-induced vertigo. *Radiology, 226,* 337–343.

Bennett, M. (2008). The vertigo case history. In G. P. Jacobson & N. T. Shepard (Eds.), *Balance function assessment and management* (pp. 45–62). San Diego, CA: Plural Publishing.

Benson, D., McCaslin, D. L., Shepard, N. T., & McPherson, J. (2019, March). *The effect of disease duration on tests of hearing and balance in patients with Ménière's disease.* Presented at the annual meeting of the American Balance Society, Scottsdale, AZ.

Beraneck, M., McKee, J. L., Aleisa, M., & Cullen, K. E. (2008). Asymmetric recovery in cerebellar-deficient mice following unilateral labyrinthectomy. *Journal of Neurophysiology, 100,* 945–958.

Bertholon, P., Bronstein, A. M., Davies, R. A., Rudge, P., & Thilo, K. V. (2002). Positional down beating nystagmus in 50 patients: Cerebellar disorders and possible anterior semicircular canalithiasis. *Journal of Neurology, Neurosurgery and Psychiatry, 72,* 366–372.

Berthoz, A. (1996). How does the cerebral cortex process and utilize vestibular signals? In R. W. Baloh & G. M. Halmagyi (Eds.), *Disorders of the vestibular system* (pp. 113–125). New York, NY: Oxford University Press.

Bhattacharyya, N., Baugh, R. F., Orvidas, L., Barrs, D., Bronston, L. J., Cass, S., . . . Haidari, J. (2008). Clinical practice guideline: Benign paroxysmal positional vertigo. *Otolaryngology-Head and Neck Surgery, 139*(5 Suppl. 4), S47–S81.

Bisdorff, A.R., Staab, J. P., & Newman-Toker, D. E. (2015). Overview of the International Classification of Vestibular Disorders. *Neurology Clinics, 3,* 541–550.

Bock, O., & Zangemeister, W. H. (1978). A mathematical model of air and water caloric nystagmus. *Biological Cybernetics, 24,* 91–95.

Bojrab, D. I., & McFeely, W. J. (2001). Taking the history: The nature of the spell. In J. A. Goebel (Ed.), *Practical management of the dizzy patient* (pp. 17–22). Philadelphia, PA: Lippincott Williams & Wilkins.

Brandt, T. (1990). Positional and positioning vertigo and nystagmus. *Journal of the Neurological Sciences, 95,* 3–28.

Brandt, T. (1993). Background, technique, interpretation, and usefulness of positional and positioning testing. In G. P. Jacobson, C. W. Newmand, & J. M. Kartush (Eds.), *Handbook of balance function testing* (pp. 123–155). New York, NY: Elsevier.

Brandt, T., & Daroff, R. B. (1980). Physical therapy of benign paroxysmal positional vertigo. *Archives of Otolaryngology, 106,* 484–485.

Brandt, T., Dieterich, M., & Strupp, M. (2005). *Vertigo and dizziness. Common complaints.* London, UK: Springer.

Brandt, T., Zwergal, A., & Strupp, M. (2009). Medical treatment of vestibular disorders, *Expert Opinions in Pharmacotherapy, 10,* 1537–1548.

Brantberg, K., Bergenius, J., Mendel, L., Witt, H., Tribukait, A., & Ygge J. (2001). Symptoms, findings and treatment in patients with dehiscence of the superior semicircular canal. *Acta Otolaryngologica, 121,* 68–75.

Brantberg, K., Bergenius, J., & Tribukait, A. (1999). Vestibular-evoked myogenic potentials in patients with dehiscence of the superior semicircular canal. *Acta Otolaryngologica, 119,* 633–640.

Brichta, A. M., & Goldberg, J. M. (1996). Afferent and efferent responses from morphological fiber classes in the turtle posterior crista. *Annals of the New York Academy of Sciences, 78,* 183–195.

Brickner, R. M. (1936). Oscillopsia: A new symptom commonly occurring in multiple sclerosis. *Archives of Neurological Psychiatry, 36,* 586–589.

British Society of Audiology (BSA). (2010). *Recommended procedure: The caloric test.* UK: Author.

British Society of Audiology (BSA), Balance Interest Group. (1999). Caloric test protocol. *British Journal of Audiology, 33*(3), 179–184.

Bruns, L. (1908). *Geschwulste des nervensystems.* Berlin, Germany: S. Karger.

Cakir, B. O., Ercan, I., Cakir, Z. A., Civelek, S., Sayin, I., & Turgut, S. (2006). What is the true incidence of horizontal semicircular canal benign paroxysmal positional vertigo? *Otolaryngology-Head and Neck Surgery, 134,* 451–454.

Carl, J. R. (1997). Principles and techniques of electrooculography. In G. P. Jacobson, C. W. Newman, & J. M. Kartush (Eds.), *Handbook of balance function testing* (pp. 69–82). San Diego, CA: Singular Publishing.

Caruso, G., & Nuti, D. (2005). Epidemiological data from 2270 PPV patients. *Audiological Medicine, 3,* 7–11.

Casani, A., Giovanni, V., Bruno, F., & Luigi, G. P. (1997). Positional vertigo and ageotropic bidirectional nystagmus. *Laryngoscope, 107,* 807–813.

Casani, A. P., Nacci, A., Dallan, I., Panicucci, E., Gufoni, M., & Sellari-Franceschini, S. (2011). Horizontal semicircular canal benign paroxysmal positional vertigo: Effectiveness of two different methods of treatment. *Audiology and Neurotology, 16,* 175–184.

Casani, A. P., Vannucci, G., Fattori, B., & Berrettini, S. (2002). The treatment of horizontal canal positional vertigo: Our experience in 66 cases. *Laryngoscope, 112,* 172–178.

Cass, S. P., Furman, J. M., Ankerstjerne, J. K. P, Balaban, C., Yetiser, S., & Aydogan, B. (1997). Migraine-related vestibulopathy. *Annals of Otology, Rhinology, and Laryngology, 106,* 182–189.

Cawthorne, T. (1944). The physiological basis for head exercises. *Chartered Society of Physiotherapy, 30,* 106–107.

Chiou, W. Y., Lee, H. L., Tsai, S. C., Yu, T. H., & Lee X. X. (2005). A single therapy for all subtypes of horizontal canal positional vertigo. *Laryngoscope, 115,* 1432–1435.

Choung, Y. H., Shin, Y. R., Kahng, H., Park, K., & Choi, S. J. (2006). "Bow and lean test" to determine the affected ear of horizontal canal benign paroxysmal positional vertigo. *Laryngoscope, 116*(10), 1776–1781.

Ciuffreda, K. J., Kenyon, R. V., & Stark, L. (1978). Increased saccadic latencies in amblyopic eyes. *Investigative Ophthalmology and Vision Science, 17,* 697–702.

Coats, A. C. (1993). Computer-quantified positional nystagmus in normals. *American Journal of Otolaryngology, 14,* 314–326.

Coats, A. C., Herbert, F., & Atwood, G. R. (1976). The air caloric test. *Archives of Otolaryngology, 102,* 343–354.

Coats, A. C., & Smith, S. Y. (1967). Body position and the intensity of caloric nystagmus. *Acta Otolaryngologica, 63,* 515–532.

Cohen, H. S., & Jerabek, J. (1999). Efficacy of treatments for posterior canal benign paroxysmal positional vertigo. *Laryngoscope, 109*(4), 584–590.

Cohen, H. S., & Kimball, K. T. (2005). Effectiveness of treatments for benign paroxysmal positional vertigo of the posterior canal. *Otology and Neurotology, 26,* 1034–1040.

Committee on Hearing, Bioacoustics, and Biomechanics (CHABA). (1992). Evaluation of tests for vestibular function. *Aviation, Space, and Environmental Medicine, 63*(2, Suppl.), A1–A34.

Crevits, L. (2004). Treatment of anterior canal benign paroxysmal positional vertigo by a prolonged forced position procedure. *Journal of Neurology Neurosurgery and Psychiatry, 75,* 779–781.

Croxson, G. R., Moffat, D. A., & Baguley, D. (1988). Bruns bidirectional nystagmus in cerebellopontine angle tumours. *Clinical Otolaryngololgy and Allied Science, 13*(2), 153–157.

Curthoys, I. S. (2002). Generation of the quick phase of horizontal vestibular nystagmus. *Experimental Brain Research, 143,* 397–405.

Curthoys, I. S., & Halmagyi G. M. (1996). How does the brain compensate for vestibular lesions? In R. W. Baloh & G. M. Halmagyi (Eds.), *Disorders of the vestibular system* (pp.145–154). New York, NY: Oxford University Press.

Cutrer, F. M., & Baloh, R. W. (1992). Migraine-associated dizziness. *Headache, 32,* 300–304.

Davis, R. I., & Mann, R. C. (1987). The effects of alerting tasks on caloric induced nystagmus. *Ear and Hearing, 8,* 58–60.

De la Meilleure, G., Dehaene, I., Depondt, M., Damman, W., Crevits, L., & Vanhooren, G. (1996). Benign paroxysmal positional vertigo of the horizontal canal. *Journal of Neurology, Neurosurgery, and Psychiatry, 60,* 68–71.

Demanez, J. P., & Ledoux, A. (1970). Automatic fixation mechanisms and vestibular stimulation. Their study in central pathology with ocular fixation index during caloric tests. *Advances in Oto-Rhino-Laryngology, 17,* 90–98.

Dieterich, M., & Brandt, T. (1999). Episodic vertigo related to migraine (90 cases): Vestibular migraine? *Journal of Neurology, 246,* 883–892.

Dix, M. R., & Hallpike, C. S. (1952). The pathology, symptomology, and diagnosis of certain common disorders of the vestibular system. *Annals of Otology, Rhinology, and Laryngology, 61,* 987–1016.

Dow, R. S. (1938). Effect of lesions in the vestibular part of the cerebellum in primates. *Archives of Neuropsychology, 40,* 500–520.

Drachman, D. A. (1998). A 69-year-old man with chronic dizziness. *Journal of the American Medical Association, 280,* 2111–2118.

Edelman, S., Mahoney, A. E., & Cremer, P.D. (2012). Cognitive behavior therapy for chronic subjective dizziness: A randomized, controlled trial. *American Journal of Otolaryngology, 33,* 395–401.

Eggers, S. D. Z., & Zee, D. S. (Eds). (2010). Overview of vestibular and balance disorders. In *Vertigo and imbalance: Clinical neurophysiology of the vestibular system* (pp. 3–4*)*. New York, NY: Elsevier.

Enloe, L. J., & Shields, R. K. (1997). Evaluation of health-related quality of life in individuals with vestibular disease using disease-specific and general outcome measures. *Physical Therapy, 77,* 890–903.

Enticott, J. C., Dowell, R. C., & O'Leary, S. J. (2003). A comparison of the monothermal and bithermal caloric tests. *Journal of Vestibular Research, 13,* 113–119.

Epley, J. M. (1992). The canalith repositioning procedure: For treatment of benign paroxysmal positional vertigo. *Otolaryngology-Head and Neck Surgery, 107,* 399–404.

Ewald, R. (1892). *Physiologische untersuchungen über das endorgan des nervous octavus.* Weisbaden, Germany: Bergmann.

Fasold, O., von Brevern, M., Kuhberg, M., Ploner, C. J., Villringer, A., Lempert, T., & Wenzel, R. (2002). Human vestibular cortex as identified with caloric stimulation in functional magnetic resonance imaging. *NeuroImage, 17,* 1384–1393.

Fernández, C., Alzate, R., & Lindsay, J. R. (1960). Experimental observations on postural nystagmus. II. Lesions of the nodulus. *Annals of Otology, Rhinology, and Laryngology, 69,* 94–114.

Fernández, C., & Goldberg, J. M. (1976). Physiology of peripheral neurons innervating otolith organs of the squirrel monkey. I. Response to static tilts and to long-duration centrifugal force. *Journal of Neurophysiology, 39,* 970–984.

Fetter, M., & Dichgans, J. (1996). Vestibular neuritis spares the inferior division of the vestibular nerve. *Brain, 119,* 755–763.

Fettiplace, R., & Fuchs, P. A. (1999). Mechanisms of hair cell tuning. *Annual Review of Physiology, 61,* 809–834.

Fife, T. D. (1998). Recognition and management of horizontal canal benign positional vertigo. *American Journal of Otology, 19,* 345–351.

Fife, T. D. (2009). Overview of anatomy and physiology of the vestibular system. In S. D. Z. Eggers & D. S. Zee (Eds.), *Vertigo and imbalance, clinical neurophysiology of the vestibular system* (pp. 5–17). New York, NY: Elsevier.

Filipo, R., Lazzari, R., Barbara, M., Franzese, A., & Petuzzellis, M. C. (1988). Psychologic evolution of patients with Meniere's disease in relation to therapy. *American Journal of Otology, 9*(4), 306–309.

Fitzgerald, G., & Hallpike, C. S. (1942). Studies in human vestibular function. I. Observations of the directional preponderance of caloric nystagmus resulting from cerebral lesions. *Brain, 65,* 115–137.

Fletcher, W. A., & Sharpe, J. A. (1986). Saccadic eye movement dysfunction in Alzheimer's disease. *Annals of Neurology, 20,* 464–471.

Foster, C. A., & Baloh, R. W. (1996). Drug therapy for vertigo. In R. W. Baloh & G. W. Halmagyi (Eds.), *Disorders of the vestibular system* (pp. 541–550). New York, NY: Oxford University Press.

Fredrickson, J. M., & Fernández, C. (1964). Vestibular disorders in fourth ventricle lesions. Experimental studies in the cat. *Archives of Otolaryngology, 80,* 521–540.

Froehling, D. A., Silverstein, M. D., Mohr, D. N., Beatty, C. W., Offord, K. P., & Ballard, D. J. (1991). Benign positional vertigo: Incidence and prognosis in a population-based study in Olmsted County, Minnesota. *Mayo Clinic Proceedings, 66,* 596–601.

Furman, J. M., & Cass, S. P. (1999). Benign paroxysmal positional vertigo. *New England Journal of Medicine, 341,* 1590–1596.

Furman, J. M., Cass, S. P., & Whitney, S. L. (2010). *Vestibular disorders* (3rd ed.). New York, NY: Oxford University Press.

Furman, J. M., & Hain, T. C. (2004). "Do try this at home": Self-treatment of BPPV. *Neurology, 63*(1), 8–9.

Furman, J. M., & Jacob, R. G. (2001). A clinical taxonomy of dizziness and anxiety in the otoneurological setting. *Journal of Anxiety Disorders, 15*(1–2), 9–26.

Furman, J. M., Marcus, D. A., & Balaban, C. D. (2003). Migrainous vertigo: Development of a pathogenetic model and structured diagnostic interview. *Current Opinions in Neurology, 16,* 5–13. Review.

Furman, J. M., Marcus, D. A., & Balaban, C. D. (2013). Vestibular migraine: Clinical aspects and pathophysiology. *Lancet Neurology, 12,* 706–715.

Furman, J. M., Wall, C., & Pang, D. L. (1990). Vestibular function in periodic alternating nystagmus. *Brain, 113,* 1425–1439.

Furman, J. M., & Whitney, S. (2016). Neurologic origins of dizziness and vertigo. In G. P. Jacobson & N. T. Shepard (Eds.), *Balance function assessment and management* (2nd ed., pp. 719–728). San Diego, CA: Plural Publishing.

Gacek, R. R., & Gacek, M. R. (2002). Vestibular neuronitis: A viral neuropathy. *Advances in Otorhinolaryngology, 60,* 54–66.

Gay, A. J., Newman, N. M., Keltner, J. L., & Stroud, M. H. (1974). *Eye movement disorders.* St. Louis, MO: C.V. Mosby.

Glaser, J. S. (1999). *Neuro-ophthalmology* (3rd ed.). Philadelphia, PA: Lippincott Williams & Wilkins.

Goebel, J. A., O'Mara, W, & Gianoli, G. (2001). Anatomic considerations in vestibular neuritis, *Otology and Neurotology, 22,* 512–518.

Goldberg, J. M. (2000). Afferent diversity and the organization of central vestibular pathways. *Experimental Brain Research, 130,* 277.

Goldberg, J. M., & Fernandez, C. (1971a). Physiology of peripheral neurons innervating semicircular canals of the squirrel monkey. I. Resting discharge and response to constant angular accelerations. *Journal of Neurophysiology, 34,* 635–660.

Goldberg, J. M., & Fernandez, C. (1971b). Physiology of peripheral neurons innervating semicircular canals of the squirrel monkey. 3. Variations among units in their discharge properties. *Journal of Neurophysiology, 34,* 676–684.

Goldberg, J. M., Highstein, S. M., Moschovakis, A. K., & Fernandez, C. (1987). Inputs from regularly and irregularly discharging vestibular nerve afferents to secondary neurons in the vestibular nuclei of the squirrel monkey. I. An electrophysiological analysis. *Journal of Neurophysiology, 58,* 700–718.

Greven, A. J., Oosterveld, W. J., Rademakers, W. J., & Voorhoeve, R. (1979). Caloric vestibular test with the use of air. *Annals of Otology, Rhinology, and Laryngolology, 88,* 31–35.

Gufoni, M., Mastrosimone, L., & Di Nasso, F. (1998). Repositioning maneuver in benign paroxysmal vertigo of horizontal semicircular canal. *Acta Otorhinolaryngolica Italy, 18,* 363–367.

Hain, T. C. (1992). Oculomotor testing: Interpretation. In G. P. Jacobson, C. W. Newman, & J. M. Kartush (Eds.), *Handbook of balance function testing* (pp. 83–122). St. Louis, MO: Mosby.

Hain, T. C., & Rudisill, H. (2008). Practical anatomy and physiology of the ocular motor system. In G. P. Jacobson & N. T. Shepard (Eds.), *Balance function assessment and management* (pp. 13–26). San Diego, CA: Plural Publishing.

Hajioff, D., Barr-Hamilton, R. M., Colledge, N. R., Lewis, S. J., & Wilson, J. A. (2000). Re-evaluation of normative electronystagmography data in healthy ageing. *Clinical Otolaryngology and Allied Sciences, 25,* 249–252.

Halmagyi, G. M., Cremer, P. D., Anderson, J., Murofushi, T., & Curthoys, I. S. (2000). Isolated directional preponderance of caloric nystagmus: I. Clinical significance. *American Journal of Otology, 21,* 559–567.

Halmagyi, G. M., & Curthoys, I. S. (1988). A clinical sign of canal paresis. *Archives of Neurology, 45,* 737–739.

Halmagyi, G. M., & Gresty, M. A. (1979). Clinical signs of visual-vestibular interaction. *Journal of Neurology Neurosurgery and Psychiatry, 42,* 934–939.

Han, B. I., Oh, H. J., & Kim, J. S. (2006). Nystagmus while recumbent in horizontal canal benign paroxysmal positional vertigo. *Neurology, 66,* 706–710.

Harrington, J. W. (1969). Caloric stimulation of the labyrinth experimental observations. *Laryngoscope, 79,* 777–793.

Heide, W., Kurzidim, K., & Kömpf, D. (1996). Deficits of smooth pursuit eye movements after frontal and parietal lesions. *Brain, 119,* 1951–1969.

Herdman, S. J., & Tusa, R. J. (1996). Complications of the canalith repositioning procedure. *Archives of Otolaryngology-Head Neck Surgery, 122,* 281–286.

Herdman, S. J., & Tusa, R. J. (2007). Assessment and treatment of patients with benign paroxysmal positional vertigo. In Susan J. Herdman (Ed.), *Vestibular rehabilitation* (pp. 451–475). Philadelphia, PA: F. A. Davis.

Herdman, S., Tusa, R., & Clendaniel, R. (1994). Eye movement signs in vertical canal benign paroxysmal positional vertigo. In A. Fuchs, T. Brandt, U. Büttner, & D. Zee, (Eds.), *Contemporary ocular motor and vestibular research: A tribute to David A. Robinson* (pp. 385–387). Stuttgart, Germany: Georg Thieme-Verlag.

Herdman, S. J., Tusa, R. J., Zee, D. S., Proctor, L. R., & Mattox, D. E. (1993). Single treatment approaches to benign paroxysmal positional vertigo. *Archives of Otolaryngology-Head and Neck Surgery, 119,* 450–454.

Heywood, S., & Churcher, J. (1981). Direction-specific and position-specific effects upon detection of displacements during saccadic eye movements. *Vision Research, 21,* 255–261.

Hilton, M., & Pinder, D. (2014). The Epley (canalith repositioning) maneuver for benign paroxysmal positional vertigo. *Cochrane Database Systematic Review, 2014*(2), CD003162.

Hirata, Y., Sugita, T., Gyo, K., & Yanagihara, N. (1993). Experimental vestibular neuritis induced by herpes simplex virus, *Acta Otolaryngologica Supplement, 503,* 79–81.

Honrubia, V., Baloh, R. W., Harris, M. R., & Jacobson, K. M. (1999). Paroxysmal positional vertigo syndrome. *American Journal of Otology, 20,* 465–470.

Hood, J. D. (1989). Evidence of direct thermal action upon the vestibular receptors in the caloric test. A reinterpretation of the data of Coats and Smith. *Acta Otolaryngologica, 107,* 161–165.

Horii, A., Mitani, K., Kitahara, T., Uno, A., Takeda, N., & Kubo, T. (2004). Paroxetine, a selective serotonin reuptake inhibitor, reduces depressive symptoms and subjective handicaps in patients with dizziness. *Otology and Neurotology, 25,* 536–543.

Hotson, J. R., & Baloh, R. W. (1998). Acute vestibular syndrome. *New England Journal of Medicine, 339*(10), 680–685.

Hudspeth, A. J. (1982). Extracellular current flow and the site of transduction by vertebrate hair cells. *Journal of Neuroscience, 2,* 1–10.

Hudspeth, A. J., & Corey, D. P. (1977). Sensitivity, polarity, and conductance change in the response of vertebrate hair cells to controlled mechanical stimuli. *Proceedings of the National Academy of Sciences, 74,* 2407–2411.

Humphriss, R. L., Baguley, D. M., Sparkes,V., Peerman, S. E., & Moffat, D. A. (2003). Contraindications to the Dix-Hallpike manoeuvre: A multidisciplinary review. *International Journal of Audiology, 42,* 166–173.

Imai, T., Ito M., Takeda, N., Uno, A., Matsunaga, T., Sekine, K., & Kubo, T. (2005). Natural course of the remission of vertigo in patients with benign paroxysmal positional vertigo. *Neurology, 64,* 920–921.

Isaacson, J. E., & Rubin, A. M. (1999). Otolaryngologic management of dizziness in the older patient. *Clinical Geriatric Medicine, 1,* 179–191.

Ishiyama, G., Finn, M., Lopez, I., Tang, Y., Baloh, R. W., & Ishiyama, A. (2005). Unbiased quantification of Scarpa's ganglion neurons in aminoglycoside ototoxicity. *Journal of Vestibular Research, 15,* 197–202.

Ishiyama, A., Lopez, I., Ishiyama, G., & Tang, Y. (2004). Unbiased quantification of the microdissected human Scarpa's ganglion neurons. *Laryngoscope, 114,* 1496–1499.

Isotalo, E., Pyykkö, I., Juhola, M., & Aalto, H. (1995). Predictable and pseudo random saccades in patients with acoustic neuroma. *Acta Otolaryngolica, 1*(Suppl. 520), 22–24.

Ito, M. (1993). Neurophysiology of the nodulofloccular system. *Revue Neurologique, 149,* 692–697.

Ito, M., Nisimaru, N., & Yamamoto, M. (1977). Specific patterns of neuronal connexions involved in the control of the rabbit's vestibule-ocular reflexes by the cerebellar flocculus. *Journal of Physiology* (London), *265,* 833–854.

Jackson, L., Morgan, B., Fletcher, J., & Krueger, W. (2007). Anterior canal benign paroxysmal positional vertigo: An underappreciated entity. *Otology and Neurotology, 28,* 218–222.

Jacobson, G. P., & Calder, J. H. (1998). A screening version of the Dizziness Handicap Inventory (DHI-S). *American Journal of Otology, 19*(6), 804–808.

Jacobson, G. P., Calder, J. A., Shepherd, V. A., Rupp, K. A., & Newman, C. W. (1995). Reappraisal of the monothermal warm caloric screening test. *Annals of Otology, Rhinology, and Laryngology, 104,* 942–945.

Jacobson, G. P., & McCaslin, D. L. (2004). Detection of ophthalmic impairments indirectly with electronystagmography. *Journal of the American Academy of Audiology, 15,* 258–263.

Jacobson G. P., McCaslin D. L., Grantham S. L., & Piker E. G. (2008). Significant vestibular system impairment is common in a cohort of elderly patients referred for assessment of falls risk. *Journal of the American Academy of Audiology, 19*(10), 799–807.

Jacobson, G. P., & Means, E. D. (1985). Efficacy of a monothermal warm water caloric screening test.

Annals of Otology, Rhinology, and Laryngology, 4(Part 1), 377–381.

Jacobson, G. P., & Newman, C. W. (1990). The development of the Dizziness Handicap Inventory. *Archives of Otolaryngology-Head and Neck Surgery, 116*, 424–427.

Jacobson, G. P., & Newman, C. W. (1993). Background and technique of caloric testing. In G. P. Jacobson, C. W. Newman, & J. M. Kartush (Eds.), *Handbook of balance function testing* (pp. 157–192). St. Louis, MO: Mosby Year Book.

Jacobson, G. P., Newman, C. W., Hunter, L., & Balzer, G. K. (1991). Balance function test correlates of the Dizziness Handicap Inventory. *Journal of the American Academy of Audiology, 2*, 253–260.

Jacobson, G. P., Newman, C. W., & Peterson, E. L. (1993). Interpretation and usefulness of caloric testing. In G.P. Jacobson, C. W. Newman, & J. M. Kartush (Eds.), *Handbook of balance function testing* (pp.156–192). St. Louis, MO: Mosby Year Book.

Jacobson, G. P., Pearlstein, R., Henderson, J., Calder, J. H., & Rock, J. (1998). Recovery nystagmus revisited. *Journal of the American Academy of Audiology, 9*, 263–271.

Jacobson, G. P., Piker, E. G., Hatton, K., Watford, K. E., Trone, T., McCaslin, D. L., & Roberts R. A. (2018). Development and preliminary findings of the dizziness symptom profile. *Ear and Hearing, 40*(3), 568-576.

Jacobson, G. P., Shepard, N. T., Dundas, J. A., McCaslin, D. L., & Piker, E. P. (2008). In G. P. Jacobson & N. T. Shepard (Eds.), *Balance function assessment and management.* San Diego, CA: Plural Publishing.

Jaeger, R., & Haslwanter, T. (2004). Otolith responses to dynamical stimuli: Results of a numerical investigation. *Biological Cybernetics., 90*(3), 165–175.

Johnson, G. D. (1998). Medical management of migraine-related dizziness and vertigo. *Laryngoscope, 108*, 1–28.

Jones, G. M., Berthoz, A., & Segal, B. (1984). Adaptive modification of the vestibulo-ocular reflex by mental effort in darkness. *Experimental Brain Research, 56*, 149–153.

Jongkees, L. B., & Philipszoon, A. J. (1964). Electronystagmography. *Acta Otolaryngologica,* (Suppl. 189), 189–191.

Jung, R., & Mittermaier, R. (1939). Zur objektiven registrierung und analyse verschiedener nystagmusformen: vestibularer, optokinetischer und spontaner nystagmus in ihren wechselbeziehungen. *European Archives of Otorhinolaryngology, 146*, 410–439.

Kamei, T., & Kornhuber, H. H. (1964). Spontaneous and head-shaking nystagmus in normals and in patients with central lesions. *Canadian Journal of Otolaryngology, 3*, 372–380.

Kandel, E. R., Schwartz, J. H., & Jessell, T. M. (2000). *Principles of neural science* (4th ed.). New York, NY: McGraw-Hill.

Kang, S., & Shaikh, A.G. (2017). Acquired pendular nystagmus. *Journal of Neurological Science, 375*, 8–17.

Kato, I., Kimura, Y., Aoyagi, M., Mizukoshi, K., & Kawasaki, T. (1977). Visual suppression of caloric nystagmus in normal individuals. *Acta Otolaryngolica, 83*, 245–251.

Kayan, A., & Hood, J. D. (1984). Neuro-otological manifestations of migraine. *Brain, 107*(Pt. 4), 1123–1142.

Kerber, K. A., Meurer, W. J., West, B. T., & Fendrick, A. M. (2008). Dizziness presentations in U.S. emergency departments, 1995–2004. *Academy of Emergency Medicine, 15*, 744–750.

Kileny, P., McCabe, B. F., & Ryu, J. H. (1980). Effects of attention-requiring tasks on vestibular nystagmus. *Annals of Otology, Rhinology, and Laryngology, 89*, 9–12.

Kim, H. J., & Kim, J. S. (2017) The patterns of recurrences in idiopathic benign paroxysmal positional vertigo and self-treatment evaluation. *Frontiers in Neurology, 8*, 690.

Kim, Y. K., Shin, J. E., & Chung, J. W. (2005). The effect of canalith repositioning for anterior semicircular canal canalithiasis. *Journal of Otorhinolaryngology and Related Specialties, 67*, 56–60.

Kimura, R. S. (1967). Experimental blockage of the endolymphatic sac and duct and its effect on the inner ear of the guinea pig. *Annals of Otology, Rhinology, and Laryngology, 76*, 4664–4687.

Kinney, S. E., Sandridge, S. A., & Newman, C. W. (1997). Long-term effects of Ménière's disease on hearing and quality of life. *American Journal of Otology, 18*, 67.

Kitahara, M. (1991). Bilateral aspects of Meniére's disease. Ménière's disease with bilateral fluctuant hearing loss. *Acta Otolaryngologica Supplement, 485*, 74–77.

Koo, J. W., Moon, I. J., Shim, W. S., Moon, S. Y., & Kim, J. S. (2006). Value of lying-down nystagmus in the lateralization of horizontal semicircular canal benign paroxysmal positional vertigo. *Otology and Neurotology, 27*, 367–371.

Korres, S., & Balatsouras, D. (2004). Diagnostic, pathophysiologic, and therapeutic aspects of benign paroxysmal positional vertigo. *Otolaryngology-Head and Neck Surgery, 131*, 438–444.

Korres, S., Balatsouras, D. G., Kaberos, A., Economou, C., Kandiloros, D., & Ferekidis, E. (2002). Occurrence of semicircular canal involvement in benign paroxysmal positional vertigo. *Otology and Neurotology, 23*, 926–932.

Korres, S., Riga, M., Balatsouras, D. G., & Sandris, V. (2008). Benign paroxysmal positional vertigo of the anterior semicifcular canal:atypical clinical findigns and possible underlying mechanisms. *International Journal of Audiology, 47*, 276-282.

Kroenke, K., & Price, R. K. (1993). Symptoms in the community. Prevalence, classification, and psychiatric comorbidity. *Archives of Internal Medicine, 153*(21), 2474–2480.

Lee, K. S., & Kimura, R. S. (1992). Ischemia of the endolymphatic sac. *Acta Otolaryngologica, 112*(4), 658–666.

Leigh, R. J., & Zee, D. S. (2006). *The neurology of eye movements* (4th ed.). New York, NY: Oxford University Press.

Lempert, T. (1994). Horizontal benign positional vertigo. *Neurology, 44*, 2213–2214.

Lempert, T., Olesen, J., Furman, J., Waterston, J., Seemungal, B., Carey, J., . . . David Newman-Toker (2012). Consensus document of the Bárány Society and the International Headache Society, Vestibular migraine: Diagnostic criteria, *Journal of Vestibular Research, 22*, 167–172.

Leveque, M., Labrousse, M., & Seidermann, L., & Chays, A. (2007). Surgical therapy in intractable benign paroxysmal positional vertigo. *Otolaryngology-Head and Neck Surgery, 13*, 693–698.

Lightfoot, G. R. (2004). The origin of order effects in the results of the bi-thermal caloric test. *International Journal of Audiology, 43*, 276–282.

Limb, C. J., Carey, J. P., Srireddy, S., & Minor L. B. (2006). Auditory function in patients with surgically treated superior semicircular canal dehiscence. *Otololgy and Neurotology, 27*(7), 969–980.

Lin, C. Y., & Young, Y. H. (1999). Clinical significance of rebound nystagmus. *Laryngoscope, 109*, 1803–1805.

Lloyd, S. K., Baguley, D. M., Butler, K., Donnelly, N., & Moffat, D. A. (2009). Bruns' nystagmus in patients with vestibular schwannoma. *Otology and Neurotology, 30*(5), 625–628.

Lopez-Escamez, J. A., Molina, M. I., & Gamiz, M. J. (2006). Anterior semicircular canal benign paroxysmal positional vertigo and positional downbeating nystagmus. *American Journal of Otolaryngology, 27*, 173–178.

Lopez, I., Ishiyama, G., Tang, Y., Tokita, J., Baloh, R.W., & Ishiyama A. (2005). Regional estimates of hair cells and supporting cells in the human crista ampullaris. *Journal of Neuroscience Research, 82*(3), 421–431.

Lopez-Escamez, J. A., Carey, J., Chung, W. H., Goebel, J. A., Magnusson, M., Mandalà, M., & Bisdorff, A. (2015). Classification Committee of the Barany Society; Japan Society for Equilibrium Research; European Academy of Otology and Neurotology (EAONO); Equilibrium Committee of the American Academy of Otolaryngology-Head and Neck Sur-

gery (AAO-HNS); Korean Balance Society, Diagnostic criteria for Ménière's disease. *Journal of Vestibular Research, 25*, 1–7.

Lysakowski, A. (2005). Anatomy of the vestibular end organs and neural pathways. In W. Cummings (Ed.), *Cummings otolaryngology head and neck surgery* (pp. 3089–3114). Philadelphia, PA: Elsevier.

Mahoney, E. G., Edelman, A., & Cremer, P. (2013). Cognitive behavior therapy for chronic subjective dizziness: longer-term gains and predictors of disability. *American Journal of Otolaryngology, 34*, 115–120.

Maione, A. (2006) Migraine-related vertigo: diagnostic criteria and prophylactic treatment. *Laryngoscope, 116*, 1782–1786.

Mark, A. S. (1994). Contrast-enhanced magnetic resonance imaging of the temporal bone. *Neuroimaging Clinics of North America, 4*, 117–131. Review.

Marmor, M. F., & Zrenner, E. (1993). Standard for clinical electro-oculography. International Society for Electrophysiology of Vision. *Archives of Ophthalmology, 111*, 601–604.

Martens, C., Goplen, F. K., Nordfalk, K. F., Aasen, T., & Nordahl, S. H. (2016). Prevalence and characteristics of positional nystagmus in normal subjects. *Otolaryngology-Head and Neck Surgery, 154*, 861–867.

Marti, S., Palla, A., & Straumann, D. (2002). Gravity dependence of ocular drift in patients with cerebellar downbeat nystagmus. *Annals of Neurology, 52*, 712–721.

Massoud, E. A., & Ireland, D. J. (1996). Post-treatment instructions in the nonsurgical management of benign paroxysmal positional vertigo. *Journal of Otolaryngology, 25*, 121–125.

Mazzoni, A. (1969). Internal auditory canal arterial relations at the porus acusticus. *Annals of Otology, Rhinology, and Laryngology, 78*, 797–814.

McAuley, J. R., Dickman, J. D., Mustain, W., & Anand, V. K. (1996). Positional nystagmus in asymptomatic human subjects. *Otolaryngology-Head and Neck Surgery, 114*, 545–553.

McCaslin, D. L., & Jacobson, G. P. (2009). Current role of the videonystagmography examination in the context of the multidimensional balance function test battery. *Seminars in Hearing, 30*, 242–253.

McCaslin, D. L., Jacobson, G. P., Grantham, S. L., Piker, D. G., & Verghese, S. (2011). The influence of unilateral saccular impairment on functional balance performance and self-report dizziness. *Journal of the American Academy of Audiology, 22*(8), 542–549; quiz 560–561.

McCaslin, D. L., Jacobson, G. P., Lambert, W., English, L. N., & Kemph, A. J. (2015). The development of the Vanderbilt Pediatric Dizziness Handicap inventory for patient caregivers (DHI-PC). *International Journal of Pediatric Otorhinolaryngololgy, 79*(10), 1662–1666.

McCaslin, D. L., Rivas, A., Jacobson, G. P., & Bennett, M. L. (2015). The dissociation of video head impulse test (vHIT) and bithermal caloric test results provide topological localization of vestibular system impairment in patients with "definite" Ménière's disease. *American Journal of Audiology, 24*(1), 1–10.

McKenna, L., Hallam, R. S., & Hinchcliffe, R. (1991). The prevalence of psychological disturbance in neurotology outpatients. *Clinical Otolaryngology and Allied Sciences, 16*, 452–456.

McLaren, J. W., & Hillman, D. E. (1979). Displacement of the semicircular canal cupula during sinusoidal rotation. *Neuroscience, 4*, 2001–2008.

Melagrana, A., D'Agostino, R., Pasquale, G., & Taborelli, G. (1996). Study of labyrinthine function in children using the caloric test: Our results. *International Journal of Pediatric Otorhinolaryngology, 37*(1), 1-8.

Minor, L. B. (2005). Clinical manifestations of superior semicircular canal dehiscence. *Laryngoscope, 115*(10), 1717–1727.

Minor, L. B., Solomon, D., Zinreich, J. S., & Zee, D. S. (1998). Sound- and/or pressure-induced vertigo due to bone dehiscence of the superior semicircular canal. *Archives of Otolaryngology Head and Neck Surgery, 124*, 249.

Minor, L. B., Cremer, P. D., Carey, J. P., Della Santina, C. C., Streubel, S. O., & Weg, N. (2001). Symptoms and signs in superior canal dehiscence syndrome. *Annals of the New York Academy of Sciences, 942*, 259–273.

Mizukoshi, K., Watanabe, Y., Shojaku, H., Okubo, J., & Watanabe I. (1988). Epidemiological studies on benign paroxysmal position vertigo in Japan. *Acta Otolaryngolica, 447*, 67–72.

Money, K. E., Bonen, L., Beatty, J. D., Kuehn, L. A., Sokoloff, M., & Weaver, R. S. (1971). Physical properties of fluids and structures of vestibular apparatus of the pigeon. *American Journal of Physiology, 220*, 140–147.

Moon, S. Y., Kim, J. S., Kim, B. K., Kim, J. I., Lee, H., Son, S. I., . . . Lee, W. S. (2006). Clinical characteristics of benign paroxysmal positional vertigo in Korea: A multicenter study. *Journal of Korean Medical Science, 21*, 539–543.

Murnane, O. D., Akin, F. W., Lynn, S. G., & Cyr, D. G. (2009). Monothermal caloric screening test performance: A relative operating characteristic curve analysis. *Ear and Hearing, 30*, 313–329.

Musiek, F. D., Baran, J. A., Shinn, J. B., & Jones, R. O. (2012). *Disorders of the auditory system.* San Diego, CA: Plural Publishing.

Nedzelski, J. M. (1983). Cerebellopontine angle tumors: Bilateral flocculus compression as cause of associated oculomotor abnormalities. *Laryngoscope, 93*, 1251–1260.

Neff, B., & Wiet, S. R. (2016). Medical management of vertigo that is otologic in origin. In G. P. Jacobson & N. T. Shepard (Eds.), *Balance function assessment and management* (2nd ed., pp. 685–698). San Diego, CA: Plural Publishing.

Neuhauser, H., Leopold, M., von Brevern, M., Arnold, G., & Lempert, T. (2001). The interrelations of migraine, vertigo, and migrainous vertigo. *Neurology, 27*, 436–441.

Neuhauser, H. K., Radtke, A., von Brevern, M., Feldmann, M., Lezius, F., Ziese, T., & Lempert, T. (2006). Migrainous vertigo: Prevalence and impact on quality of life. *Neurology, 67*, 1028–1033.

Noaksson, L., Schulin, M., Kovacsovics, B., & Ledin, T. (1998). Temperature order effects in the caloric reaction. *International Tinnitus Journal 4*(1), 71–73.

Nunez, R. A., Cass, S. P., & Furman, J. M. (2000). Short- and long-term outcomes of canalith repositioning for benign paroxysmal positional vertigo. *Otolaryngology-Head and Neck Surgery, 122*, 647–652.

Nuti, D., Agus, G., Barbieri, M. T., & Passali, D. (1998). The management of horizontal-canal paroxysmal positional vertigo. *Acta Otolaryngolica, 118*, 455–460.

Nuti, D., Nati, C., & Passali, D. (2000). Treatment of benign paroxysmal positional vertigo: No need for postmaneuver restrictions. *Otolaryngology-Head and Neck Surgery, 122*, 440–444.

Nuti, D., Vannucchi, P., & Pagnini, P. (1992). Benign paroxysmal vertigo of the horizontal canal: A form of canalithiasis with variable clinical features. *Journal of Vestibular Research, 6*, 173–184.

Odman, M., & Maire, R. (2008). Chronic subjective dizziness. *Acta Otolaryngolica, 128*, 1085–1088.

Oghalai, J. S., Manolidis, S., Barth, J. L., Stewart, M. G., & Jenkins, H. A. (2000). Unrecognized benign paroxysmal positional vertigo in elderly patients. *Otolaryngology-Head and Neck Surgery, 122*, 630–634.

Oh, S. Y., Kim, J. S., Jeong, S. H., Oh, Y. M., Choi, K. D., Kim, B. K., . . . Lee, J. J. (2009). Treatment of apogeotropic benign positional vertigo: Comparison of therapeutic head-shaking and modified Semont maneuver. *Journal of Neurology, 256*, 1330–1336.

Okada, Y., Takahashi, M., Saito, A., & Kanzaki, J. (1991). Electronystagmographic findings in 147 patients with acoustic neuroma. *Acta Otolaryngolica, 487*, 150–156.

Olsson, J (1991). Neurotologic findings in basilar migraine. *Laryngoscope, 101*, 1–41.

Paparella, M. M., & Mancini, F. (1985). Vestibular Meniere's disease. *Otolaryngology-Head and Neck Surgery, 93*(2), 148–151.

Parnes, L. S., Agrawal, S. K., & Atlas, J. (2003). Diagnosis and management of benign paroxysmal positional vertigo (BPPV). *Canadian Medical Association Journal, 169*, 681–693.

Parnes, L. S., & McClure, J. A. (1991). Posterior semicircular canal occlusion in the normal hearing ear. *Otolaryngology-Head and Neck Surgery, 104*, 52–57.

Parnes, L. S., & McClure, J. A. (1992). Free-floating endolymph particles: A new operative finding during posterior semicircular canal occlusion. *Laryngoscope, 102*, 988–992.

Parnes, L. S., & Price-Jones, R. G. (1993). Particle repositioning maneuver for benign paroxysmal positional vertigo. *Annals of Otology, Rhinology, and Laryngology, 102*(5), 325–331.

Pender, J. D. (1992). *Practical otology.* Philadelphia, PA: J. B. Lippincott.

Pierrot-Deseilligny, C., & Milea, D. (2005). Vertical nystagmus: Clinical facts and hypotheses. *Brain, 128*, 1237–1246.

Popper, A.N., & Fay, R. R. (1973). Sound detection and processing by teleost fishes: A critical review. *Journal of the Acoustical Society of America, 53*, 14–38.

Pournaras, I., Kos, I., & Guyot, J. P. (2008). Benign paroxysmal positional vertigo: A series of eight singular neurectomies, *Acta Otolaryngogica, 128*, 5–8.

Proctor, L. R. (1992). The ice water caloric test. *The ENG Report Archives* (pp. 69–72). Denmark: ICS Medical.

Radtke, A., Lempert, T., Gresty, M. A., Brookes, G. B., Bronstein, A. M., & Neuhauser, H. (2002). Migraine and Ménière's disease: Is there a link? *Neurology, 59*(11), 1700–1704.

Radtke, A., Neuhauser, H., von Brevern, M., & Lempert, T. (1999). A modified Epley's procedure for self-treatment of benign paroxysmal positional vertigo. *Neurology, 53*, 1358–1360.

Radtke, A., von Brevern, M., Tiel-Wilck, K., Mainz-Perchalla, A., Neuhauser, H., & Lempert, T. (2004). Self-treatment of benign paroxysmal positional vertigo: Semont maneuver vs Epley procedure. *Neurology, 63*, 150–152.

Rahko, T. (2002). The test and treatment methods of benign paroxysmal positional vertigo and an addition to the management of vertigo due to the superior vestibular canal (BPPV-SC). *Clinical Otolaryngology and Allied Sciences, 27*, 392–395.

Raphan, T., Matsuo, V., & Cohen, B. (1979). Velocity storage in the vestibulo-ocular reflex arc (VOR). *Experimental Brain Research, 35*, 229–248.

Rasmussen, A. T. (1940). Studies of the VIIIth cranial nerve of man. *Laryngoscope, 50*, 67–83.

Rasmussen, B. K., Jensen, R., & Olesen, J. (1991). A population-based analysis of the diagnostic criteria of the International Headache Society. *Cephalalgia, 11*(3), 129–134.

Rauch, S. D., San Martin, J. E., Moscicki, R. A., & Bloch, K. J. (1995). Serum antibodies against heat shock protein 70 in Ménière's disease. *American Journal of Otology, 16*(5), 648–652.

Roberts, R., & Gans, R. (2008). Background, technique, interpretation, and usefulness of positional/positioning testing. In G. P. Jacobson & N. T. Shepard (Eds.), *Balance function assessment and management* (pp.171–196). San Diego, CA: Plural Publishing.

Robinson, D. A. (1964). The mechanics of human saccadic eye movement. *Journal of Physiology, 174*, 245–264.

Rosenhall, U. (1973). Degenerative patterns in the aging human vestibular neuro-epithelia. *Acta Otolaryngologica, 76*, 208–220.

Ross, M. D., Donovan, K., & Chee O. (1985). Otoconial morphology in space-flown rats. *Physiologist, 28*, 219–220.

Ruckenstein, M. (2001). Therapeutic efficacy of the Epley canalith repositioning maneuver. *Laryngoscope, 111*, 940–945.

Ruckenstein, M. J., & Staab, J. P. (2009). Chronic subjective dizziness. *Otolaryngology Clinics of North America, 42*, 71–77.

Rucker, J. C. (2010) Overview of anatomy and physiology of the ocular motor system. In S. D. Z. Eggers & D. S. Zee (Eds.), *Vertigo and imbalance: Clinical neurophysiology of the vestibular system* (pp. 18–42). New York, NY: Elsevier.

Sakaida, M., Takeuchi, K., Ishinaga, H., Adachi, M., & Majima, Y. (2003). Long-term outcome of benign paroxysmal positional vertigo, *Neurology, 60*, 1532–1534.

Salt, A. N. & Rask-Andersen, H. (2004). Responses of the endolymphatic sac to perilymphatic injections and withdrawals: Evidence for the presence of a one-way valve. *Hearing Research, 191*, 90–100.

Salvinelli, F., Firrisi, L., Casale, M., Trivelli, M., D'Ascanio, L., Lamanna, F., . . . Costantino, S. (2004). Benign paroxysmal positional vertigo: Diagnosis and treatment. *La Clinica Terapeutica, 155*, 395–400.

Sato, H., Ohkawa, T., Uchino, Y., & Wilson, V. J. (1997). Excitatory connections between neurons of the central cervical nucleus and vestibular neurons in the cat. *Experimental Brain Research, 115*, 381–386.

Scherer, H., Brandt, U., Clarke, A. H., Merbold, U., & Parker, R. (1986). European vestibular experiments on the Spacelab-1 mission: 3. Caloric nystagmus in microgravity. *Experimental Brain Research, 64*, 255–263.

Schor, C. M. (2003). Neural control of eye movements. In P. L. Kaufman, & A. Alm (Eds.), *Adler's physiol-

ogy of the eye (10th ed., pp. 830–858). St. Louis, MO: Mosby.

Schuknecht, H. F. (1962). Positional vertigo. Clinical and experimental observations. *Transactions of the American Academy of Ophthalmology and Otolaryngology, 66*, 319–331.

Schuknecht, H. F. (1969). Cupulothiasis. *Archives of Otolaryngology, 90*, 765–778.

Schuknecht, H. F., & Igarashi, M. (1964). Pathology of slowly progressive sensori-neural deafness. *Trans–American Academy of Ophthalmology and Otolaryngology, 68*, 222–242.

Schuknecht, H. F., & Ruby, R. R. (1973). Cupulothiasis. *Advances in Otorhinolaryngology, 20*, 434–443.

Schwarz, D. W. F., & Tomlinson, R. D. (2005). Physiology of the vestibular system. In R. K. Jackler & D. E. Brackman (Eds.), *Neurotology* (2nd ed., pp. 91–121). Philadelphia, PA: Elsevier Mosby.

Sekitani, T., Imate, Y, Noguchi, T., & Inokuma, T. (1993). Vestibular neuronitis: Epidemiological survey by questionnaire in Japan. *Acta Otolaryngologica Supplementum* (Stockh.), *503*, 9–12.

Semont, A., Freyss, G., & Vitte, E. (1988). Curing the BPPV with a liberatory maneuver. *Advances in Otorhinolaryngology, 42*, 290–293.

Seok, J. I., Lee, H. M., Yoo, J. H., & Lee D. K. (2008). Residual dizziness after successful repositioning treatment in patients with benign paroxysmal positional vertigo. *Journal of Clinical Neurophysiology, 4*, 107–110.

Shepard, N. T. (2006). Differentiation of Ménière's disease and migraine-associated dizziness: A review. *Journal of the American Academy of Audiology, 17*, 69–80.

Shepard, N. T., & Schubert, M. (2008). Interpretation and usefulness of ocular motility testing. In G. P. Jacobson & N. T. Shepard (Eds.), *Balance function assessment and management* (pp. 45–62). San Diego, CA: Plural Publishing.

Sherrington, C. S. (1947). *The integrative action of the nervous system.* New Haven, CT: Yale University Press.

Silverstein, H., Smouha, E., & Jones, R. (1989). Natural history vs. surgery for Ménière's disease. *Otolaryngology-Head and Neck Surgery, 100*(1), 6–16.

Sloane, P. D. (1989). Dizziness in primary care. Results from the National Ambulatory Medical Care Survey. *Journal of Family Practice, 29*, 33–38.

Söhsten, E., Bittar, R. S., & Staab, J. P. (2016). Posturographic profile of patients with persistent postural-perceptual dizziness on the sensory organization test. *Journal of Vestibular Research, 26*, 319–326.

Soper, J., McCaslin, D. L., McPherson, J., Anderson, A., Stoelb, C., Goulson, A., . . . Shepard, N. (2018, March). *Clinical utility of vibration induced nystagmus (VIN).* Presentation at the American Balance Society, Scottsdale, AZ.

Staab, J. P. (2011). Clinical clues to a dizzying headache. *Journal of Vestibular Research, 21*(6), 331–340

Staab, J. P. (2012). Chronic subjective dizziness. *Continuum, 18*, 1118–1141.

Staab J. P., Eckhardt-Henn A., Horii A., Jacob R., Strupp M., Brandt T., & Bronstein A., (2017). Diagnostic criteria for persistent postural-perceptual dizziness (PPPD): Consensus document of the committee for the Classification of Vestibular Disorders of the Bárány Society. *Journal of Vestibular Research, 27*(4), 191–208.

Staab, J. P., & Ruckenstein, M. J. (2005). Chronic dizziness and anxiety: Effect of course of illness on treatment outcome. *Archives of Otolaryngology-Head and Neck Surgery, 131*, 675–679.

Staab, J. P., & Ruckenstein, M. J. (2007). Expanding the differential diagnosis of chronic dizziness. *Archives of Otolaryngology-Head and Neck Surgery, 133*, 170–176.

Staab, J. P., Ruckenstein, M. J., & Amsterdam, J. D. (2004). A prospective trial of sertraline for chronic subjective dizziness. *Laryngoscope, 114*, 1637–1641.

Straka, H., Biesdorf, S., & Dieringer, N. (2000). Spatial distribution of semicircular canal nerve evoked monosynaptic response components in frog vestibular nuclei. *Brain Research, 880*, 70–83.

Strupp, M., & Brandt, T. (2013). Vestibular neuritis. In A. M. Bronstein (Ed.), *Vertigo and imbalance* (pp 207–213). Oxford, UK: University Press.

Strupp, M., Brandt, T., & Steddin, S. (1995). Horizontal canal benign paroxysmal positional vertigo: Reversible ipsilateral caloric hypoexcitability caused by canalolithiasis? *Neurology, 45*, 2072–2076.

Sugaya, N., Arai, M., & Goto, F. (2017). Is the headache in patients with vestibular migraine attenuated by vestibular rehabilitation? *Frontiers in Neurology, 8*, 124.

Sylvestre, P. A., & Cullen, K. E. (1999). Quantitative analysis of abducens neuron discharge dynamics during saccadic and slow eye movements. *Journal of Neurophysiology, 82*, 2612–2632.

Takemori, S., & Cohen, B. (1974). Loss of visual suppression of vestibular nystagmus after flocculus lesions. *Brain Research, 72*, 213–224.

Tanimoto, H., Doi, K., Katata, K., & Nibu, K. I. (2005). Self-treatment for benign paroxysmal positional vertigo of the posterior semicircular canal. *Neurology, 65*, 1299–1300.

Thompson , K. J., Goetting, J. C., Staab, J. P., & Shepard, N. T. (2015). Retrospective review and telephone follow-up to evaluate a physical therapy protocol for treating persistent postural-perceptual dizziness: A pilot study. *Journal of Vestibular Research, 25*, 97–103.

Timmerman, H. (1994). Pharmacotherapy of vertigo: Any news to be expected? *Acta Otolaryngolica, 513*, 28–32.

Tomlinson, R. D., & Robinson, D. A. (1981). Is the vestibule-ocular reflex cancelled by smooth pursuit? In A. Fuchs & W. Becker (Eds.), *Progress in oculomotor research* (pp. 533–539). New York, NY: Elsevier.

Torok, N. (1979). Pitfalls in detecting vestibular decruitment with air calorics. *Journal of Otorhinolaryngology and Related Specialties, 4*, 143–146.

Uzun-Coruhlu, H., Curthoys, I. S., & Jones, A. S. (2007). Attachment of the utricular and saccular maculae to the temporal bone. *Hearing Research, 233*, 77–85.

Van Der Stappen, A., Wuyts, F. L., & Van De Heyning, P. H. (2000). Computerized electronystagmography: Normative data revisited. *Acta Otolaryngolica, 120*, 724–730.

Van Ombergen A., Heine L., & Jillings S. (2017). Altered functional brain connectivity in patients with visually induced dizziness. *Neuroimage Clinics, 14*, 538–545.

Vannucchi, P., Giannoni, B., & Pagnini, P. (1997). Treatment of horizontal semicircular canal benign paroxysmal positional vertigo. *Journal of Vestibular Research, 7*, 1–6.

Versino, M., Sances, G., Anghileri, E., Colnaghi, S., Albizzati, C., Bono, G., & Cos, V. (2003). Dizziness and migraine: A causal relationship? *Functional Neurology, 18*, 97–101.

von Brevern, M., Radtke, A., Lezius, F., Feldmann, M., Ziese, T., Lempert, T., & Neuhauser, H. (2007). Epidemiology of benign paroxysmal positional vertigo: A population-based study. *Journal of Neurology, Neurosurgery, and Psychiatry, 78*, 710–715.

von Brevern, M., Schmidt, T., Schönfeld, U., Lempert, T., & Clarke, A. H. (2006). Utricular dysfunction in patients with benign paroxysmal positional vertigo. *Otology and Neurotology, 27*, 92–96.

von Brevern, M., Zeise, D., Neuhauser, H., Clarke, A. H., & Lempert, T. (2005). Acute migrainous vertigo: Clinical and oculographic findings. *Brain, 128*, 365–374.

Westheimer, G., & McKee, S. P. (1975). Visual acuity in the presence of retinal image motion. *Journal of Optometry Society of America, 65*, 847–850.

White, J. A., Coale, K. D., Catalano, P. J., & Oas J. G. (2005). Diagnosis and management of lateral semicircular canal benign paroxysmal positional vertigo, *Otolaryngology-Head and Neck Surgery, 133*, 278–284.

Whitney, S. L., Marchetti, G. F., & Morris, L. O. (2005). Usefulness of the dizziness handicap inventory in the screening for benign paroxysmal positional vertigo. *Otology and Neurotology, 26*, 1027–1033.

Wladislavosky-Waserman, P., Facer, G. W., Mokri, B., & Kurland, L. T. (1984). Meniere's disease: A 30-year epidemiologic and clinical study in Rochester, MN, 1951–1980. *Laryngoscope, 94*, 1098–1102.

Wolf, J., Boyev, K., Manokey, B., & Mattox, D. (1999). Success of the modified Epley maneuver in treating benign paroxysmal positional vertigo. *Laryngoscope, 113*, 659–662.

Wong, A. M. F. (2008). *Eye movement disorders.* New York, NY: Oxford University Press.

World Health Organization (WHO). (2002). *Towards a common language for functioning, disability, and health. ICF* (pp. 1–22). Geneva, Switzerland: Author.

Yacovino, D. A., Hain, T. C., & Gualtieri, F. (2009). New therapeutic maneuver for anterior canal benign paroxysmal positional vertigo. *Journal of Neurology, 256*, 1851–1855.

Yuen, H. W., Boeddinghaus, R., Eikelboom, R. H., & Atlas, M. D. (2009). The relationship between the air-bone gap and the size of superior semicircular canal dehiscence. *Otolaryngology-Head and Neck Surgery, 141*, 689–694.

Zangemeister, W. H., & Bock, O. (1980). Air versus water caloric test. *Clinical Otolaryngololgy and Allied Science, 5*, 379–387.

Zapala, D. A., Olsholt, K. F., & Lundy, L. B. (2008). A comparison of water and air caloric responses and their ability to distinguish between patients with normal and impaired ears. *Ear and Hearing, 29*, 585–600.

Zigmond, A. S., & Snaith, R. P. (1983). The hospital anxiety and depression scale. *Acta Psychiatrica Scandinavica, 67*, 361–370.

Index

Note: Numbers in **bold** reference non-text material.